Research
in Nursing Practice

DONNA DIERS, R.N., M.S.N., F.A.A.N.

Professor and Dean
Yale University School of Nursing
New Haven, Connecticut

J. B. Lippincott Company

PHILADELPHIA   NEW YORK   TORONTO

Copyright © 1979 by J. B. Lippincott Company

ISBN 0-397-54221-6

Library of Congress Catalog Card Number 79-878

PRINTED IN THE UNITED STATES OF AMERICA

2 4 6 8 9 7 5 3 1

Library of Congress Cataloging in Publication Data
Diers, Donna.
  Research in nursing practice.
  Bibliography.
  Includes index.
  1. Nursing—Research.   I. Title.
RT81.5.D53   610.73′07′2   79-878
ISBN 0-397-54221-6

for ILENE *and* DON DIERS
with love, respect and admiration

Acknowledgments

During the years this book took shape, many persons contributed to my thinking and growing.

One person started it all: Robert C. Leonard, now Professor of Sociology, University of Arizona, but formerly teacher and colleague at Yale. His inspiration and encouragement, research sophistication and real respect for nursing made him a dynamic teacher, and a true friend in developing clinical studies of direct patient care.

Ruth Schmidt, as student, colleague and scholar pushed and prodded and finally criticized the finished product with insight and intellect, and the fact that it finally exists owes much to her constancy.

I was privileged to work with and learn from James Dickoff and Patricia James, gifted teachers and elegant thinkers. Much of the conceptual work was developed from ideas generated by Dickoff and James, Ernestine Wiedenbach, Lucy Conant and Joyce Semradek in the nursing theory seminars at Yale in the 1960s. Any misunderstanding of practice theory is, unfortunately, all mine. Several faculty colleagues deserve special mention: John A. Wolfer, for long and stimulating discussions and lovely arguments about experimentation and exploratory studies; Nancy Hedlund for clarity and comprehension of social science and patient care; Susan Molde, for exquisite clinical insights, and "systems of care"; Florence Wald for faith, vision, wisdom and the purest kind of conceptual ability; Beth Strutzel, Eileen Hodgman and Barbara Geach for excellent thoughts, believing and pushing; the classes of 1968–1978 of the Yale University School of Nursing for making me finally sit down and do it.

I wish to acknowledge the powerful effect of the mentors in nursing I have been fortunate enough to know: Ada Jacox, Carol A. Lindeman, and Ingeborg Mauksch. And for role models in university life and the potential of women, Hanna Holborn Gray and Ellen Ash Peters teach the balance of discipline and compassion, ambition and dedication to excellence.

Long as the period of manuscript preparation has been, its eventual publication was significantly hastened by David Miller of J. B. Lippincott Company, a good friend and trusted editor.

Years of random conversations with friends and fellow academics are reflected in these pages: Powhatan Wooldridge on reliability; Judy Krauss, Ann Slavinsky and Judy Tierney on intervention and social competence; the late Margaret Arnstein on nurses and research, and on cohort studies; Rhetaugh Dumas on experimentation, power and many other things; John D. Thompson on clinical research to change the health care system; Barbara Johnson and Jean Johnson on measurement; Jeanne Benoliel on exploratory studies and patient participation; Jane Dixon on evaluation. Doris Banchick helped review the literature for early chapters and throughout the work, counseled, supported, complained and complimented. Special thanks go to Judy Krauss for taking over the dean's work so I could have the sabbatical leave to write.

Finally, Laraine Werstler's interest in the work as she typed early drafts spurred me on. The work of Patricia McCormick Moore in preparing the final drafts and catching all the errors and omissions made all the difference in the world.

Contents

Prologue

There's a danger in telling how a book came to be written. The tale can be mistaken for the author's cop-out—see how hard I've worked, don't be too critical of me. Take my word for it—the work was hard. The motivation for writing and the process this manuscript went through need to be described to give some perspective.

I began teaching research methods to graduate students in nursing in 1964. That was a time when the idea of research in nursing practice was beginning to gain some visibility. But the texts available at the time were unsatisfying. I was teaching in an institution with a defined commitment to research in patient care (1), and the available references at that time dealt superficially, if at all, with research into direct nursing services.

After a couple of years of hunting for references for students, one student group suggested I write my own syllabus for the research course and a faculty colleague encouraged me. I tape-recorded my lectures that year and the first draft of the book came out of those lectures. That first version became the text for the course the following year and experiences in using it made redrafting imperative. The second draft became the text for the course for two years, then a reference after that. Thus, several classes of graduate students have used the draft manuscript, criticized it, supplemented it, quoted it, and when copies ran low, even stolen it. At the same time, faculty colleagues have read and dissected it, as have colleagues in other universities and in clinical settings. In the meantime, nursing practice research has assumed an increasingly strong place in the profession, and as our experience with doing it has grown, so have our ideas about its problems (2).

Much of what was written in that first draft now seems either naive or outdated. (Some of it, of course, seems visionary!) The early drafts were full of polemics and pleadings for nursing *practice* research as valid content area, when most of the research being done was curriculum study or studies of nurses. Readers of this volume are spared those arguments (3). Indeed, the point is no longer arguable—the National Commission for the Study of Nursing and Nursing Education put as its first recommended priority the

1

study of nursing practice problems (4). But this kind of research is still new and this book is a picture of the state of the art at a particular point.

For purposes of this volume, "nursing practice research" means research on problems in patient care. Deliberately excluded are studies of nurses, of curricula, historical studies and certain kinds of administrative studies when they do not deal with issues of nursing practice directly. But nursing practice research is broadly construed and may include studies of indirect care (for example, care given through other people not defined as the patient, like parents of children, siblings and so on), studies of systems of care when their effect on patients is at issue and so on. The intention is not to exclude curriculum studies or other nonpractice research as illegitimate for the profession; rather this book concentrates on clinical research in nursing practice as the content area within which now the majority of nursing research should be conducted.

The book is meant to be read chronologically, for the most part. For example, the research process is discussed in Chapter 3, but the discussion of some of the more practical issues in data collection is left for a later chapter after study designs have been covered. While it is clear that as process, research doesn't move all that logically from problem to study design to data collection to data analysis to conclusions, the order established by the organization of the book promotes the ideal state—that research is, above anything, logical.

The device of notes at the end of chapters has been used rather than references or bibliographies. Writing about research is no less a human process than research is, with all the human tendencies to tangential thinking and irrelevancy. Those thoughts, as well as the more orthodox references and citations, are combined in the notes, along with elaboration of some points the advanced reader may wish to pursue. An attempt has been made to make the literature citations as complete as possible, with no pretensions of exhaustiveness.

This book is written for an audience of nurses—undergraduate and graduate students, nurse faculty, practicing clinicians.

Research examples will range from studies of problems in patient care as perceived by staff nurses, through problems in special settings or with patients with specific kinds of illness, through problems perceived by nurses in various kinds of "expanded roles," as nurse clinicians, clinical nurse specialists, nurse practitioners or nurse midwives.

It is only partly a how-to-do-it text. How to do research isn't all that difficult—there are rules and conventions and well-tried techniques that are not arbitrary, but based in tested knowledge. What is harder is why do it, and when and where and with whom and with what end in mind. And how to fit research and nursing together.

The basic assumption that lies under all of these pages is that *all* nurses can, and should, do research (5). The old dichotomy that nursing practice is doing and research is thinking, is just that—old. The essence of research is contained in the everyday practice of nursing (6). Suppose a nurse has charge of a patient she's never met before. She may gather information about him before she goes into his room, from the chart, or from morning report or from her colleagues. That's data collection. She approaches the patient and assesses his needs. From what he tells her and what she observes, she comes to some formulation of his needs. That's taxonomy—naming. Based on this nursing diagnosis, she puts into effect a plan to meet his needs, a plan based on the prediction that the actions will have their intended effect. That's prediction. Then she observes or questions to evaluate the effect and changes the plan as new evidence comes in. The practicing nurse in this sequence has to worry about the same problems a researcher does: is the information gained from or about the patient reliable? Is it valid? What are the alternative explanations for the results of the treatment? What other variables might be operating? Most of the basic principles of research are contained in thoughtful nursing practice.

But there is a prevailing myth that research is clean and pure and uncontaminated by human hands. To the beginning nurse-researcher, "research" conjures up images of the cold, clinical scientist in a dirty lab coat, perfectly objective, totally controlled, unemotional, slightly mad though clever with statistics. The idea of "nursing research" may modify the image only by changing the gender.

When a Nobel Prize winner writes that

> . . . science seldom proceeds in the straightforward logical manner imagined by outsiders. Instead, its steps are often very human events in which personalities and cultural traditions play major roles. . . . Styles of scientific research vary almost as much as human personalities. . . . I do not believe that the way DNA came out constitutes an odd exception to a scientific world complicated by the contradictory pulls of ambition and the sense of fair play. (7)

he is revealing the real inside story of research and researchers. Dr. Watson apparently embarrassed some of his colleagues by publishing the human side of the story of the discovery of the structure of DNA and he certainly dumfounded some laymen.

The image of the "pure" scientist is so pervasive that it has become almost a stereotype. Another Nobel laureate has written

> You've seen him in the movies: the scientist who is infallible, insensitive and coldly objective—little more than an animated computer. . . . He takes measurements and records results as if the collection of data were his sole object in life; and if a meaningful pattern emerges it comes as a blinding surprise. The assumption is that if one gathers enough facts about something the relationships between those facts will spontaneously reveal themselves. Nonsense. (8)

If research isn't just fact-gathering and researchers are as human as anyone else, what is it really like? The same author writes, "The heart of scientific inquiry and the source of excitement it engenders in its practitioners lies not in the doing of experiments nor in the gathering of facts but in the application of imagination and intelligence to a problem." (9) And apparently the ideas of geneticists like Beadle and biochemists like Watson are shared by some members of the behavioral sciences, too. For example, a group of psychologists writes, "The process of doing research is a rather informal, often illogical and sometimes messy-looking affair. It includes a great deal of floundering around in the empirical world. . . ." (10) If research is all this messy, how does it ever contribute anything?

In the first place, research is neither all messy nor all coldly factual, but some kind of balance of both. Second, some of the perceptions of science and scientists as being objective are true, in that researchers make use of certain tools or methods to assure that the facts gathered and the inferences made truly represent reality.

Still it is not surprising that most nurses approach the idea of research with trepidation, if not downright antipathy. Nursing education has not, until recently, been preparing undergraduates for research, nor has much of the content taught been research-based. The former is changing, with some interesting effects (11), and the latter will change, too, as more nursing practice research is done, and as we gradually recover from our traditional paranoia about medicine and isolation from the rest of the world and begin to use literature from other fields. Nursing students are often given the traditional humanistic orientation to their "calling," a view which if true militates against a research orientation.

Similarly, nursing practice settings have not supported research in nursing and that, too, is changing (12).

No amount of research can ever destroy the personal satisfaction that comes from giving excellent patient care, nor can any amount of research ever predict or prescribe all of nursing care for an individual patient. But research can provide information on which to base decisions about patient care. As we learn more about what in nursing brings about the desired effects for patients, the patient care gets better and better, and that's the whole purpose for nursing research. When we know what in nursing practice works, we can design curricula to teach that, or invent nursing administrations to foster it.

Nursing is considerably ahead of other disciplines in the scientific examination of its practices. The bulk of the research in medicine is basic science research, which may or may not have immediate relevance to clinical problems. Dr. Alvan Feinstein has written eloquently about the need for a science of "doctoring," the science of the practice of medicine (13). Despite nursing's relative youth in research, we have the advantage of a professional, national commitment to research in nursing practice, and we have not had to contend quite so much with a professional academic value system that rewards activities unrelated to practice, and degrades those closest to patient care. As nursing matures rapidly in these days of human liberation, we need not go the direction of other professions, as we have so often in the past. If nurses don't do nursing research, no one else is going to do it for us; no one else can. It's our special privilege and obligation.

Examination of one's work can be a painful experience especially since nurses are taught, like doctors, that they are infallible, if not omnipotent. Perhaps part of the reason many nurses are uneasy with the thought of research is that to question what is not being done amounts to criticism. Yet nurses are constantly modifying their own practice in the light of new information, whether based on continued experiences or on more formally gathered knowledge. Research simply helps the modification process along, and if carefully constructed, makes appropriate use of clinical experience in designing and conducting studies that have maximum potential for improving practice. In fact, the closer the relationship between nursing practice and nursing research, the better the research and the better the practice.

To do nursing research requires not only curiosity, a questioning attitude and a bent toward systematic study, but also a more important attitude: before one launches into the study of nursing one must believe nursing is important enough to study. There's more than a little depressing questioning in the air about whether nursing is worth anything. That questioning may be, in part, an effect of the lack of nursing research, for how can one successfully argue that nursing makes a difference without data? The peculiar problems of nursing's self-concept are beyond the scope of this book (14). But as nursing moves ever more rapidly into its rightful place in health care delivery, as nurses take on increasing responsibility and authority for patient care, and as we go beyond nursing responsibilities into some traditionally medical functions, the demand for proof of our contributions will become more and more severe. We will lose the protection of our mostly female (read "nonthinking") composition, and of our peculiar attire. We will have to bring our intuition to conscious instead of unconscious intelligence, and defend our decisions with facts.

It's an exciting time for nursing, and nursing research is still new enough that every new researcher is a pioneer.

NOTES

1. The point of view that changes in nursing education and administration must follow from, rather than precede, examination of the nature and effect of nursing practice was controversial at that time. The philosophy and history of the development of the notion of research in nursing practice are reported in:

   Wald, Florence S. and Robert C. Leonard: Toward development of nursing practice theory. *Nursing Research*, 13:309–313, Fall 1964. Also reprinted in Fox, David J. and Ruth Kelly (eds.): *Research Process in Nursing*. New York: Appleton-Century-Crofts, 1967, pp. 50–60, and in Folta, Jeannette R. and Edith Deck (eds.): *A Sociological Framework for Patient Care*. New York: John Wiley & Sons, 1966, pp. 315–323.

   Wald, Florence S. and Robert C. Leonard: Faculty development for research in nursing— practical problems at the operational level. In *Development of Faculty Competence in Research*. Report of the 17th Conference of the Council of Member Agencies of the Department of Baccalaureate and Higher Degree Programs, National League for Nursing, Boston, Mass., April 1–3, 1964. New York: National League for Nursing, 1964, pp. 16–29.

   Diers, Donna: Faculty research development at Yale. *Nursing Research*, 19:64–71, January–February 1970.

Leonard, Robert C.: Developing research in a practice oriented discipline. *American Journal of Nursing*, 67:1472–1475, July 1967.

Wooldridge, Powhatan, Robert C. Leonard and James K. Skipper, Jr.: *Clinical Experimentation to Improve Practice*. St. Louis: C.V. Mosby, 1978, pp. 173–184.

2. *Nursing Research*, celebrating its 25th Anniversary, published a very good series of summary articles on the recent development of research in nursing in which the point is often made that the trend toward more research in nursing practice is clear. See *Nursing Research*, 26(1–4), January–August 1977 especially.

3. Those who might wish to read more about various points of view regarding what kind of reseach should be done in nursing might begin with the following:

Adama, Appolonia: Research—the "R" in nursing. *Journal of the American Medical Association*, 178:49–52, May 7, 1960.

Dilworth, Ava S.: The need for patient oriented studies. *Nursing Research*, 5:134–135, February 1957.

Folta, Jannette R. and Leonard Schatzman: Education in research for nurses. In Folta and Deck (eds.): *A Sociological Framework for Patient Care*, pp. 309–315.

Henderson, Virginia: An overview of nursing research. *Nursing Research*, 6:61–71, October 1956.

McManus, R. Louis: Nursing research—its evolution. *American Journal of Nursing*, 61:76–79, 1961.

Simmons, Leo and Virginia Henderson: *Nursing Research*. New York: Appleton-Century-Crofts, 1964, especially pp. 1–31.

Whaley, Paul J.: Nursing research: limbo or liberty. *American Journal of Nursing*, 67:1675–1677, August 1967.

Ellison, Margaret, et al.: Uses of behavioral science in nursing: further comment. *Nursing Research*, 13:71–72, Winter 1964.

Symposium: Research—how will nursing define it. *Nursing Research*, 16:108–130, Spring 1967.

Wald, Florence S. and Robert C. Leonard, see Note 1.

Notter, Lucille: Editorials, *Nursing Research*. Many of Notter's editorials have dealt with priorities for nursing research. Among the best are: 20:3, January–February 1971; 20:99, March–April 1971; 20:195, May–June 1971.

A.N.A. Research Conferences. Published annually since 1965, this series provides an excellent overview of the development of research, and some of the arguments about what should be done. New York: American Nurses Association, 1965–1976.

Rogers, Martha E.: Nursing research: relevant to practice? 5th Nursing Research Conference, A.N.A., New Orleans, March 3–5, 1969, pp. 352–359.

Lindeman, Carol A.: Nurse practice research: what's it all about? *Journal of Nursing Administration*, 5(3):5–7, March–April 1975.

Gortner, Susan: Contributions of nursing research to patient care. *Journal of Nursing Administration*, 6:22-28, March–April 1976.

Gortner, Susan: Research for a practice profession. *Nursing Research*, 24:193–197, May–June 1975.

Notter, Lucille: The case for nursing research. *Nursing Outlook*, 23:760–763, December 1975.

Jacox, Ada: Theory construction in nursing: an overview. *Nursing Research*, 23(1):4–13, January–February 1974.

Taylor has compiled a bibliography of over 1,000 references in English on nursing research. Included are 144 articles on development, status, trends, problems, issues and need for nursing research. See Taylor, Susan D.: Bibliography on nursing research, 1950–74. *Nursing Research,* 24:207–225, May–June 1975.

4. The complete quotation is

. . . we believe that [our] many suggestions for change in nursing practice and education should be seen in terms of three basic priorities. These are the needs for: (a) increased research into both the practice of nursing and the education of nurses; (b) enhanced educational systems and curriculum based on the results of that research; (c) increased financial support for nurses and for nursing to ensure adequate career opportunities that will attract and retain the number of individuals required for quality health care in the coming years.

(p 285) National Commission for the Study of Nursing and Nursing Education, Summary Report and Recommendations. *American Journal of Nursing,* 70:279–294, February 1970.

But see Donaldson, Sue K. and Dorothy M. Crowley: The discipline of nursing. *Nursing Outlook,* 26:113–120, February 1978.

5. The seminal work on the point that all nurses can and should do research is Dickoff, James, Patricia James and Joyce Semradek: 8–4 research: a stance for nursing research—tenacity or inquiry (Part I). *Nursing Research* 24:84–88, March–April 1975; and the continuation of their article: Designing nursing research—eight points of encounter. *Nursing Research,* 24:164–176, May–June 1975. See also letters to the editor in subsequent issues, especially letters by Suzanne Hall Johnson and Beverly Volicer, *Nursing Research,* 25:63–66, January–February 1976 and the responses of Dickoff, James and Semradek that follow the Volicer letter.

For a particularly clear and clever statement of the dilemmas in clinical nursing research, see Semradek, Joyce and Carolyn Williams (eds): *Resolving Dilemmas in Practice Research: Decisions for Practice.* Proceedings of a Symposium of the School of Nursing, University of North Carolina at Chapel Hill, March 1974. Chapel Hill: University of North Carolina School of Nursing, 1976. See especially the brilliantly reasoned section by James Dickoff and Patricia James: From dilemmas to presets through design, pp. 1–19.

For additional background on this point see the following:

Abdellah, Faye G. and Eugene Levine: *Better Patient Care Through Nursing Research.* New York: Macmillan, 1965, especially Chapters 1–4.

Diers, Donna: This I believe—about nursing research. *Nursing Outlook,* 18:50–54, November 1970.

Leonard, see Note 1.

Norris, Catherine M.: Delusions that trap nurses. *Nursing Outlook,* 21:18–21, January 1973.

Werley, Harriet H.: This I believe—about clinical nursing research. *Nursing Outlook,* 20:718–722, November 1972.

Hanson, Robert L.: Research—a necessity in nursing service. *Journal of Nursing Administration,* 3:61–62, May–June 1973.

Hanson, Robert L.: Research in nursing service. *Nursing Outlook,* 19:520–523, August 1971.

Diers, Donna: Research for nursing. *Journal of Nursing Administration,* 2:8, January–February 1972; 2:7, March–April 1972.

Henderson, Virginia: Research in nursing practice—when? *Nursing Research,* 4:99, 1956.

Dickoff, James and Patricia James. A theory of theories. *Nursing Research,* 17:197–203, September–October 1968.

Hassenplug, Lulu W.: This I believe—about university nursing education. *Nursing Outlook*, 18:38–40, May 1970.

Lindeman, Carol A.: Nursing research: a visible, viable component of nursing practice. *Journal of Nursing Administration*, 3:18–20, March–April 1973.

Nuckolls, Katherine B.: Nursing research—good for what? *Nursing Forum*, 11(4):374–384, 1972.

6. See for example: Wooldridge, Powhatan et al.: *Behavioral Science, Social Practice and the Nursing Profession.* Cleveland: The Press of Case Western Reserve University, 1958, pp. 55–56. See also, for a parallel point of view in medicine, Feinstein, Alvan: *Clinical Judgment.* Baltimore: Williams & Wilkins, 1967, especially the Prologue.

7. Watson, James D.: *The Double Helix.* New York: Atheneum, 1968, pp. xi–xii.

8. Beadle, George and Muriel: *The Language of Life.* New York: Doubleday, 1966, p. 54.

9. *Ibid.*, p. viii.

10. Taylor, Donald W. et al.: Education for research in psychology. *The American Psychologist*, 14:167–179, 1959.

11. Martocchio, Benita, et al.: Developing a research attitude in nursing students. *Nursing Outlook*, 19:384–386, June 1971.

Verhonick, Phyllis J.: Research awareness at the undergraduate level. *Nursing Research*, 20:261–264, May–June 1971.

Voda, Anna M., et al.: On the process of involving nurses in research. *Nursing Research*, 20:302–308, July–August 1971.

Passos, Joyce Y. and Alice A. Stallings: Introduction of concepts of measurement and statistics to sophomore nursing students. *Nursing Research*, 22:249–253, May–June 1973.

Kreuger, Janelle C.: The value of summer research for undergraduate nursing students. *Nursing Research*, 21:159–160, March–April 1972.

Werley, Harriet H. and Fredericka P. Shea: The first center for research in nursing. *Nursing Research*, 22:217–231, May–June 1973.

Johnson, Jean E., et al.: Research projects for teaching methodology. *Nursing Outlook*, 16:27–30, November 1968.

Oram, Phyllis and Wilda R. Routhier: Research as inservice education. *Nursing Outlook*, 16:20–22, September 1968.

Hawley, Janet: Reconciling nursing with research. *Nursing Outlook*, 16:34–35, June 1968.

12. Stetler, Carol and Gwen Marram: Evaluating research findings for applicability in practice. *Nursing Outlook*, 24:559–563, September 1976.

Jacox, Ada: Nursing research and the clinician. *Nursing Outlook*, 22:382–385, June 1974.

Ellis, Rosemary: Practitioner as theorist. *American Journal of Nursing*, 69:1434–1438, July 1969.

Abraham, Gertrude E.: Promoting nursing research in an organized nursing service. *American Journal of Nursing*, 68:818–821, April 1968.

Cross, Deana: Nursing research in the Veterans Administration. *Nursing Research*, 26:250–252, July–August 1977.

Spector, Audry F.: Regional action and nursing research in the South. *Nursing Research*, 26:272–276, July–August 1977.

Elliott, Jo Eleanor: Nursing research through WICHEN. *Nursing Research*, 26:277–280, July–August 1977.

13. Feinstein, See Note 6.

    See also almost any article of Dr. Feinstein's, as well as his continuing series in the *Journal of Clinical Pharmacology and Therapeutics* called "Clinical Biostatistics," beginning with Vol. 11, No. 1, pp. 135–148, January–February 1970.

14. Nursing's odd self-concept is discussed in the series of articles and audience participation under the title Nursing leadership–problems and possibilities, *American Journal of Nursing*, 72:1445–1456, August 1972.

    A number of interesting articles have reported nurses' experiences in a changing self-concept as they go into research:

    Conant, Lucy: On becoming a nurse researcher. *Nursing Research*, 17:69–70, January–February 1968.

    Davis, Marcella Z.: Some problems in identity in becoming a nurse researcher. *Nursing Research*, 17:166–168, March–April 1968.

    Malone, Mary: Research as viewed by researcher and practitioner. *Nursing Forum*, 1(2):39–55, Spring 1962.

    Ellis, Rosemary: Values and vicissitudes of the scientist nurse. *Nursing Research*, 19:440–445, September–October 1970.

    Eisler, Jeanne: Research is fun. *Nursing Forum*, 11(4):385–394, 1972.

    Nehring, Virginia and Barbara Geach. Patients' evaluation of their care: why they don't complain. *Nursing Outlook*, 21:317–321, May 1973.

    Eisler, Jeanne et al.: Strangers in computerland. *American Journal of Nursing*, 72:1120–1122, June 1972.

    McBride, M. Angela, et al.: Nurse-researcher: the crucial hyphen. *American Journal of Nursing*, 70:1256–1260, June 1970.

1

Research Problems

Research always begins with a problem, and research in nursing practice begins with problems in nursing practice.

FINDING NURSING PROBLEMS

There is no great scarcity of clinical nursing problems (1). One cannot help but stumble over things to wonder about in any clinical situation. But the problem with problems is that there can be so many of them that they become simply overwhelming without inspiring action. Or else one is spurred to action too quickly without really investigating the problem.

A graduate student was reporting on her research project to a group of staff nurses. The conversation turned to things that had happened during the data collection period. The graduate student was talking about how she was curious about some of the incidents she saw and hadn't had a chance to check out, when one of the staff nurses suddenly said, "There's something I've been wondering about too. I work nights mostly and I've noticed that an awful lot of men who have had prostatectomies get confused the second night after surgery. Sometimes they don't seem to know where they are, and if you don't watch carefully, they'll get up out of bed and pull out their catheters or CBIs. I spend half my shift just keeping a watch on them. Why do you suppose this happens?"

The temptation is to respond automatically to this nurse, suggesting possible explanations—age of the patient, length of surgery, complicated internal psychic states involving the patient's perception of his manhood, lack of nursing time on the night shift, perhaps poor preoperative preparation or medical follow-up, sedative effects and so on. But the point is, without study the answer will be just guesswork. That the nurse was wondering—curious— means that she was standing in the right place for a research idea to find her. She could have been merely annoyed.

The "I wonder why . . ." problems are one type of research topic. Another type is, "I wonder what would happen if. . . ."

A young nurse was working in the prenatal clinic of a large urban hospital. Like many clinics, this one was overpopulated and understaffed, and there was a very high attrition of patients. Pregnant women were not registering for the clinic until very late in their pregnancies, and women who had delivered were not returning for their six-week checkup. With her public health background, the new staff nurse was concerned about preventive care. She began wondering, What would happen if we kept the clinic open in the evening and on weekends? What would happen if the clinic nurses each carried a case load of their own and followed-up with patients to see that they got care? What would happen if the nurses took an ombudsman role and helped ease patients through the clinic morass? Any or all of these if's could and should be studied systematically. It is all too easy to institute a procedural change in the happy hope that it will do some good, but without planning and evaluating to be sure that it will.

These research problems were just lurking about waiting to be discovered, but curiosity is a condition that has to exist before a problem for research can be seen for what it is.

There is another precondition to research buried in these examples that is even more important than curiosity. To see a problem as a possible research problem, one must be able to make mental connections between incidents or cases. A nurse can observe one postoperative patient who becomes confused and pulls out his catheter and think of it only as an isolated happening. When she begins to see this happening as an example of a whole class of cases or incidents, she is in effect conceptualizing the problem at a higher level of abstraction. Problems for research must be moved to a higher level to be investigated so that they will have generality beyond the merely immediate, isolated instance.

Sometimes, too, it takes a new pair of eyes to see research possibilities. For example, a nurse going to work in the intensive care unit for the first time was struck with the incredible amount of noise. Solutions were bubbling, gasses were hissing, people were talking loudly, equipment clanked, patients moaned. The staff who worked there seemed not to notice, but the patients appeared exhausted when they were finally transferred back to floor care. The new nurse wondered just how much rest patients got in the intensive care unit and what effect their stay had on them. (This story has a happy ending. The nurse did investigate sleep and rest in the intensive care unit and established the fact that patients were deprived of rest. Her findings came to the attention of the chief of surgery who subsequently instituted changes in the standing orders for the unit to provide uninterrupted rest periods for patients.) (2)

Another good source of ideas for research may be found in the practice of older nurses with the wisdom of years of experience. Listen to one of them talk about her practice sometime; they all have invented ways to help patients better or to simplify routines. Can their techniques be generalized so that other nurses can practice them too? The story of the legendary pediatric nurse who gives shots to children and they never cry may be apocryphal, but wouldn't it be interesting to find out if it is true? And how she does it?

It is not hard at all to find researchable problems in nursing. The possibilities are almost overwhelming and hardly any of them have been studied enough. But it is hard to find problems if you aren't looking for them, if you aren't standing in the right place or if you aren't in the right frame of mind to let them find you.

A "problem" is something that seems wrong (3). It is a difference between two states of affairs, a *discrepancy* between the way things are and the way they ought to be, or between what one knows and what one needs to know to eliminate the problem. A problem makes itself known as a feeling of discomfort. Sometimes the feeling is expressed as a gripe: We're short staffed again. Why are gyn. patients so hard to take? I can't seem to get through to Mr. Smith that he doesn't need so much pain medication. What's wrong with him anyhow? If we only had a little more time, we could really prepare patients for surgery better. It makes me mad that patients won't come back for their postpartum appointments when we've told them how important it is. Those emergency room nurses are great when it comes to machines and techniques, but they don't do a thing with the patient's emotional feelings. It's idiotic that we have to give medications always at 8-12-4-8 when, with report and all, we never get them done on time and then we mess up the patient's meal time. Mrs. Brown knows she has to take her insulin regularly, but she just won't.

Similarly, research problems may come from professional wishes or desires, the need to improve something, born out of the altruism of professional practice that means developing new and better ways to help patients cope better, or feel better, or recover faster, or live more fully. For example, a group of coronary care nurses was concerned with its inability to predict when a patient might be about to experience cardiac tamponade, clearly a medical disaster. The nurses felt that there must be some way besides constant monitoring and watchfulness, some signs in either physiological responses or nursing observations, that would signal approaching catastrophe (4). This problem called for a study of the variables associated with incidence of tamponade—variables in the patients themselves, the surgical procedure, anesthesia, recovery room and intensive care routines and so forth.

Another group of nurses, nurse midwives this time, were convinced that there must be better ways to help low-income patients with restricted means and access to health care to have better babies, since they knew that infant birth weight is the best predictor of later pediatric development. This called for a study to test the effect of a new program of antepartum care and nutritional counseling, including patient advocacy, patient participation and home visits on infant and maternal outcome. A series of studies has now documented improved outcomes for mothers who receive these kinds of services (5).

Primary nursing itself grew out of a series of studies (stimulated, oddly enough, by a need to define the role of the unit manager.) (6) In the course of doing those studies, Manthey and others were drawn to the concern that nurses were not practicing to the full extent of their capacity or training, and, thus, patient care was suffering. The desire to improve patient care then led to the development of primary nursing as a new system of care, and to several studies of its effect (7).

Two relatively more recent sources of problems for clinical nursing research come from the two most powerful recent advances in health care—the increasing use of technology and the expanding role of nurses. For example, nurses may profitably do studies to prepare patients better for complicated diagnostic procedures or treatments, examine the ways to increase the reliability of measures taken from new equipment or study ways to help patients cope with the experience of monitoring or intensive care.

Similarly, as nurses more consciously take on more responsible roles in health care, new topics for investigation come up naturally. The easiest to feel, of course, are the problems that call for evaluation of the services offered by nurses in expanded roles. But equally prevalent now are studies dealing with certain aspects of care for which nurses have long been responsible, but haven't formally studied, such as discharge planning, nutrition counseling, patient teaching and the like.

These studies, like the ones that flow from gripes or wishes, have their own psychological motivation. In the case of technology studies, it is often the desire to counter the depersonalization nurses believe patients experience, or the desire to see that the new technology does not rule the patient's experience.

In the case of expanded role studies, the motivation is often a political one, in the sense of documenting that nurses can do as well as physicians, or that nurses deserve to be treated more equitably because of the excellence of the services they offer.

As motivations, these are as powerful and as effective as the motivation to correct something wrong, stated as a gripe, or the more altruistic wish to improve patient care. Political motivations, however, have the inherent danger that the research becomes merely documentation of the obvious, or is badly designed in order to bias the case. This is discussed later in the chapters on methodology.

Many gripes and wishes might be sources of research problems, but not all of the problems are going to be researchable, and some will not even need research for their solution. Three qualities make discrepancies into potential research problems. The first criterion is that the potential research problem is a *difference that matters*. There are numberless differences in the real world but not all of them may be problems. Some physicians prefer to have their patients take rectal temperatures, others have no expressed preference. This difference may not matter if it has no particular effect on either the patient or the nursing staff, and if whatever the temperature procedure is, it produces accurate information. Similarly, some nurses prefer pediatric nursing and others like geriatrics. If nurses are able to work in their preferred setting, this difference may not matter either. If not, they may not be happy or care for patients adequately. What makes a difference matter, first of all, is its consequence in patient care. The appropriate focus for research in nursing practice is the systematic study of problems in patient care.

The second criterion that makes a problem a research problem is its *relationship to more general, conceptual issues*. Given that research in nursing has two goals—improvement of patient care (thus, the first criterion for research problems) and development of professional practice knowledge, problems for research have to have the potential of contributing to nursing theory development (nursing knowledge). This means that a problem has to be seen as an instance of a larger class of events, concepts and so on.

It is quite possible to solve important patient care problems without doing research and developing theory. The nursing literature is full of case reports of a nurse solving one patient's care problem by trial and error or by more systematic methods. A brief report of how a nurse discovered that the cause of one pregnant patient's severe hypotension was the supine position in which the pregnant uterus pressed against the inferior vena cava, cured by turning the patient on her side, is a good example (8). One could develop that clinical problem in theoretical terms, but it really isn't necessary when the answer is already available in the knowledge of physiology and physics.

Research in nursing practice is hard work, and, therefore, should be done when and where it will realistically have the most payoff. To use research to solve problems whose answers are already available isn't the most efficient use of scarce professional resources. Similarly, to use research methods to establish the existence of a problem may have political benefit, but doesn't contribute much to the development of professional knowledge. Research is more than merely the systematic collection of facts from which to argue. For example, a nurse who had had abdominal surgery returned to the surgical clinic a week or so after surgery to have a drain removed. She discovered that in this clinic, all patients were given appointments for the same hour and she found herself at the end of a long line of fellow sufferers, in a waiting area with too few chairs and benches. A little questioning provided the information that the surgeons liked to have all patients come at the same time to make sure that they didn't have to waste any of their time waiting for a patient to show up. It would be tempting to do some simple collecting of data to document the length of waiting time, the number of patients who pass out or have untoward symptoms from waiting and so on. But there's no theoretical problem here—just a practical one, solved easily by changing the appointment system and buying some chairs. It may be necessary in such situations to collect that kind of information to argue one's case with the chief of surgery or the nursing office, but that isn't really research—it's data collection. What makes an activity research, as described here, is its reference to theory—its obligation to produce generalized information that can go beyond data immediately collected through development of theories that can guide practices in other situations. From the beginning of analyzing a nursing problem to turn it into a research problem, the notion that the clinical problem is an *instance* of a class of related problems has to be kept in mind.

The third criterion that makes a problem a nursing research problem is whether nurses (or nursing) have *access* to and *control* over the phenomenon in question (9). Even if nurses do not have direct access to or control over a phenomenon in a given setting, is it still something that sometime, somewhere, it is reasonable to think would be important to nurses? For instance, generally nurses do not have legal access to or control over the prescribing of medications, though they may in some settings and under certain conditions alter the dosage or manipulate the timing. Thus, problems about a patient's tolerance or liking for a particular medication are not really something over which nursing has control, and, therefore, might better be studied by others. However, access and control are interpreted broadly. Nurses have access to and control over a number of things that they may not consciously contemplate, for example: the physician's behavior, administrative decisions, policy and procedures, patients' feelings, equipment, tools, papers, charts. Any of these could be appropriately incorporated into research questions. If the research is to have implications beyond the merely immediate situation, one should consider also what nurses might have access to or control over in the future, if not at present. For example, some years ago nurses were not allowed to insert intravenous needles. It would have been nice in those days if someone had investigated different methods of insertion, preparing for the day that nurses would have that responsibility. Nowadays with the increasing expansion of the nursing role into traditionally medical functions, it is almost incumbent on us to begin developing the body of knowledge that will lie under that practice of nurse practitioners in areas not now normally a part of "nursing" practice. The mind can consider a very large scope of potential nursing research questions that involve things nursing might soon have access to or control over, or things that nursing should, knowing, of course, that there may be administrative or other limitations put on the investigator's freedom to explore some questions.

With the expanding nursing role, it is more and more difficult to think of clinical phenomena that are completely closed to nursing's access, and impervious to nursing's impact. Even the medication example does not hold in certain nurse practitioner situations. There is a recent report in the nursing literature of a study which tested the effect of topical insulin on decubitus ulcers and which apparently had no physician input (10).

ANALYZING CLINICAL PROBLEMS

Once a problem has been tagged a discrepancy that matters and once one perceives that it has a conceptual relationship to like problems, the problem has to be turned into a form that will make it researchable. The steps in that process are outlined in Figure 1-1.

The first step is to examine the discomfort or the gripe or wish more

Figure 1-1. *Guide for Analysis of Clinical Problems*

1. Identify and state the discrepancy.
   A. Why, or how, do you know there is a discrepancy? How did you come to feel it as a discrepancy?
   B. How do you know it's a difference *that matters?*
   C. If the discrepancy were removed, what would the result look like? What are the implications of removing the discrepancy? Of not removing it?
2. Describe the significance of the discrepancy to practice and theory.
   A. How big is it? How big a gap is there between what is and what should be, or what's known and needs to be known?
   B. What is this problem an instance of?
3. Analyze the nature of the discrepancy.
   A. What are the two conditions?
   B. What factors are involved in each?
   C. How are the factors related? How do you know?
4. State the questions that need to be answered to remove the discrepancy.
   A. What are the most important questions? Why?
   B. How practical will obtaining the answers be? Consider your own resources—energy, time, money, interest, experience.
   C. Select the questions to be answered.
5. Specify the type of study that is appropriate.
   A. Have you identified factors? Relationships?
   B. Do you have hypotheses or predictions or are you looking for them?
   C. If you have hypotheses, what form do they take?

closely. It usually consists of two parts—a statement of facts as they are now and an implicit indication of what they ought to be. Something is wrong, and it shouldn't be. For example, the gripe, We never have enough time to really *nurse,* can become, We never have enough time and we ought to because the patients need good nursing care. The next step then is to take this discrepancy between what is and what ought to be apart. What exactly is really nurse? How much time does that take? Is time the only important thing or is it energy, commitment, competing demands, rewards or what? What effect does the frustration of too little time have on nurses and on patients? How do you know? How long is never? Is it true that nurses never have enough time or that only certain aspects of patient care are being neglected? What do nurses do with their time? What would happen with more time? What is good patient care and what would it look like? In the best of all possible worlds, how should the time be alloted? How do you know?

Following is a clinical problem that arose not as a gripe but as a critical observation:

A nurse observed wide differences in the nursing care given on a medical ward. Certain patients received the epitome of care and attention, while others seemed to be unattended, uncomfortable and dissatisfied. . . . Nurses working on this ward appeared to voice favorable or unfavorable feelings about many of their patients. (11)

In this case, the discrepancy is between what is and what might be or ought to be. Patients were getting different kinds of care and their care seemed to be related to how nurses felt about them. However, patient care should not depend on how well the nurse likes the patient. Incidentally, this same discrepancy can be felt from sources other than direct observation. Duff and Hollingshead's book contains the same discrepancy culled from their study of hospitalized patients (12).

Problems may come from observations or secondhand observations about practice. They may also come from the experiences of others (such as Duff and Hollingshead), from previous research reported in the literature or from theories. Theories in other disciplines may be a source for nursing studies, as, for example, in trying to find out if a psychological theory that predicts how certain types of patients will fare after surgery will hold up when a nurse tries to be guided by that theory in her practice.

In the case of problems that arise from theories in other disciplines, the problem is experienced as, Gee, that's an interesting idea. I wonder if it will work in (or help explain) this clinical problem I see. For instance, the theory of locus of control—the extent to which people believe that they personally are in control of what happens to them or are influenced by factors outside themselves (13) might occur to a nurse as something that might be operating to explain why stress-reducing preoperative preparation seems to work better for some patients than for others. Or theories about altered states of consciousness, derived from neurophysiology and psychiatry might help the nurse mentioned earlier figure out why patients are confused following prostrate surgery.

Referring back to the clinical problem quoted above, the nurse notices that patients seemed to be getting different kinds of care and that nurses had different feelings about different patients. In this step of the analysis of the problem, she might go more deeply into her original observation and ask what "epitome of care" looked like, how she knew some patients were uncomfortable or neglected. She might think of examples of things nurses had said about patients that led her to think nurses had different feelings about different patients. She might think about her experience on this ward and remember certain kinds of patients who particularly seemed to be neglected, or certain kinds who were not. If the problem had come from the literature instead of from practice, the nurse might reread the evidence that led her to feel the discrepancy. She might ask how good the evidence was and how it fits with her own experience. This step really means getting clear about what that feeling called discrepancy is.

Sometimes problems are felt not so much as discrepancies between what is and what ought to be as between facts, or between what one knows and what one needs to know. (These can have the ought feeling too—How come there are two different sets of facts here when there ought to be one? I ought to know more than I do.) In either case, the first step in analyzing the clinical problem is the same: think through and state both conditions in the discrepancy. The examination of patient care rituals illustrates these kinds of discrepancies nicely. Nurses have been doing catheter irrigations as a nursing procedure for a very long time. Why? Do we know what the procedure is supposed to do, and, therefore, how to evaluate whether it accomplishes its purpose? Does it work at all? Are there ways to make it work better? Here the clinical problem, the state of discomfort, stems from realizing the ritual of doing something without knowing why, and the consequent need to know (14).

Another instance: a graduate student in psychiatric nursing had her clinical experiences in two different settings, one that used seclusion liberally, another which never used it. Both settings argued heatedly for the virtue of their position. Here is a discrepancy between two sets of facts, in this case, opinions. Nurses are often confronted with the need to help patients reconcile discrepancies between two sets of facts: some nutritional literature says pregnant women should drink lots of milk; other writing says milk is dangerously high in cholesterol and should be avoided after puberty. Some physicians will prescribe, even order, pregnant patients to abstain from intercourse for varying lengths of time before delivery. Others will not. Some nurses will insist that intramuscular injections should always be given in the hip; others will use hip, thigh or arm. The nurse faced with the patient's question about these contradictions has stumbled into a research problem.

Sometimes this first step in analyzing a discrepancy—stating the two conditions—leads to removing the problem as a problem. For example, one nurse was concerned with the high "no show" rate among the postpartum mothers she cared for who did not keep their clinical appointments. When she came to look at the "keeping clinic appointments" end of the discrepancy, she discovered that a very high proportion of the mothers were getting their care elsewhere, through the VNA well-child conferences, private physicians, or other sources, even though they didn't come back to clinic. While it may be nice to have a patient care problem "solved" so easily, if you're a graduate student in search of a researchable problem for a thesis, some ambivalence is natural!

The first step in analyzing the problem—stating the discrepancy—is crucial because every other step in the research process will follow from this one. The mental work involved in beginning to characterize an empirical, singular event in abstract, conceptual terms is using a way of thinking that is not common nursing practice. We are so used to "individualizing patient care" that to conceptualize an instance with a particular patient as only a part of a class of events seems almost perverted. But that's the essence of the circular relationship between research and practice, or more particularly, between abstraction and data. One moves from the instance to the concept that names that class of events, then back to gather data on like events, then back to reconceptualizing, inferring, interpreting again in conceptual terms. Even the language changes. One changes from thinking my patient, Mr. Jones, who has pain . . . to patients who have pain. . . .

The questions under the main headings in Figure 1-1 are just different ways to think about discrepancies in order to state them clearly. They are intended to alert one to the often unstated and implicit values—the shoulds and oughts that make up the discrepancy. They also lead one's thinking naturally forward into professional judgement—what makes a difference *matter?* This point is trickier than it looks because in nursing, as in other professions, there are no guidelines that help define a problem as a high priority. While classes of problems have been identified for the profession to investigate (15), the choice of an actual empirical problem is the investigator's own. A problem that matters to one investigator may seem trivial to another. But it is important to identify and state why any given problem is a problem worth putting the time and effort into investigating.

(Parenthetically, one often sees in the nursing literature reference to someone's "theory of nursing," or more accurately, someone's treatise or point of view on nursing as justification for studying a given problem. Since deciding what matters and what doesn't is partly a problem of professional judgment, referring to a thoughtful statement on the nature of nursing is a helpful addition, and in the long run may assist in developing actual theory derived from what have often been philosophical notions.) (16)

Stating the discrepancy is harder than it looks. Few nursing problems are tiny and simple, and when one begins to think about what the two ends of the discrepancy are—the *is* end and the *ought to be* end—one can easily stray off into humanistic grandiosity on the latter end, or into increasingly convoluted description on the former. But the purpose of analyzing a clinical problem to turn it into a research problem is to narrow it down to a manageable handful. That handful has to have a relationship to the larger world of nursing goals, however, and they too have to be stated clearly, even if the research is to deal with only a small fragment of the reality.

The second major heading on the outline for analysis of the problem is to begin to focus on the clinical problem in conceptual terms. Describing the significance of the problem is tightening up the reasoning on what makes the difference matter. It also means beginning to refer to what is already known, and that means beginning to conceive of the problem in words that are concepts. The question, How big is the discrepancy? is not used literally so much as imaginatively—how much research distance, time and space is there between the two conditions in the discrepancy? For example, is this a problem on which nothing has ever been done? Or is the discrepancy one that something is known about, but not enough? Is it a problem that lies at the very heart of patient care, or is it one somewhat removed or peripheral? Part of the answer to how big the discrepancy is comes from the first step in analyzing the problem in which the implications of removing it were considered. The other part begins to come out of reviewing previous work and previous experience outside of research in the area. And here the most important question in the whole analysis of the problem occurs—what is this problem an *instance of?*

At this stage, the researcher is forced to start to name the concepts revealed in the discrepancy. That process of "conceptualizing" is critical for it will lead into the review of literature, into the study design itself, into the methods of measurement and data collection, and will be the framework in which the results are eventually interpreted. This step in analyzing the problem can feel very frustrating since problems are capable of being named or conceptualized in an almost infinite variety of ways. For example, the clinical problem that certain patients do not seem to follow their prescribed treatment regimen at home can be an instance of compliance theory to one investigator, an example of alienation to another, a case of communicator congruence to a third, social distance to a fourth, lack of information to a fifth and so on. The choice of how to conceptualize a problem follows no real rules. Concepts are adopted out of familiarity or intrigue, because they seem to fit, because they're investigatable or just because one likes them.

It is also at this stage that the beginning nurse-researcher may start to feel the discomfort that comes from having to narrow one's view to only a piece of the action, and seeming to have to lose sight of the particular patient (a view so highly valued in nursing) to put her/his problem in some larger, academic framework. That's the nature of research, however, and the nature of the professional need to be able to relate one event to another in order to learn and improve care for more than one patient at a time. Conceptualizing gives the glue that holds the one deeply felt personal event from which the problem sprang to the class of events that can be investigated.

The third step in analyzing clinical problems is to name and define the factors or concepts involved in both conditions of the discrepancy. Here the researcher makes specific the orginal observations and tries to isolate the factors that made it. In the clinical problem cited, the researchers began to wonder not only how nurses felt about patients, but how they felt about themselves. They also focused on what felt meant and decided they really wanted to know how nurses accepted themselves and how that related to their acceptance of patients. Then they turned to patients and wondered if there were certain factors in patiency that might be important in patient acceptance—the length of stay in the hospital, patient age, condition, illness and so forth. They might also have analyzed the other end of the discrepancy and looked at what they meant by good care as it should be given. What factors might be involved in the ought condition of the discrepancy? They might have chosen something like patient satisfaction or comfort or rapid recovery as the important factors. In effect, this step means specifying the variables to be investigated. At this point, the process of analyzing a problem is isolating the factors. And it is about here that ideas about study design start to swim into consciousness. If the factors in the discrepancy cannot be named, or the available names are unsatisfactory, it may be that a factor searching study is called for—to provide a way of naming the variables. If the factors can be named but there is not enough information available to predict relationships among them (or if such relationships haven't ever been studied), a relation searching study may be the one. If the factors are named and enough is known to allow one to hypothesize a relationship, an association-testing or causal hypothesis-testing study may be in order. But the selection of study design is still premature until the next step is done: state the questions that need to be answered to remove the discrepancy.

Given that one thing research does is answer questions, which ones need answering for the clinical problem chosen? For example, this briefly stated clinical problem:

> When (the author), a nurse, was a patient in a medical center, she was disappointed in the nursing care she received and blamed the intercom system used by the hospital for her disappointment. (She) thought that the intercom was too impersonal and that at times it was embarrassing to use. (She) also thought that the intercom tended to isolate (patients) from the nurse because the nurses rarely entered (her) room unless a request was made via the intercom. (17)

The following list of possible questions to pursue was then developed:
1. How do nurses perceive the use of the intercom?
2. How do nurses perceive patient requests made via the intercom?
3. When patients make requests via the intercom, do nurses follow them up to find out what the need is?
4. Is the number of patient requests related to nurse-patient ratio, or the kind of hospital accommodation (private, semiprivate)?
5. How do patients perceive the intercom?
6. What kinds of requests do they make?
7. Do patients feel inhibited in the kinds of requests they make?
8. Does the request the patient makes via the intercom really indicate his need?

Note the range of questions here—from nurse feelings to patient feelings, from requests to needs, from possible relationships between intercom use and some framework variables to documentation of nursing activities. The range is not unusual (and in this case the number of questions has been cut considerably from the original). The point here is to list all the possible questions that need to be answered, without, at first, any regard for whether they are answerable, whether answers are already available or any other consideration. This step has the effect of rounding out the problem, which is now almost completely converted from a clinical problem to a research problem. The naming of variables provides the skeleton; the list of questions adds the "guts" of the research.

Once the questions are listed, which can be creative and enjoyable exercise, the hard work starts again in choosing which ones to tackle in any one study. Thus, the next task is to decide what are the most important, or most feasible, questions. Often some questions will logically precede others; some will be obviously interrelated so that the answer to one provides the answer to others. Some will be impractical in a given time period, with given resources in energy, time, money, interest, experience. Some questions will be demonstrably trivial. Some will not be empirical questions at all (see later section of this chapter).

In the intercom example, the investigator decided to concentrate on the patient's perception of the intercom and the relationship between patient request and patient need, reasoning that studying the nurse's perception of her activities was not really patient care research. (Incidentally, she found that indeed, patient requests did not necessarily indicate their need, that patients were not inhibited by the intercom, but they were inhibited by the busy nurses.)

In the last analysis, selecting research questions to be answered is a matter only in part of professional judgment; it's also a matter of personal preference and interest, as well as a practical problem. Especially in artificially time (and budget) limited student research, the most interesting problems may be the ones that would take ten years to investigate and one has to settle for something less than earth-shaking. Other times the real research questions are outside the limits of the nurse's capacity to control the situation enough to provide the answers. For example, the gripe listed earlier about medication scheduling could well lead to a question like, What would happen if we changed the medication schedule to 9-1-5-9? But a student or a staff nurse is unlikely to have the kind of clout in the system to direct such a change and study it.

There is also a practical limit to the number of questions that can usefully be tackled in one study. There is no magic number because the number depends in part on the specificity of the questions and their relationship with one another, and to what extent they require different study designs to answer. Which leads to the last step in the analysis of a clinical problem.

Given the pared-down list of questions, what sorts of answers do they require? If they pose relationships between factors, they can be converted into hypotheses and tested by one of the available hypothesis-testing designs (see Chapters 6 and 7). If they are questions trying to discover relationships, they must be investigated differently (see Chapter 5). And if they are still at the What's going on here? level, a still different approach is indicated. (Actually, the need for a factor-searching study will probably have become clear before this last step.)

It is very often the case that patient care problems mysteriously turn into problems about nurses. It is very difficult somehow to retain the focus on patient care, as well as the sense of anger that prompts many research problems in patient care, and not convert that into quasi-studies of why nurses don't act the way they're supposed to. But it cannot be emphasized enough that it is a misuse of research simply to accuse the system when there is not a relationship to theory that advances the state of knowledge of the profession. Consider the following discrepancy:

> In the course of his treatment (hemigastrectomy and vagotomy) Mr. A. had been given several intravenous and intramuscular injections of antibiotics. The administration of the intramuscular injections caused Mr. A. excessive physical and emotional discomfort which were reflected in his vital signs and general agitation. He complained that his buttocks and hips were sore. For ten days the injection sites had not been rotated beyond these areas. Rotation of injection sites to anterior and lateral thighs were instituted but it was discovered that rotation of injection sites could not be instituted without a doctor's order. Hospital policy mandated

that the safe area for intramuscular injections was the buttock and hip area. An incident report with nursing rationale was submitted to the nursing supervisor, indicating the need to rotate sites for optimum medication absorption and minimum tissue damage. Although the nursing rationale was well based, hospital policy did not recognize this intervention as being in the realm of the nurse. (18)

Clearly, this problem could be converted into a research project on decision-making in hospital systems, or authority structures in patient care institutions, or even interpersonal dynamics within a nursing organization. But these studies would not be patient care research as it is being discussed here. Rather, a study could be designed to test the effect of different medications given in different sites (indeed, such studies have probably already been done).

It all depends on how the problem is conceptualized. The above discrepancy could be a political problem, not a research problem at all, solved by organizing the nurses as a force for change in administrative policy. Or it could be conceived of as a research project in systems or interpersonal sociology. Or it could be a patient care problem.

If one keeps always in mind the goal of nursing research, or of any individual study, as providing information on which to base improvements in practice, the temptation to convert patient care problems into problems about nurses is curtailed. One way to keep that focus is always to ask "so what?" about the potential answers to the research questions. So what is not taken cynically, and in this context does not mean prove it to me. Rather, so what should be translated as, So what will happen if I follow this line of inquiry to its logical conclusion and imagine the findings that might be produced? What will it all mean to the improvement of patient care? (19)

For example, the following perceived discrepancy: "From observations while working for three years in an emergency room, I have concluded the emotional needs of families of patients are not being met as adequately as they could be." (20)

This can be framed as a question about nurses: what factors contribute to nurses not meeting emotional needs (nursing education, personality, time, interest and so on? But suppose one pursues that line of inquiry and does the study. So what? If one discovers that certain kinds of nurses with certain personalities are less likely to be oriented to the emotional needs of families, what does one do with that information? Select other kinds of nurses to work in emergency rooms? Make personality an admission criterion for nursing school?

The position taken in this book is that studies of nurses, and of their training, curriculum, experience and so on, are necessary and interesting—for nursing education. For nursing practice, such studies may be too remote from the pressing need to change services for the better, and, thus, a higher priority is assigned to studies which have the potential of having direct impact on patient care. In the emergency room example, the patient care problems that might be studied might include a descriptive study of the specific kinds of needs families have, or an experimental study that placed a psychiatric nurse clinician in the setting to assist families, and tested the effect of her–his work on some family and patient variables.

That's the problem with problems—they are capable of being translated in an almost infinite number of possible ways, each calling for different attacks. A good part of the reason why problems become so problematic is the nature of the knowledge that underlies the practice of nursing itself, as well as the social context in which the practice of patient care occurs. Nursing knowledge, in the sense of tested information on which patient care can be based, lies at the intersection of concepts and theories, from the social to the physical sciences, the humanities and performing arts and the clinical sciences. And the practice of the profession takes place these days in such a complicated social arena that problems initially perceived as patient care problems almost automatically have ramifications in other realms, especially when the problem is initially seen by a sensitive, aware nurse.

The only point to be stressed here is that it takes some mental discipline to convert the kinds of emotion-provoking incidents cited above into something that can be systematically and unemotionally investigated.

In real life, the process of analyzing a problem proceeds much faster than does writing about it or reading about it. The steps naturally meld into each other and overlap—indeed, they are devised to do just that by providing different ways of looking at discrepancies and picking them apart.

The analysis of the problem leads directly into the study design because, as indicated earlier, different kinds of questions require different ways of providing answers. The clearer the analysis and statement of the problem, the easier the whole research process will be. The more fully each step of the process is done, the more satisfying the research process will be.

The guide for analyzing clinical problems is quite deliberately not the way one writes up the results of such an analysis, but is a guide to thinking it through. Nevertheless, it is a useful exercise to write out each step because in the writing, the problem gets clearer and clearer. The written statement of the problem then becomes a greatly condensed version that should include, however, how the investigator came to see the problem, how important it is, and in what conceptual framework (very briefly stated) the problem is housed, and what sort of a research problem it is at what level of inquiry.

RESOURCES FOR ANALYSIS OF PROBLEMS

In general there are two categories of resources for analyzing clinical problems (or finding them, for that matter)—the experiences of others, reported in the literature or less formally, and one's own experience of nursing.

It has been said that in the clinical wisdom of nurses there is a goldmine of information. It has also been said that that wisdom is inarticulate. Both are true. The guide to analyzing nursing problems is in part intended to force the articulation of what is already *known*, so that it can be written, summarized, and in short, *used* by others. The first resource for analyzing nursing problems, then, is the unanalyzed experience of oneself or others. The nursing literature is full of such accounts, often very moving and highly descriptive. The theory or concepts behind the innovations or experiences reported are unstated, sometimes even unhinted. But in that accumulated experience are nuggets to be dug out, and then named and related to one's own experience and one's beginning analysis of nursing problems. In using this kind of literature, it is up to the researcher to provide the labels, names, or concepts, and in doing so, even before one does a research project, one may already be contributing to the accumulation of knowledge that makes science. Gathering the experiences of others under one common heading helps build up a body of common events into a fuller description, and using that description, ideas for measurement, for interventions, for study designs may come out. It is too easy to ignore this kind of nursing literature as "unscientific" or "too nursey," but that is a disservice. Nursing is, after all, the care of patients, and that can be very intellectually stimulating, as well as personally moving. And it can be used as background to developing research.

The more technical research literature is an obvious source of information for analyzing nursing problems.

The published literature should be treated as a goldmine in the same way that nursing experience is. Reading others' work doesn't stop when the problem is defined and the concepts outlined and made operational. The essence of science is its cumulative nature, and that means more than just repeated studies of the same thing to confirm findings. The literature should be reviewed not only for previous work on the problem itself, but for measurements, statistics, interpretations, suggestions for implementing the results, in other words, any stage in the research process.

Finally, the best resource, and the one handiest, is one's own experience of nursing. Note the order of words—"nursing experience" is too narrow. Lucy Conant once wrote about how in the course of her very large study she found herself using some of her own life experiences, such as building a home, as well as her formal nursing work at various points in the study (21). Even before one gets deeply into conducting a research project, one's own experience of nursing should be thoughtfully probed. Even the casual conversations nurses have over coffee—I once had a patient who . . . or That reminds me of . . . are clues to conceptualizing aspects of nursing. What ties these stories together? A little thought may well produce a concept on which whole studies can hang.

There is a more personal side of experience that is rarely discussed but may be valuable as well. Clinical problems are not chosen by accident—they have very real, personal meaning. Some introspection on the part of the budding investigator may well produce insights into the nature of the problem that would not otherwise occur. Of course, there is the danger of finding a problem to study in order to prove one's own idiosyncratic belief.

But short of that, the intrapersonal reasons that prompt one to study any given problem may well be a resource for research not often tapped (22).

Discussing one's flowering research idea with carefully selected others often leads to new insights or twists on the problem. One can search out the very experienced, acknowledged excellent nurse and ask for her/his view. One can turn to the very new people on the ward—the interns who change every July, the new student nurses or the graduate students. Families of patients and patients themselves are resources far too infrequently tapped for their "clinical knowledge." Indeed, one aspect of the significance of any research problem is how significant it is for the consumers themselves. As professionals, we may think that the real patient care problem is that no one will deal with the patients' feelings about his illness, surgery, or the like, when what the patient is most concerned about is whether his call light will be answered on time or whether he will be helped to be comfortable.

The emphasis here on the less formal sources of input for analyzing nursing problems and making research problems out of them does not in any way suggest that these resources can substitute for a thorough and systematic review of the literature. But because these resources are often neglected (23) they deserve a little attention.

RESEARCHABLE AND NONRESEARCHABLE PROBLEMS

The questions that spark research activities, besides being carefully determined from the problem and being clearly at certain levels of inquiry, have one more characteristic. They must be answerable by research. Questions of value, or policy questions, are not researchable.

If one asks a random group of nurses for a question they might be interested in pursuing as a research study, they often come up with something like, What should the nurse's role be? It sometimes is a nasty shock that such a question can never be answered by research. It is a question of value. One could interview several thousand nurses and ask them what they think a nurse's role ought to be, but the results might indicate only how much agreement there is on opinions, which still doesn't answer the question. Opinions are *facts; should* questions are policy questions and cannot be answered by any amount of research. Questions about the kinds of values people hold are researchable, but these are not the same as unresearchable questions about the kinds of values people *should* hold.

This is not to say that values never enter into research. Obviously, in the analysis of the problem step that asks what the two conditions are, the real and ideal, there is some conception of the ideal. Without the ideal, the real cannot be judged for how close it comes to what is valued. Unless there is some sort of theory or some set of values we don't even know where to look for the facts.

Research deals with questions of fact, statements of what is, predictions of what could be and comparisons between things. However, the researcher's values or the values of a particular profession in which the research is being carried out dictate in some ways the kinds of fact-gathering that are considered appropriate or meaningful. For instance, in this book, the purpose of nursing research is stated as the improvement of nursing practice through the development of prescriptive theory. This is a policy statement and one which may guide or set as priority some research efforts. Whether or not this is a legitimate (valid, useful, effective) purpose for nursing research is a matter of opinion and philosophy and cannot be answered by conventional research methods. The consequence of adhering to this philosophy can be examined, but the "goodness" of the philosophy is still a value judgment.

Even questions such as which nursing treatment is better for a patient cannot be answered specifically by research. What research can do is to provide data on what the different effects of two treatments are. But the question of betterness still remains one of judgment and such judgment is dictated by values. A study might find that because of one kind of treatment, patients experience more relief from pain than they do with a different kind of treatment. But that study does not answer the question of whether relief from pain is a good thing to have happen to patients or not. Though it may seem overly cynical to question the goodness of relief from pain, one can think of situations in which relief from pain might not be considered a desirable thing to achieve. For instance, if the spinal cord is severed, the patient feels no pain below the level of the cut. The patient is also paralyzed below that level. Does this mean to relieve the patient's pain in the lower extremities, cut the spinal cord? Of course not. Questions of betterness of one treatment over another or questions of shouldness are not answerable by research.

Even though such questions are not answerable by research, research can provide evidence which can be used to improve the services to patients, if implemented in practice. Research may help build up the knowledge base upon which patient care depends. And, research can provide evidence which may enable people in a position to make decisions to make decisions on firmer ground (24). For instance, the question, What should a nurse's role be? might be reworded and lead to a series of studies in which various kinds of roles are compared with respect to their effect both on the nurse and on the patient. The decision-maker could compare the evidence and decide to implement those roles that had effects judged good.

The beauty of systematic study—research—is its dependence on facts or data as opposed to the other available methods of solving practice problems (25). Yet simply gathering facts is not research. Public opinion polls regularly tell us what a sample of people think about political issues, but this is only research in the sense that it abides by regularity and rules. At the risk of redundancy, research makes its contribution through the development of knowledge, not just the acquisition of numbers. Thus, there are problems that may be solved, by political means, through arguing on the basis of data. On the whole, that is a better argument than unsupported opinion. But it isn't research.

NOTES

1. Some of the material in this chapter is taken from Diers, Donna: Finding clinical problems for study. *Journal of Nursing Administration*, 1:15–18, November–December 1971, and Diers, Donna: Research for nursing. *Journal of Nursing Administration*, 2:7,61, May–June 1972. Used by permission.

2. Dowd, Kathleen: A study of sleep and rest in postoperative cardiovascular patients. Unpublished Master's Thesis, Yale University School of Nursing, 1968.

3. For a similar conception of nursing problems see Wandelt, Mable: *Guide for the Beginning Researcher*. New York: Appleton-Century-Crofts, 1970, especially pp. 1–100.

4. I am grateful to Carol Stetler, Director of Staff Development, Massachusetts General Hospital for this example. The nurses involved are Carolyn Anderson, Sally Keck and Janice Rieth, all head nurses.

5. McDonaugh, Helena: Retrospective study to determine factors influencing perinatal outcome. Unpublished Master's Thesis, Yale University School of Nursing, 1975; Wirth, Victoria H.: Effect of nurse midwifery services in a neighborhood clinic on differences in perinatal outcome. Unpublished Master's Thesis, Yale University School of Nursing, 1976; Harrison, Debra: A replication study: effectiveness of nurse midwifery service in a neighborhood health clinic. Unpublished Master's Thesis, Yale University School of Nursing, 1978. McDonaugh's study provided the baseline data from which Wirth was able to compare the effects of a nurse midwifery service in an impoverished setting. Harrison replicated Wirth's study and added another group of cases. Comparisons are made both with the baseline data and with samples drawn from the University medical center clinics during the same time periods.

6. Marie Manthey, personal communication. Ms. Manthey's story of how primary nursing came to be has not yet been published. Some of the conceptual background is contained in Manthey, Marie, et al.: Primary nursing: a return to the concept of "my nurse" and "my patient." *Nursing Forum*, 9(1):65–83, 1970. Manthey, Marie and Marlene Kramer: A dialogue on primary nursing. *Nursing Forum* 9(4):366–379, 1970. Manthey, Marie: Primary care is alive and well in the hospital. *American Journal of Nursing*, 73:83–87, January 1973.

7. Daeffler, R.J.: Patients perceptions of care under team and primary nursing. *Journal of Nursing Administration*, 5(3):20–26, 1975.

   Felton, Geraldine: Increasing the quality of nursing care by introducing the concept of primary nursing: a model project. *Nursing Research*, 24:27–32, January–February 1975.

   Williams, I.: Evaluation of nursing care: a primary nursing project–Part I, report of the controlled study. *Supervisor Nurse*, 6(1):32–39, 1975.

   Marram, Gwen, et al.: *Cost Effectiveness of Primary and Team Nursing*. Wakefield, Mass: Contemporary Publishing, Inc., 1976.

   Jones, Katherine: Study documents effect of primary nursing on renal transplant patients. *Hospitals* (JCAH), 16(49):85–89, 1975.

8. Langhorne, Florence: Supine hypotension syndrome. *American Journal of Nursing*, 70:1260, June 1970.

9. For two excellent examples of studies where serious concern with access and control determined design and measurements, see the following:

   Jacox, Ada and Mary Stewart: *Psychosocial Contingencies of the Pain Experience*. Iowa City, Iowa: University of Iowa College of Nursing, 1973; also, Jacox, Ada: Development of a rationale for practice: a study of pain experiences. In Semradek, Joyce and Carolyn Williams (eds.): *Resolving Dilemmas in Practice Research: Decisions for Practice*. Proceedings of a symposium of the School of Nursing, University of North Carolina, Chapel Hill, March 1974. Chapel Hill: University of North Carolina School of Nursing, 1976, especially pp. 63 and 73.

Lindeman, Carol A. and Betty Van Aernam: Nursing intervention with the presurgical patient—the effects of structured and unstructured preoperative teaching. *Nursing Research,* 20:319–332, July–August 1971.

See also, Lindeman, Carol A.: Case studies of practitioner research. In Semradek and Williams, (eds.): *Resolving Dilemmas in Practice Research,* pp. 86–100.

And finally, see Diers, Donna and Ruth L. Schmidt: Interaction analysis in nursing research. In Verhonick, Phyllis J. (ed.): *Nursing Research.* Boston: Little, Brown, 1976, pp. 77–132.

10. Van Ort, Suzanne and Rose M. Gerber: Topical application of insulin in the treatment of decubitus ulcers. *Nursing Research,* 25:9–12, January–February 1976.

11. Dee, Frances Schutt, et al.: Self-acceptance of nurses and acceptance of patients: an exploratory investigation. *Nursing Research,* 14:345–350, Fall 1965, especially pp. 345–346.

This article is an excellent example of research evolving from nursing observation. It is also a good example of how the original idea for a study may have to be revised when it becomes clear that basic information is needed before proceeding to develop the original project.

12. Duff, Raymond and August Hollingshead: *Sickness and Society.* New York: Harper & Row, 1968.

13. Rotter, Julius B.: Generalized expectancies for internal versus external control of reinforcement. *Psychological Monograph,* 80(1), 1966, whole issue # 609.

14. For one excellent study on this problem, see Cleland, Virginia, et al.: Prevention of bacteriuria in female patients with indwelling catheters, *Nursing Research,* 20:309–318, July–August 1971.

See also, Cleland, Virginia: Investigations in the clinical setting. In Verhonick (ed.): *Nursing Research,* especially pp. 53–75.

For a somewhat similar example, see Champion, Victoria: Clean techniques for intermittent self-catheterization. *Nursing Research,* 25:13–15, January–February 1976. In this study, the "ritual" of automatic installation of indwelling catheters for patients with paraplegia or neurological damage is successfully questioned.

15. Lindeman, Carol A.: *Delphi Survey of Clinical Nursing Research Priorities.* Boulder, Colorado: Western Interstate Commission for Higher Education, August 1974.

Abdellah, Faye G.: Overview of nursing research, Part I. *Nursing Research,* 19:6–17, January–February 1970.

Abdellah, Faye G.: U.S. Public Health Service's contribution to nursing research—past, present, future. *Nursing Research,* 22:244–249, July–August 1977.

16. Frequently cited nursing theorists include:

Peplau, Hildegard: *Interpersonal Relations in Nursing.* New York: G.P. Putnam's Sons, 1952; Orlando, Ida Jean: *The Dynamic Nurse-Patient Relationship.* New York: G.P. Putnam's Sons, 1961; Wiedenbach, Ernestine: *Clinical Nursing: A Helping Art.* New York: Springer, 1964; Rogers, Martha: *An Introduction to the Theoretical Basis of Nursing.* Philadelphia: F.A. Davis, 1970; King, Imogene: *Toward a Theory for Nursing: General Concepts in Human Behavior.* New York: John Wiley & Sons, 1971; Orem, Dorothea: *Nursing: Concepts of Practice.* New York: McGraw-Hill, 1971; Riehl, J.P. and Sr. Callista Roy: *Conceptual Models for Nursing Practice.* Englewood Cliffs, New Jersey: Appleton-Century-Crofts, Division of Prentice-Hall, 1974; Roy, Sr. Callista: Adaptation: a basis for nursing practice. *Nursing Outlook, 19:254–257,* April 1971; Roy, Sr. Callista: *Comment: the Roy adaptation model. Nursing Outlook,* 24:690–691, November 1976.

17. Hogan, Marjorie: Needs and requests of patients via the intercom. Unpublished Master's Thesis, Yale University School of Nursing, 1966.

18. This problem was identified as a class assignment by Ruth Churley in Introduction to Nursing Research. Yale School of Nursing, 1974. Used by permission.

19. This clarification is intended to forestall the too-prevalent tendency of criticizing any and all research as only confirming the obvious—"so what?" In the first place, the obvious is not all that obvious. In the second, this cynical "so what" can be sour grapes, a disgusted exclamation based on private knowledge, not shared, so not known by others. Painful experience has been that presenting clinical research results to nursing audiences often invokes this kind of "so what" response, often followed by, "But we already knew that." We didn't know that, or at least we didn't know it with certainty, with objectivity, without intrusive bias. This kind of response is a kind of backhanded compliment, testifying that the research evokes a response and must have been meaningful, in tune with the practice problem, for it to have sparked such reply. But it is disconcerting to have five years of one's professional work dismissed so off-handedly!

20. See Note 18. Problem identified by Jane Sulya. Used by permission.

21. Conant, Lucy: Closing the practice-theory gap. *Nursing Outlook,* 15:37–39, November 1967.

22. See, for example, Hammond, Phillip: *Sociologists at Work.* New York: Basic Books, 1964, for some "inside" descriptions of how research in sociology works.

23. For one example of what happens with such neglect, see Bermosk, Loretta and Raymond Corsini: *Critical Incidents in Nursing.* Philadelphia: W.B. Saunders, 1973, pp. 86–93.

24. The phenomenal growth of interest in the "policy sciences" attests to the concern that decisions be made in the most thoughtful and careful manner, on the best available information. Early examples of this interest can be seen in ethical questions, the examination of which drew together physicians, lawyers, the clergy, and others to study decision-making in defining death and in treating chronic renal disease with dialysis. Other examples include the moral principles to guide university endowment investment as well as the obvious questioning about political and military decisions. See Simon, John G.: *The Ethical Investor.* New Haven: Yale University Press, 1972.

    The National Science Foundation regularly advertises several contracts to institutions who will pull together the relevant literature and experience in a given area and develop "policy recommendations," presumably to be fed to Congressional committees and other branches of government.

25. See Diers, Donna: Research for nursing. *Journal of Nursing Administration,* 2:94, September–October 1972.

    The other methods are the "method of tenacity"—clinging doggedly to a belief without question; the "method of authority"—reference to a power for justification; and the "method of intuition"—"feeling" one is correct.

2

Knowledge for Clinical Judgment

INTRODUCTION

In the Prologue and Chapter 1, the purpose of clinical nursing research, or research in nursing practice, was stated as the improvement of patient care, through providing new knowledge to guide patient care practices. What this means, more specifically, is that research in nursing has as its aim improving *clinical judgment* —the artful and scientific process nurses use to arrive at decisions about how, when, where, with what means, why and toward what end any nursing act is done. In a later chapter (Chapter 8), clinical judgment has a broader meaning as well, but for now, we are interested in what the kinds of knowledge are that need to be provided to improve clinical judgment (1).

Two important assumptions are stated now, one having to do with nursing as a practice, one having to do with nursing as a profession. First, it is assumed that nursing practice is done consciously, if not always with a formal plan, that it is not done mindlessly. Further, the practice of nursing implies accountability for one's own acts, authority over one's activities, and responsibility, and while it may involve carrying out the plans of others (physicians, primary nurses), it is not simply following rigid rules of procedure without analysis. This assumption is important because unless there is some conception that nursing is like this, there is no particular reason for spending the effort to continue to develop the bases on which nurses make decisions about their practice with patients.

Second, nursing is a *practice profession*. It exists to bring about changes in the real world, given a general societal charge, reinforced by formal regulations and enabling legislation. As a practice profession, nursing joins the other practice professions like medicine, the ministry, the practice of law, social work and so on. And as a practice profession, it is unlike academic sociology, psychology or the liberal arts in which knowledge is valued for its own sake, not for the use to which it may be put in a real world of decisions and human encounter (2).

31

Further, as a practice profession, the activities of nursing are purposeful and goal-directed (even if those goals are not stated out loud). Unlike the basic sciences, social sciences or humanities in which discoveries may by themselves be the end point of research, and it's up to someone else to decide what to do with the new information, knowledge in practice professions is *for* something, here stated as improving the services given to the consumers of those services.

Because the use to which the knowledge generated from research is to be put is different in a practice profession, the techniques, rules and point of view derived from the physical sciences as research method content are not sufficient for nursing's needs, nor entirely on target for nursing's goals (3). Research in a practice profession requires new ways of thinking about information derived from research and new ways of generating that information so that it will truly be useful in enhancing clinical judgment (4).

Before proceeding with an in-depth description of these new ways of thinking, it may be well to state what the traditions of research are from which the new material departs.

Nursing research acquires its mystique from its connection with science—that marvelous, arcane set of activities that produces the knowledge of the world. Jacox (5) usefully distinguishes between science as a product and science as a process. The former usage means the accumulated body of knowledge of a discipline, the latter

> . . . the systematic attempt to understand and comprehend the natural world. It is a determination to enter deeply into the natural world, not just superficially, but to achieve a rational expression in language and mathematical symbolism of the order and beauty of operation that lies behind the external world. . . . all aspects of our own experience of ourselves—all perception, imaginings, emotions and actions—everything properly comes into the purview of science. (6)

In the physical sciences, the accumulated body of knowledge comes closer to approaching the ideal of a set of unvarying explanations for phenomena. In the behavioral and social sciences, the science consists more often of inter-related theories, at various levels of abstraction, that attempt to put together direct or indirect observations of the real world in order first to understand and then control nature. In the physical sciences, control over natural phenomena has reached a high point as the rapidly developing disciplines of genetics, immunology, biofeedback and nuclear physics testify. In the social sciences, until recently, the researchers were said to "watch the world go by—*rigorously.*" (7) Recent applications of social science theory to human problems, for example, combining political science, psychology and sociology with law in experiments in jury selection (8), show the potential for developing a field of practice for what have been traditionally academic, nonpracticing social sciences.

It is revealing that the above exercise of using social science knowledge in service was done in connection with one of the "learned professions"—law.

Law, medicine, ministry, teaching and nursing, among others, all carry a societal mandate that goes beyond an obligation to *understand* the world into an obligation to *change* it for the better. Thus, the kind of knowledge the practicing professions need, and need to create and test through research, is of a different order.

The physical science model of research is familiar from grade school on. Chemistry experiments with candles and bottles to show that oxygen is consumed, physics experiments with the sound of trains coming and going illustrate the method and the findings. The model is the experimental design: observe something, introduce a new something and see what happens, making sure that what is introduced is the only difference from whatever the naturally occurring event is. Or, select a situation and divide instances of it into two parts. Use one as the control, introduce something in the other, and see what the difference is. In the experimental model, there is always a formally stated prediction of what will happen if the thing is introduced, and there is formal evaluation of the effect of it. The canons of science are such that it is then possible to claim that the thing one introduced really *caused* the effects one found.

The physical science model is also "value-free." Since in the physical sciences, the purpose of research is to generate new knowledge, it is not necessary to think in terms of values. That is, until quite recently, it was considered all right to study anything, and build any kind of new information, even if the information sought had potentially dangerous consequences. The moratorium on recombinant DNA research represents one of the few times the issue of the goodness of information has been faced directly in the physical sciences (9).

While the DNA example is dramatic, the value-free position of the physical science model is more pervasive. In the model, the values of the scientist are to be deliberately controlled so that they do not affect the findings. That is, the scientist must design her–his experiments in such a way that any conscious or unconscious biases toward finding one thing over another are ruled out. Rigor of design and method are the ultimate values. Social science and medical research derived from this model have occasionally carried the value-free notion to extremes when the consequences to the person under study (the patient) were ignored. While the ethics of research will be discussed in a later chapter, it is important to point out here the distinction between values which are biases in a negative sense and values which are positive in order to increase the meaningfulness of the information to be sought. Particularly in a practice profession, it is not enough simply to have found a wonderful clinical situation in which to look at measures of stress, for example. As it happens, labor and delivery make a very good situation in which to do certain kinds of behavioral measures of stress (and perhaps certain kinds of physiological measures as well). And to the medical scientist, having good measures of stress is a good all in itself. On the other hand, approaching research problems with the idea that in a practice profession, the knowledge obtained has to be meaningful, not just precise, might direct the researcher to particular kinds of measures of stress in labor and delivery, the kinds that will produce the most meaningful information that nurses in that situation can use. The notion of meaningfulness is in itself a value, quite different from the kind of bias that precise experimentation attempts to rule out. And meaningfulness comes from the commitment to excellence in practice, and from the realization that informed bias—meaningfulness—enhances the quality of the research, rather than detracting from it.

In conventional science, including social science, which has borrowed the model from the physical sciences, the value-free, experimental model is the one taken as the most desirable, the most powerful for research. In some social sciences, particularly sociology, in which it is not possible to control the phenomena of interest in order to introduce an experimental variable, the research model is one of correlation—trying to see if two things vary together (co-relate)—with the desire to then make statements about which one causes the other one. The experimental model is so well established that in some writing it is taken to mean the same thing as science or scientific method.

Nursing has borrowed the model and used it as the definition of the ideal in research, adopting at the same time some of the conventions of physical science—control, objectivity, precision, rigor and so on—all of them carefully spelled out in detail to be applied in any one study (10).

There is no question that the experimental method is the best and only one for answering needs for certain kinds of knowledge, including some knowledge to improve clinical judgment. The more we know about what in nursing practice affects what in patient condition, the better off we are in implementing improvements in patient care. But to depend on the experimental model and the un-thought-through conventions of modern physical science is to do a great disservice to the needs of the nursing profession for all kinds of information to guide clinical judgment. For not all needs for information are capable of being provided by experimentation alone. And further, experimentation alone is not enough; it is not the only form of knowledge for a field in which knowledge must be translated into action. As Annie W. Goodrich said, many years ago,

> . . . To the nurse, working in the different levels of the social structure, in touch with the fundamentals of human experience, is given a unique opportunity to relate the adventure of thought to the adventure of action—this to the end that the new social order to which we are committed by our forefathers may be realized. To effectively interpret the truly great role that has been assigned her, neither a liberal education nor a high degree of technical skill will suffice. She must also be master of two tongues, the tongue of science and that of the people. (11)

The "tongue of science" is where most research stops. The "tongue of the people," in this case research which addresses meaningful clinical problems in meaningful ways in order to produce meaningful results to improve clinical practice, requires some new language and some different ways to see both research problems or questions, and their potential answers.

KINDS OF QUESTIONS

The experimental method has been put to good use in nursing to address such problems as how to prepare patients for surgery or hospitalization or treatment (12), how to relieve patients' pain (13), whether nurse practitioners are as safe and effective as community physicians (14), and any number of other problems. These kinds of problems are all the same in one sense. All of them took the form of making a prediction that if some new treatment or procedure were introduced, certain consequences for the patient would result. For instance, one set of studies predicted that if patients who were facing a sophisticated and new diagnostic precedure were informed not only about what would happen to them, but what it would feel like, they would tolerate the procedure better than if they weren't (15). It is possible to state a problem this way when there is enough information available to suspect that the prediction will work out, and there are ways to measure whether it does. But suppose that there weren't any handy ways to measure whether patients would tolerate the procedure? Suppose the nurse wasn't even sure what tolerating or not tolerating (or tolerating more or less well) looked like? Then a different kind of problem would be stated, and it would be studied differently.

Or, put a different way, these studies are alike in the kind of research question that is asked. In all the cases given above, the question is, What will happen if . . . ? For example, What will happen if the nurse explains not only what the patient will experience, but what he will feel? Or, I think patients will be less anxious upon hospitalization if the nurse who admits them explores their feelings as well as gives information. Will it really happen this way?

This type of question is typical of the kinds of questions posed in the usual way of thinking about scientific research. For example, What will happen if penicillin is given for this identified organism, will it kill the bacillus? Or, What will happen if I fire electrons at the nucleus of this atom. Will certain kinds of subnuclear particles appear? If I cut off the air supply to a burning candle by lowering a jar over it, will the flame go out? Or, If I give massive doses of saccharine to these rats, will they develop bladder cancer? All these questions call for experimental designs so that the cause-and-effect relationship can be established (or at least so the lack of it can be dismissed).

But there are four kinds of questions that can be identified:
1. What *is* this?
2. What's happening here?
3. What will happen if . . . ?
4. How can I make . . . happen?

There is an order to the questions based on the kind of question that is posed, and, therefore, the kind of answer that is needed. And that order then calls up the kind of study design best suited to provide the answer needed.

What Is This?

Take the What *is* this? kind of question. This comes up when there are available no ways (or no very good ways) to describe a given phenomenon or situation. It may be because the situation itself is a new one, or because the usual ways the situation is described do not help nurses use the description to improve clinical judgment, or because nobody has ever bothered to study it before. For example, a nurse elected to involve herself in a community action agency. There was at the time nothing in nursing or other literature that described this kind of nontraditional setting or role, so she decided to develop a study to answer the question, What *is* this? meaning, What is it for a nurse to get involved with a community action agency? (16)

Or another nurse, wanting to figure out how to measure whether nursing support during labor helped the patient, characterized the problem as the lack of a way to describe patient behavior in labor. So her question became, What *is* this? meaning, What is the patient's behavior in labor? (17)

The best known What *is* this? studies in nursing came out of the question, "What is it, dying in hospitals?" and the sociologists Barney Glaser and Anselm Strauss went on to find ways of characterizing what the situation of dying was like for patients, for the institution, for the personnel, and so on (18).

And Marguerite Kay, troubled by not understanding how to help chicano patients in a neighborhood health setting, asked, "What is this, the patient's concept of disease?" and found ways to describe those concepts (19).

Notice what ties all these examples together. In all of them, the answer to the question is simply description, whether it comes in a narrative account, or in something more technical like a set of categories. The community action agency study produced a narrative description, as did parts of the death and dying study. The support in labor study produced more formal categories of facial expression—ways of classifying what the various parts of the face looked like (forehead, brow, eyelids, eyes, nose, and mouth). The forehead could be smooth, wrinkled horizontally, smooth on the sides and crinkled in the middle, creased vertically, or a combination of signs. Each description had its own symbol for easy recording when observing a patient. The disease concepts study produced concepts, short descriptive words or phrases, but not ordered in any way as categories are.

There is no formal attempt to introduce change and try to measure its effects, not even in the community action agency study. There, though the nurse joining the setting might be called introducing a change, the study did not attempt to measure that change at all, but rather to describe what it was like to enter a nontraditional setting, function there as a nurse, and leave (20).

What also ties these studies together is their absence of *a priori* definitions, hypotheses, theories, categories or concepts. Studies of the What *is* this? variety are the most basic that can be done (though not the easiest, as we shall see later). They begin with a problem, perhaps a general point of view or focus, but since they are called for when there aren't available previous studies, theories or hypotheses, their purpose is simply to describe, not to predict yet or even to attempt to relate, factors discovered to each other.

But notice also that the question, What *is* this? implies more than mere *reporting*. By analogy, newspaper accounts of an event or series of events are reporting, but political scientists or psychologists may analyze those reports to develop more abstract understanding, in the form of theories and hypotheses. Collecting data in studies like these is not an end in itself but serves to stimulate the intellectual work of giving new names to clusters of observations, taking the empirical reality to the level of "idea." The actual events of Watergate are well recorded and reported in any number of accounts. But the concept of corruption of power is a way to join those events together to make a different order of knowledge.

Diagnosis (nursing or medical) is a good example of the distinction between data and concept. The doctor may collect data—temperature elevation, diaphoresis, cells in the urine, reported flank pain, reported urinary urgency and frequency. By themselves, these are simply observations, or reports. But the diagnosis of urinary tract infection is a way to bring all of them together in one meaningful phrase. Or, the nurse may observe oozing of liquid stool, absence of formed stool for three consecutive days, hard formed fecal mass in rectum and abdominal distension, connect all these observations and decide impaction (21). Impaction is a concept, not an observation.

Research produces knowledge, not simply facts. Indeed, as the above examples hint, facts by themselves are not all that useful in improving clinical judgment. It still takes a mental effort to put the facts together and raise them to a higher level of abstraction upon which action may be based, even if the action is only communication of the abstraction to others.

Another word for knowledge is *theory*. For the layman, the word theory tends to have a connotation of tentativeness, as opposed to the word *law* or even *principle*, both of which somehow sound more final and confirmed. Here, theory is simply, "a mental invention to some purpose." In the case of studies of the What *is* this? variety, the purpose of the theory (description, categorization, conceptualization) is simply to describe, to characterize in words what the situation is, in as full a way as possible so that the reader has a picture of the event or situation he can relate to.

To even think of theory having a purpose, instead of just existing, is a different point of view from that of the physical or social sciences, liberal arts, or humanities. In the most general sense, all theories, of whatever kind, have the purpose of explaining. Some may explain by describing, some by predicting, some by prescribing. The use to which the desired theory, understanding or explanation is to be put determines the study design, data collection procedures, sampling, analysis and interpretation of findings, and conditions the implementation as well. Thus, there are different kinds of theories for different purposes, the predictive theory of modern science being just one kind. Studies of the What *is* this? variety produce a different kind of theory, as we shall see later—a theory intended not at all to predict, but simply to describe by attaching names to observations or other data. These studies are done when, quite literally, one doesn't know what a situation is, or when the available ways of understanding or depicting a situation are inaccurate, incomplete or otherwise wanting.

What's Happening Here?

When one has at least names for the factors involved in a situation, one can do another kind of study, to develop a different kind of theory, with a different purpose. These studies are the What's happening here? kind, and they assume that the variables or factors elected to be studied are already named satisfactorily. The effort then is to see how, if at all, the factors are related to each other, or to one important other factor, usually called a "criterion variable."

For example, suppose one were interested in what is related to how smooth a patient's recovery from surgery is. A nurse might be interested in doing this kind of a study with the ultimate purpose of figuring out when and how to introduce change—nursing intervention—to improve the recovery for patients. In this kind of study, the names for the variables and the variables themselves are already available, so the researcher selects those that are of interest. Often these studies use a "shotgun" approach, trying to include as many variables as possible, so that one can have the fullest possible understanding of what's happening. In the recovery from surgery study (22), the researcher might include variables related to the patient's own person and background—age, sex, race, social class, previous experience with surgery, diagnosis and so on. Things such as psychological states might be included—fear level, preoperative anxiety, psychological preparation for surgery, social resources (family, etc.). Some physiological variables might be included, such as pain tolerance or previous health state. And some treatment factors might be collected, such as operative procedure, number and kinds of diagnostic tests, length of time in the recovery room and so on.

Notice that in this kind of study, the researcher already has some notions of at least what variables are or might be involved, in contrast to the What is this? kind of study in which not even the variables are known.

When the variables are selected, ways to collect data on them are invented, data are collected and analyzed and the end product is a description of what is related to what, in this case, how all the variables are related to recovery from surgery. Modern statistical procedures will even allow one to figure out which variables in combination are most strongly related to recovery.

What's happening here? studies may or may not have been preceded by a formal What *is* this? study. Most often they aren't. The research may draw on previous studies of surgical patients, on one's own clinical knowledge, or on the knowledge of others to decide what interesting and perhaps relevant factors to include. In the recovery from surgery study, fear level was included on the basis of previous investigations, while pain tolerance was included on a clinical hunch.

Sometimes these studies do not have one single criterion variable to relate all the others to, yet the factors are named and the attempt is made to relate them all to each other so that a description of the situation results. For example, a study of medication taking among elderly patients in nursing homes was done to identify drug-drug interactions that might have potentially dangerous implications for the patient (23). Here, the variables to be included were known and named already—patient age, number of drugs, kinds of medications, p.r.n. medications and so on. The study then identified the most frequently occurring potential drug-drug interactions by relating numbers and kinds of drugs to each other, then checking the pattern with known drug-drug interactions. On the basis of their data, the researchers could then make suggestions about how to alter the possibilities of untoward drug interactions for patients in these situations.

The use of the particular words for naming kinds of questions is deliberate. What's happening here? is intended to convey more of the sense of dynamic movement than the question, What *is* this? The difference here is between describing a situation or circumstance at a given point in time, so as to characterize it in words or phrases, and dividing the situation or circumstance up into its components. But the question is not asking for the relationship between that circumstance and anything else. The description simply *is;* it exists, in more or less completeness and is more or less convincingly representative of a piece of reality.

In contrast, the question, What's happening here? is intended to convey a search for relationships between things already named and described. But there is still a sense of tentativeness about the question, and that, too, is deliberate because these questions are posed when not enough information exists to predict relationships. There is an order to the kinds of questions, though, that may begin to become apparent. The What's happening here? question presumes that previous What *is* this? questions have been asked and answered either in formal study or in clinical wisdom. It is not possible to proceed to a question about what's happening without having first named the components of the question.

What Will Happen If . . . ?

The third kind of question, What will happen if . . . ? becomes a natural next step. This kind of question is asked when the names of the factors or variables are known (or selected) and there is some reason for thinking that there might be a relationship among factors, and when it is possible to predict that relationship formally. In contrast to What's happening? questions, in which there is more openness to search for relationships, What will happen if . . . ? questions depend on prior study or clinical knowledge to decide that there may indeed be a relationship between the identified factors, and to design a rigorous test to see if that is so. The suspected relationship is stated in a formal way as an hypothesis, so studies to answer, What will happen if . . . ? questions are hypothesis-testing studies. What's happening here? questions imply no formal hypothesis at all; indeed, one of the expected outcomes of such studies may be the generating of new hypotheses to be tested later.

Studies with formal hypotheses presume that the factors or variables have been named and that there is some reason for thinking a predicted relationship will occur, whether there was a formal relation-searching study done previously or not.

As discussed earlier, What will happen if . . . ? questions are at the level of inquiry that calls for conventional experimental designs, or in the case of a situation in which it is not possible to manipulate the variables, for orthodox survey design procedures. The designs themselves and their logic are discussed later. For now, it is only important to understand where the experimental design and experimental model of scientific investigation fit in the larger scheme being developed here for naming and labeling different kinds of questions that require different kinds of answers from those the experimental design alone can produce.

How Can I Make . . . Happen?

Finally, there is the How can I make . . . happen? kind of question, which assumes, like the others, that there has already been identification of factors, hunches about relationships and tested hunches or hypotheses. But at this level of inquiry, there is more than simple curiosity to see what will happen if something is done. Rather, questions here make explicit goals for the nursing activity of interest, develop *prescriptions* to achieve the goals, and specify the conditions in which the relationship between activity and goal occur, thus allowing the accomplishment of the goal. In other words, unlike What will happen if . . . ? kinds of questions, questions at this level of inquiry assume the answers to the if questions, and focus attention on how to *make* a desired outcome happen. Questions like these lead to explicit statements about goals to be achieved as desirable ends, not just as potential outcomes if a given change is introduced, as is the case in predictive-type questions.

For example, a What will happen if . . . ? question might ask, What will happen if pregnant women's diets are supplemented with protein? Will they have bigger babies? Prescriptive-type questions would say, Bigger babies are a good thing to have happen (for these reasons). How can I help bigger babies happen?

How can I make . . . happen? questions are the most complicated kinds of questions to ask, and, therefore, the most complicated to try to answer, as we shall see later. But prescriptive-type questions are the ones to be raised in a practice profession where the answers needed—the knowledge or theory—have to take account of the reality of the activities of practice, and most especially have to take proper account of the fact, implicit or not, that professional practice always has *goals*. To reiterate, unlike social sciences such as sociology, in which the only goal of the profession, and, thus, of the profession's activities—teaching and research—is to develop knowledge, in a practice profession, knowledge is for something, must be put to use (24). And, therefore, the form that the knowledge takes has to be a form that fits the needs of the practicing profession, not simply descriptions, not simply tested predictions, but eventually *prescriptions* that tell how, when and under what conditions, a given activity or set of activities meets a given stated goal. The question, How can I make . . . happen? is meant to tip off the need for knowledge in a different form, knowledge of a different kind from tested hypotheses, predictions or descriptions, no matter how evocative.

As noted in Chapter 1, it may be evident that nearly all clinical problems or problems in patient care have an element of How can I make . . . happen? in them. Indeed, since clinical problems come from gripes or perceptions of inequities, or wishes and desires, there is implicit even in the perception of the problem, the need to change things so that the problem perceived doesn't happen anymore. Identifying this perception as a type of research question, leading to a particular kind of study, and eventually producing a certain kind of knowledge or theory simply makes more explicit these connections. But to tackle head-on a prescriptive question assumes quite a lot of previous knowledge, whether from research or from clinical experience. Which is why even though many clinical research problems start out as prescriptive questions, they emerge after analysis needing more work done before a prescription can be stated and tested.

It also happens that while most clinical research questions start out implicitly as prescriptive, somewhere along the line in analyzing the problem, nearly every budding researcher realizes that almost any problem could be a What *is* this? problem as well. That is, despite the incredible amount of knowledge available in the world, there's never enough of it, and in clinical research, where so few problems have been investigated with any consistency, almost any problem could profit from a new look at what the situation really is.

To the layman or the person new to research, it seems as if it is all pretty mechanical and technical and that once one has found a problem to investigate, the rest just happens. Actually, even finding a problem and deciding what kind of animal it is (what kind of question) involves some creative risk-taking. So much of the theory behind nursing practice is as yet unstated, or inarticulate, that it takes some intellectual courage to move to test an hypothesis when there has been no previous research on the question. Dumas' original study provides an interesting case in point (26). Dumas, a psychiatric nurse, "just knew" that when she talked with patients preoperatively, using a nursing approach outlined by Orlando (27), they seemed more relaxed the night before surgery, and she suspected that they went through surgery more easily and recovered more smoothly. At the time she had this idea, there were no experimental tests of nursing intervention in the literature. In fact, there was a good deal of speculation that such studies were impossible to do because the clinical situation was so cluttered with extraneous variables. Yet Dumas made the creative leap to the hypothesis that nursing could indeed reduce preoperative anxiety and have effects on postoperative recovery. She could have simply tried to describe what preoperative anxiety was (What *is* this?), or she could have tried to find out what in the preoperative course was related to postoperative recovery (What's happening here?). Instead, the question was posed as a What will happen if . . . ? question and the hypothesis that a certain kind of nursing care preoperatively would reduce postoperative vomiting was tested. To pose the question as a What will happen if . . . ? question required that the variables (nursing intervention, anxiety, preoperative time, and so on) be named and that there be some justification given for even thinking that the hypothesis was possible. That was done, relying heavily on clinical wisdom and experience, since there was no research to cite, and even the opinions of professionals were against her (28).

This study is also an interesting example of the implicit prescriptive values that often guide studies at lower levels of inquiry. The selection of postoperative vomiting was not accidental. It was selected in part because it could be justified on physiological grounds as a reasonable measurement of postoperative recovery. But more important, it was chosen because postoperative vomiting is not a good thing to have happen to patients. It is uncomfortable even when it is not dangerous, Dumas' professional judgement said. While the study is clearly not a prescription-testing study, the role of clinical judgement, even in selecting things to measure, is apparent.

The phrases chosen to label the various kinds of research questions in this section are a kind of shorthand, and as we will see later, cannot be taken too literally. For instance, there are two kinds of studies to answer What will happen if . . . ? questions, and one kind is probably more accurately stated, What happens if . . . ? Similarly, How can I make? is stated that way to get attention, when it might less personally be stated, How can . . . be made to happen?

Early in this section, the kinds of questions were listed in an order. Now it should be clear what that order is, that is, the increasing complexity of the nature of knowledge needed to answer the question. Since it is the questions themselves that lead to the studies that lead to the knowledge or theory, the questions themselves have to be listed in the same order as the theories are.

KINDS OF ANSWERS

In a technical sense, all research does is answer questions, more or less well. In a practice discipline, however, the obligation of research as part of professional responsibility is not only to answer questions by providing new information, but to produce that knowledge or information in its most usable form, and then to use the knowledge to improve the practice.

Answers to research questions are in the form of theory, that is, abstraction. It can be good theory or bad theory, useful or not, tested or not, confirmed or not, complex or simple, descriptive, predictive or prescriptive—it's all theory. In some writing on nursing research (and social science research as well), there is a drive toward the kind of confirmed theory called "law," "principle" or "axiom." (29) Certainly one of the things that drive nurses to do research is the endless search for certainty, for unfailingly accurate prediction, for complete, perfect prescription. Sometimes that drive seems to color how researchers think about the kinds of knowledge for practice, and the word theory takes on a pejorative tone, as in, It's *only* theory. . . . The position taken here is that there is nothing intrinsically bad, good or indifferent about theory as a concept in itself. But there are different kinds of theory, for different purposes, and there are more or less useable, more or less tested, more or less confirmed theories.

Here, theory means simply a mental invention to some purpose (30). To call it an invention is to emphasize that theory is not born, it is made, and is different from other kinds of amassed but not necessarily related information. And to emphasize that theory has *a* purpose is to begin to differentiate *among* different purposes of theory.

There are many ways of differentiating among kinds of theories. The philosophy of science literature emphasizes the distinction between "analytic" and "synthetic" theory; in nursing we often hear about psychological theory, sociological theory and so on—categorization by discipline. One of the more useful ways of talking about theories is proposed by Dickoff and James—to differentiate them on the basis of what they do—their purpose (31).

And to make the connection back to kinds of questions, let us say that in a technical sense, all research does is provide answers to questions—theories—and, therefore, the purpose of the research for different kinds of questions is to produce different kinds of theory. That is, What *is* this? questions provoke a particular kind of study that produces a particular kind of theory, called *naming theory*. The theory consists simply of names attached to clusters of data. Similarly, What will happen if . . . ? questions provoke particular kinds of studies which produce the kind of theory called predictive theory, the kind that states, If x, then y.

As the purposes of theory differ, so do the names for theories with different purposes. In English, words ending in –ing, when they are gerunds, convey the sense of the functional activity. For example, building as a gerund means the activity; building as a noun means the product of the activity. Thus, the names of theories in the sections to follow are factor-isolating, factor-relating, situation-relating, and situation-producing, all named according to the function or purpose they have.

Factor-isolating Theory

Factor-isolating theory or *naming theory* is the most basic kind of descriptive theory. Like all the other kinds of theory discussed here, this kind is named for its function—it describes by isolating factors and giving them names. Factors or names are conceptual handles that provide meaning in abstract terms to real-world phenomena. This kind of theory just attaches names to things, but does not in its pure form propose relationships among concepts or factors. Examples of this kind of theory are common in psychiatry, particularly in analytic psychiatry where names such as id, Oedipus complex, regression, ego strength, and so on are names of complicated phenomena described in detail. The periodic table of elements in chemistry is also naming theory, as well as the Linnean classification system in biology—phylum, genus, species and so on. Anatomy might be considered naming theory. Glaser and Strauss' "awareness contexts" (32) are an example of factor-isolating or naming theory closer to nursing. In their work they identify (name) and describe four kinds of awareness shared (or not shared) between a dying patient and others about him.

Examples of naming theory in nursing are harder to come by except in studies where attempts have been made to develop classification systems for behavior or attitudes and names attached to the various categories. A recent example is Kay's study of disease concepts in the barrio (33) which tries to classify the notions of illness expressed by Mexican Americans according to the site of symptoms and gravity of illness as well as their colloquial meaning. Holly Wilson's study of Soteria House, a nontraditional residential setting for emotionally ill people is an excellent example of both the method of study and the resulting theory. In her study, Wilson developed concepts and properties of the concepts that expressed the relationship between this setting and the outside world (34).

The mammoth nursing diagnosis project is another good example of beginning factor-isolating or naming theory (35). For instance, the Second Conference Report includes not only some nursing diagnoses derived from physiological conditions (such as decreased cardiac output), but numerous new attempts to attach names to phenomena that are of interest to nurses— impairment of parenting, fear, family coping, potential impairment of skin integrity, alterations in body image and many more. Each nursing diagnosis has a beginning list of defining characteristics and when this project is finished, it will consist of factors (diagnoses), each supplied with a definition.

The characteristic of factor-isolating theory is that it provides names or labels for things along with descriptive definitions for the terms employed (36). The descriptions may range from very formal and precisely defined categories to very large and abstract conceptualizations involving general broad descriptions without formal definition.

Note that in this kind of theory, the concepts or categories and their definitions themselves are the theory. When connections are made between concepts and other concepts, and when relationships are proposed, one has gone beyond factor-isolating theory into a higher level of theory, which will be discussed later. For example, the concept of Oedipus complex along with its formal definition is a factor isolated in theoretical terms. When Freud or others then go on to develop connections between the concept and certain symptoms of emotional disturbance in later life, a different kind of theory is in operation. Or when the nursing diagnosis project develops the concept of impaired skin integrity, that is naming or factor-isolating theory. If that concept is then related to others, nutrition, for example, a different kind of theory is being presented.

Note also that a useful product of any kind of research, whether done with the formal motivation of developing factor-isolating theory or not, is the production of concepts—isolated factors. For example, Janis' early work on psychological stress produced the notion of "fear levels" (37) in the course of studying the relationship between psychological state and recovery from surgery. Because factor-isolating theory is the most basic (in the sense of the first step) kind of theory, it is a part of every other kind of theory, and can be developed as part of many kinds of studies. But when the purpose of a study is to develop factor-isolating theory, a particular kind of study design is called for (discussed in Chapter 4).

Factor-relating Theory

Factor-relating theory (situation-depicting theory) does just that—relates factors, suggests the connection among concepts in some kind of order. This kind of theory is rarely seen in its pure form, probably because the human desire is not only to suggest relationships, but to suggest actual causes and consequences, which is the next level of theory. This kind of theory is the kind most often called *descriptive* in other disciplines.

This kind of theory is the natural next step from identifying concepts in factor-isolating theory. For example, Glaser and Strauss developed the concept "social loss" in their factor-isolating theory, then went on to try to discover if social loss was related to anything else—age of the patient, clinical setting, and so on (38). Their findings resulted in factor-relating theory about when and where social loss occurs and how it can be seen along with some hints about its consequences. The attempt was not to state an *a priori* hypothesis about the relationship of social loss to other variables, but to try to *discover* if there were some relationships.

This kind of theory is produced when one is attempting to see *if* there are any kinds of relationships among the factors one has chosen to study. The theory produced consists, therefore, of more or less formal descriptions of the relationships found along with hypotheses for future testing.

The relationships found as hypotheses constitute the "situation," hence, another name for this kind of theory: situation-depicting or situation-describing (39) to indicate that the descriptions in the theory are without time reference—descriptions of a given situation at one moment in time. The "natural history state" of theory discussed by Northrup (40) has been used as an example of this kind of theory.

Oleson and Whittacker's study of nursing students (41) might be an example of theory as factor-relating, natural history. Or, Duff and Hollingshead's controversial *Sickness and Society* (42) fits this model as well. Much of the theory produced by "ethnoscience" (43) could be considered factor-relating, as well as much of anthropological description and some historical description.

Factor-isolat*ing* and factor-relat*ing* mean both the kinds of theory—the product—and the activity of isolating or relating factors. That process can be done formally as described in later chapters when the intent of a study is to produce certain kinds of theory, or it may be done as part of studies at higher levels. For example, the review of literature and analysis of a problem (see Chapter 1) involve the process of naming or identifying factors and relationships. The kinds of theory are deliberately ordered so that each higher theory presupposes the activities as well as the end products of lower theory-making. More simply, before one can test an hypothesis (in situation-relating theory), one must first have identified the factors or variables, then identified a supposed relationship among them.

Both naming theory and descriptive theory (factor-isolating and factor-relating) can be identified as part of the "context of discovery," as opposed to the "context of verification." (44) That is, the activities to develop factor-isolating and factor-relating theory are activities of trying to discover, as opposed to trying to confirm or verify the existence of something already discovered and predicted.

Situation-relating Theory

Situation-relating theory is the name given to the kind of theory more familiarly known as predictive or explanatory theory. Here the theory is developed to the point where actual predictions of relationships among concepts or factors can be made and then tested and confirmed or not. As before, situation-relating theory makes use of the information in factor-isolating and factor-relating theories (whether formally derived or not) to propose specific kinds of relationships (causal, contributory, inhibitory, catalytic or merely covariation) among and between factors. Examples of this kind of theory are abundant, since this is the most common notion of theory in the behavioral and social sciences and in nursing. Some of the better examples occur in behavioristic psychology—learning theory, reinforcement, behavior modification and so on. Here very clear predictions of effect can be made and tested—reward behavior and it will continue; stop rewarding it and it will stop. In nursing, examples of constructed theory are beginning to appear in relation to psychological preparation (45) and in pain and nursing (46). Evidence is being built that certain nursing practices have predictable and repeatable consequences for patients about to undergo surgery or treatment or those in pain.

Other examples of this kind of theory occur almost uniformly in the medical sciences: the causes and consequences of skin breakdown, the effects of various medications on target conditions, the effect of exposure to infection on development of disease and so on.

Situation-relating or predictive theories include both causal theories—if x, then y—and correlational theories which do not include prediction of cause but merely state that x and y vary together, but x does not necessarily cause y or y cause x. The relationship between social class and mental illness is a good example. In that theory, social class is not taken as a cause of mental illness (though social class may be related to a how a clinician diagnoses, what label she–he attaches), or mental illness as a cause of social class, especially of low social class. But the reseach demonstrates some provocative relationships between the two variables (47).

Causal or correlational theories are produced by different means, and in fact are called for in different circumstances. What links the two kinds of theory together and makes them both situation-relating, or explanatory, is that in both cases, formal statements of relationship between the factors can be made and when the data are in and analyzed, formal probability statements can be made about the direction, and strength of the relationships. In certain cases, even without experimental designs, it is possible to claim a cause-and-effect relationship when it is not possible to introduce one variable and measure its effect (see Chapter 7).

Situation-producing Theory

Finally, *situation-producing theory* or *prescriptive theory* is the name given to the kind of theory that not merely predicts but actually contains prescriptions for activities to bring about the goals defined within the theory itself. Theory of this kind includes theories of other kinds in the prescriptions, but the most predominant characteristic of this kind of theory is the explicit inclusion of professionally defined goals for the prescribed activities. By definition, the goals are value-laden and their appearance in this kind of theory makes it distinctly different from situation-relating theory in which predictions simply state that if x happens, y will follow, not that y is a good thing to have happen (48).

Prescriptive theory has two aspects: the statement of goals to be achieved and the prescription of activities intended to achieve the goals. Dickoff and James have further provided a way of looking at the prescription by identifying six points of view that can be taken on any nursing activity and that must all be covered and included in a statement of a prescriptive theory. They call these elements of activity the "survey list" (49) and it includes agency—who or what performs the activity; patiency—who or what receives it; framework—within what context it is performed; procedure—how it is done; dynamics—why it is done; terminus—with what end result is the activity done.

A very simplified example may help here. Suppose you have a headache. You want to be comfortable (the goal) because pain is interfering with your composure and concentration. You (agency) give yourself (patiency) two aspirin (procedure) to relieve the pain (dynamics). You do this activity within a certain context in time and space (framework) and pretty soon your headache goes away (terminus). You then feel better and can get back to work (goal achieved). This example is oversimplified for illustration, but look at it carefully. It is a very specific instance of prescription to achieve a goal. But the aspects do not depend on very specific examples. For instance, suppose you are allergic to aspirin. Then you (agent) might take enteric-coated empirin (procedure) instead to achieve the same goal. No matter what the explicit small details of the prescription (aspirin for headache), the aspects of prescriptions in general will stand (agency, patiency and so on). Any prescription for any goal-oriented activity would include all of the aspects.

Most nursing activity is a great deal more complicated than the example given, partly because the goal contents are more complicated. *Goal content* means the articulation of that which is conceived as desirable of attainment. One frequently expressed goal of nursing goes something like this: to assist the patient to attain maximum comfort and ability to cope with his situation. Such a goal might suggest literally infinite procedures, agents, frameworks, kinds of patients and so forth. Yet the same aspects would hold, and each would have to be accounted for.

The relationship between prescriptive theory and other kinds may become clear with a few examples. A physiological theory can say that a certain drug relieves pain (predictive theory). Nursing prescriptive theory would say that pain should be relieved (for these reasons) so here is how, why, with whom, when, where and so on, to relieve it. Anatomy theory may describe the connection between the knee bone and the thigh bone, and nursing may incorporate this description into a prescription leading to full mobility for the patient. A sociological theory may suggest that lower social class patients are treated differently from higher social class patients, while nursing may set goals for all patients and take into account their socioeconomic resources in prescribing to meet the goals.

Examples of prescriptive theory have not yet appeared in the literature *as prescriptive theory* (50). So there seems yet to be a gap between activities like demonstration projects and evaluations of service, and the realization that these may be treated as attempts to test prescriptions for practice, even if as prescriptions they are not fully developed. For example, in an attempt to improve the quality of care and decrease infant mortality in Madera County in California, two nurse midwives were introduced as care givers in the clinical setting (51). Data were collected before, during and after the introduction of the nurse midwives and their form of care, and comparisons were made of infant mortality rates (among other variables) before nurse midwives, with nurse midwives and after the nurse midwives could, unfortunately, no longer be supported. (Incidentally, the results were that infant mortality went from 23.9 per 1,000 to 10.3 with the nurse midwives, then back to 32.1 per 1,000 after the project was discontinued.) In this example, the goal for the activity was fairly well stated and explicit. The prescription was not as filled-out as would be ultimately desired in a prescriptive theory, but the major details can be guessed at. In this case, the agency was nurse midwives. The patiency was the particular group of patients for whom the care was prescribed, in this case mostly medically indigent in a poor agricultural county. The framework would have included such things as the hospital relationships, the clinic structure, protocols for physician coverage, reimbursement, the acceptance of the nurse midwives and their collegial support, economic structure of the community and so on. The procedure would be the nurse midwifery care, spelled out in some detail, but assumed to include a family-centered orientation, with inclusion of the patient in decision-making, care of the normal woman, general nonintervention in normal processes of pregnancy, labor and delivery, diet counseling, health teaching and support during labor and delivery. The dynamics would be a bit harder to guess at, but would include the motivations for activity, why the nurse midwives did the work, and with what energy, money and so on the activity was performed. The terminus would include the results of care—health of the mother and baby, compliance, early registration for care and the like.

Note here that the way the activity is defined determines how the survey list aspects are labeled. In this case, the activity is nurse midwifery care, broadly construed.

Another example, even less articulate than this one might be efforts to improve the quality of care to hospitalized patients through introducing primary nursing to a given setting. Here the goals are stated in broad, philosophical terms—humanizing care, improving quality of care, increased job satisfaction, decreased nursing turnover, and so forth. The prescription is primary nursing. The agency then becomes the primary nurses, perhaps including LPNs; the patiency the patients (of specific diagnosis or treatment perhaps); the framework the time, space and psychological context of the practice of primary nursing, including such things as availability of consultation to the nurses, role of the head nurse, acceptance by physicians, money and so on. The procedure becomes primary nursing, defined in as much detail as possible, including the case method of assignment, perhaps matching the seriousness of the illness to the skill of the nurse, 24-hour responsibility, peer evaluation and monitoring, use of nursing process, problem-oriented record systems and on and on. The dynamics would include the energy sources for the activity—the motivation, satisfaction, rewards the primary nurses may need to be provided with. The terminus again is the effects of care on whatever variables make sense to the population of patients, such as length of stay, complications, and might also include some nurse variables, such as job turnover or job satisfaction.

These two examples are intended to point out the difference between the structure and function of prescriptive theory and theory at other levels of inquiry. In prescriptive theory, much more complex relationships among factors and situations must be spelled out, and the aspects of the prescription—agency, patiency and so on—defined in some detail. More important, the goal for the activity is not simply implicit as an outcome, but stated formally as a goal to be achieved, with justification for why it is a good goal.

"Professional purpose requires a commitment beyond mere understanding or describing." (52) Or predicting. In other words, theories limited to describing, predicting, and understanding are not enough for a practice profession to be satisfied; prescriptive theories are what are needed. Like all the other kinds of theory discussed here, prescriptive theories presume and include in them other kinds of theory. For example, primary nursing as prescriptive theory might make use of the factor-isolating nursing diagnosis theories so as to match patients with certain kinds of diagnosis to nursing skill levels. Or it might include theories derived in psychology about the effect defined accountability for one's own actions has on performance. Or it might include theories from organization behavior about the effects of decentralized decision-making on the ward ambience. A fully developed prescriptive theory for primary nursing would have, insofar as humanly possible, all these various theories spelled out in their relationships with one another, as the "package" that is the prescription and goal.

The two examples given above involve very large and complicated prescriptions, but the same kind of reasoning would apply to prescriptive theory for rather smaller bits of reality. For example, it might be possible to spell out a prescriptive theory including the goal to make the coronary patient's transition from intensive care to floor care as smooth and healthful as possible. Then the prescription would include the agency—who is going to do this? Intensive care nurses? Nurses and family? Floor nurses? Psychiatric liaison-consultation nurses? The patiency—what is the coronary patient like, in age, sex, family circumstances, economic level, personality and so on? The framework—what institutional and societal factors need to be taken into account? The procedure—how will the activity be done? Patient teaching? Counseling? Patient participation? Explanation? And when will it be done? The dynamics—what energy will make the activity be done? And the terminus—what effects will it have on the patient?

There may be a good deal of inarticulate prescriptive theory already in existence in nursing procedure manuals. Generally, these manuals specify a goal, for the procedure, if not in larger terms. They may be somewhat vague about who would do the procedure, whether it has to be an R.N. or whether it can be delegated. The patiency is likely to be vague as well, perhaps only specifically considering the physiological or psychological signs that indicate a need for the procedure. The dynamics is likely to be absent altogether. Some aspects of the framework may be stated—where equipment is, for example, or instructions about specific physical accommodations for the procedure. The procedure itself is spelled out in some detail, but not always with logic or scientific principles behind it. And the terminus is usually just the end of the procedure rather than anything more abstract. But all of the aspects of prescriptive theory are contained in a nursing procedure.

Prescriptive theory has been proposed as the kind of theory most needed and most desired for a practice profession because it would provide the knowledge to guide the activities of the practitioners to achieve worthwhile goals. Thus, the creation of prescriptive theory becomes, in effect, a professional goal for nursing—the development of the kind of body of knowledge on which the practice of the profession rests. And when one is aware of the goal, the activities undertaken in service of that goal look different. If the invention of prescriptive theory is a goal of theory construction efforts in nursing, and if research is one of the activities that contributes to theory construction, research in nursing practice takes on some characteristics it would not otherwise have. No longer is it enough to merely find out facts, make predictions and test them or develop knowledge for its own sake. Rather, research and theory development are essential activities in pursuit of the creation of a very special kind of nursing knowledge.

Note that throughout this discussion, the emphasis has been on *kinds* of theory for nursing, rather than the content of theories themselves, or the invention of *a* nursing theory. Nursing is far too complex to think that any one theory would ever encompass all that we call nursing. Although the notion of kinds of theory may seem overly abstract and, therefore, not immediately useful, it offers a way to transcend the territorial arguments about what constitutes nursing theory—that is, theory *by* nursing, *for* nursing, *in* nursing, *about* nursing, *around* nursing or what? Instead, we can think about the kind of theory that will help nursing do what its societal mission is—give excellent patient care and continually develop and improve its practices. That kind of theory will undoubtedly contain concepts, hypotheses, predictions, constructs, principles, even laws from other sciences, but then no one discipline owns knowledge anyhow. The idea of prescriptive theory enables us to think about classes or categories of information to guide nursing activities and where the information comes from becomes less important than whether it works to serve the improvement of patient care.

Just as questions for research form themselves in a hierarchy from the most basic, What *is* this? to the most complex, How can I make . . . happen?, the four kinds of theory discussed here are arranged parallel to the kinds of questions, and in the same order. That is, factor-isolating theory is the kind of information needed to answer a What *is* this? question. Each kind of theory has a different purpose—describing, explaining, predicting, prescribing. When the kind of questions are put to the kinds of answers—theories—the following figure results:

Figure 2-1. *Questions and Answers (Theories)*

QUESTION	KIND OF THEORY NEEDED
1. What *is* this?	Factor-isolating (naming theory)
2. What's happening here?	Factor-relating (situation-depicting, situation-describing)
3. What will happen if . . . ?	Situation-relating (predictive theory)
4. How can I make . . . happen?	Situation-producing (prescriptive theory)

A note of caution: just because this discussion has used an ordered continuum of theories for organizing this material, it doesn't mean that any given predictive theory, say, is "better" than any given descriptive theory. What makes theories good or bad is highly technical and very abstract area, with its own rules. Those rules, insofar as the technical aspects of theory construction or philosophy of science go, are beyond the scope of this book, though in later chapters the relationship between data and interpretation as theory-building will be addressed. What is important for now is to begin to think of the intellectual activity of theorizing as part of nursing and part of nursing research and to perceive that formal theory may take different forms for different purposes.

Another way to talk about the hierarchy of questions and answers is to talk in terms of "levels of inquiry." That is, certain kinds of questions are at certain levels, or stages, if you will on the route to prescriptive theory. What *is* this? questions are at the factor-isolating level of inquiry; What will happen if . . . ? questions are at the situation-relating level of inquiry, and so on. Level of inquiry is just a technical term for the kind of theory needed to answer the question, and not surprising, the levels of inquiry may be numbered 1, 2, 3, and 4, from factor-isolating to situation-producing. The theories may be discussed as third level or fourth level theories as well.

Throughout this section, it has been hinted that because questions occur at different levels of inquiry, they must be investigated differently, so as to produce the different kinds of answers needed. And it happens that just as the kinds of questions line up neatly, and the kinds of theories do, so do the kind of study designs.

LEVELS OF INQUIRY AND STUDY DESIGN

In a technical sense, all research does is develop or test theory in the form of hypotheses to answer specific kinds of questions. Research can function in the assaying or testing of a theory—or even in stimulating thought toward the production of theory. But there will be a long, long wait if anyone waits for research to invent a theory. That is, risk-taking speculation is required for the proposing of a theory or even of an hypothesis as part of a theory (53). The speculation has to come from somewhere, however, and that somewhere is data or information the researcher mines. But as discussed above, theory comes in different forms, so logically the information on which the kind of theory is based must be provided differently, according to what the purpose of the theory is. That is, data for theory which is intended to be merely descriptive is provided by different methods than is theory that is intended to test specific predictions.

Like the labels for kinds of theory, the labels for kinds of study design make use of the English –ing ending, so they are named according to what they do, in a quite literal sense.

For problems at the factor-isolating level of inquiry, the study design is called *factor-searching*—again named for its activity, literally looking for ways to name what is going on in the situation under study. For problems at the factor-relating level of inquiry, the study design is called, not surprisingly, *relation-searching*. For problems at the situation-relating level of inquiry, two kinds of study designs are possible—*casual hypothesis-testing* and *association-testing*, for the problem here is to find out if a predicted relationship really exists. And at the situation-producing level of inquiry, study design might be called *prescription-testing*.

This new terminology is used in preference over other possible ways of organizing studies or study designs because it affords the most general and abstract way of categorizing research, and emphasizes the *purpose* of theories.

In other literature, however, other terminology is used. So in Figure 2-2, the picture begun in Figure 2-1 is extended to include the study designs that go with the questions and answers, and the other names for the designs. Note that this terminology, like the terms for the kinds of theory, has no reference to the *content* of the investigations (54).

Using Figure 2-2, it can be seen that other terminology for study design fails to make some distinctions that have been made here. For example, in some writing, all studies which are not experimental are "exploratory" (55), but exploratory doesn't distinguish just *how* exploratory a study might be; that is, whether it is a truly basic, factor-searching kind of study, or is a more advanced relation-searching one.

The basic elements of the research process—sampling, data collection, data analysis, and so on—occur in all studies, at all levels of inquiry. But how they occur, and why they may be viewed differently at different levels of inquiry is what is important. Elements of research and study designs for various levels of inquiry are addressed in the next few chapters in some detail.

It is important to reemphasize one point: this method of classifying and organizing research in terms of levels of inquiry is not content-specific. That is, a nursing administration study, a patient care study, a nursing education study, a study of surgical nursing, obstetrical nursing, primary nursing, primary care could all be at the same level of inquiry, if they address the

Figure 2-2. *Questions, Study Designs, Answers*

LEVEL OF INQUIRY	KIND OF QUESTION	STUDY DESIGN	KIND OF ANSWER (THEORY)	OTHER NAMES FOR STUDY DESIGN
1	What is this?	Factor-searching	Factor-isolating (naming)	Exploratory Formulative Descriptive Situational control
2	What's happening here?	Relation-searching	Factor-relating (situation-depicting, situation-describing)	Exploratory Descriptive
3	What will happen if . . . ?	Association-testing Causal hypothesis-testing	Situation-relating (predictive)	Correlational Survey design Nonexperimental Natural experiment Experimental Explanatory Predictive
4	How can I make . . . happen?	Prescription-testing	Situation-producing (prescriptive)	

same level of problem. Thus, this framework for research shows the similarity among many different studies, as long as they are at the same level of inquiry. This makes available to the researcher methods, tools, techniques, ways of thinking about concepts, study designs, statistical procedures that might otherwise not be considered because they occurred in a study whose content was not of interest. Reviewing the literature before doing a study may then consist not only of looking for studies in the same content area as the one the researcher has picked, but also looking for studies at the same level of inquiry for new ideas, or tested ones, on how to proceed.

To reiterate (because we are dealing with very abstract material here and new and strange terminology), the organizing principle for research methods or study designs used here is the level of inquiry of the research problem, and thus, the kind of theory developed or tested. And that principle is embedded in the conviction that because nursing is a practice profession with a mission of service the kind of knowledge needed is of a particular kind.

Nursing research has as its goal the improvement of patient care (56). There is really no other justification for insisting that nurses study their practice when they have so many other competing demands. Dickoff, James and Wiedenbach write movingly of the relationship between nursing theory development and nursing practice when they list two "power sources" of motivation for nursing practice:

> One such source is the desire for the immediate, aesthetic satisfaction available to the true craftsman, pleasure felt in the very doing, because of the quality of the performance and the agent's awareness and pride in the quality. A second source, that builds on the first, is the desire for self-esteem, a desire resting on a conception of the agent's role as one worthy of fulfilling, a sense of true craftsmanship, and a sense of responsibility in fulfilling that role. (57)

They go on:

> *The more developed is the theory or conception of nursing practice, the more likely will these two power sources be available for producing and sustaining activity realizing a nursing goal.* (58)

With that purpose always in mind, one approaches the study of nursing differently than if one follows the more conventional path that research's purpose is only the discovery and testing of knowledge, sufficient unto itself. Research problems are seen differently, different considerations in data collection, study design, ethics, sample selection, measurement and interpretation of findings emerge when one knows that the eventual usefulness of nursing research must be in the improvement of practice.

NOTES

1. The material in this chapter draws heavily upon the important work of James Dickoff and Patricia James, two philosophers with many years of experience with nurses and nursing.

I was fortunate to have worked with them in the early days of their association with the profession.

See Dickoff, James and Patricia James: A theory of theories: a position paper. *Nursing Research*, 17:197–203, May–June 1968. This first paper spells out the framework for development of the kind of knowledge to guide practice professions, elaborated later in a number of papers:

Dickoff, James and Patricia James: Researching research's role in theory development. *Nursing Research*, 17:204–206, May–June 1968.

Dickoff, James, Patricia James and Ernestine Wiedenbach: Theory in a practice discipline. Practice oriented theory (Part I). Practice oriented research (Part II). *Nursing Research*, 17:415–435, September–October 1968 and 17:545–554, November–December 1968.

Dickoff, James and Patricia James. Beliefs and values: bases for curriculum design. *Nursing Research*, 19:415–427, September–October 1970. See also Wiedenbach, Ernestine: Comment on Beliefs and values: bases for curriculum design. *Nursing Research*, 19:427–428, September–October 1970, and Dickoff and James' response in a letter to the editor, 19:510, November–December 1970.

Dickoff, James, Patricia James and Joyce Semradek. 8–4 research: a stance for nursing research—tenacity or inquiry (Part I). Designing nursing research—eight points of encounter (Part II). *Nursing Research*, 24:84–92 and 24:165–176, March–April and May–June 1975. See also letters to the editor by Suzanne Hall Johnson and Beverly Volicer and Dickoff, James and Joyce Semradek's response, *Nursing Research*, 25:63–66, January–February 1976.

Dickoff, James and Patricia James. From dilemmas to presets through design. In Semradek, Joyce and Carolyn Williams (eds.): *Resolving Dilemmas in Practice Research: Decisions for Practice.* Chapel Hill: University of North Carolina School of Nursing, 1976. See also the final section of this report (pp. 101–110), the conference summary.

For an extraordinarily lucid commentary on the philosophers' own development of their ideas, as well as some of the logic behind them, see Dickoff, James and Patricia James: Theory development in nursing. In Verhonick, Phyllis J: *Nursing Research*, Vol. 1. Boston: Little Brown, 1975, pp. 45–92.

Finally, see Dickoff, James and Patricia James commentary on another paper: Clarity to what end? *Nursing Research*, 20:499–502, November–December 1971.

2. See Diers, Donna and Mary C. Dye: Situation producing theory. In *Second Nursing Theory Conference.* Kansas City: University of Kansas School of Nursing, 1969, pp 34–44. See especially the early parts of this paper where otherwise unpublished material from Dickoff and James is quoted.

3. Dickoff, James and Semradek, 8-4 research (Part II) see Note 1.

4. For an interesting point of view from an individual who is apparently a philosopher who then went into nursing, see Zbilut, Joseph Peter: Nursing research and the humanities (letter to the editor). *Nursing Research*, 26:67, January–February 1977. This is one of the few recent communications on nursing theory that has included discussion of the humanities, in addition to the social and physical sciences.

5. Jacox, Ada: Theory construction in nursing: an overview. *Nursing Research*, 23:4–13, January–February 1974.

6. Eccles, John C.: The discipline of science with specific reference to the neurosciences. *Daedalus*, 102 (2):85–86, Spring, 1973.

7. Falck, Hans, S.: Letter to the editor. *Transaction*, 5:63, June 1968.

8. Shulman, Jay; *et al.*: Recipe for a jury. *Psychology Today*, 6:37–44, 77–84, May 1973.

9. Two excellent, nontechnical books discuss the recombinant DNA problem. Wade, Nicholas: *The Ultimate Experiment.* New York: Walker, 1977; and Rogers, Michael: *Biohazard.* New

York: Knopf, 1977. For a larger perspective on the same problem see Goodfield, June: *Playing God.* New York: Random House, 1977.

10. See, for example, the discussion of Dickoff and James' paper in Symposium on theory development in nursing. *Nursing Research,* 17:223–227, May–June 1968; also Norris, Catherine M. (ed.): *Proceedings of the First, Second* and *Third Nursing Theory Conferences.* Kansas City: University of Kansas Medical Center, Department of Nursing Education, 1969–1970, especially the *Second Conference;* Walker, Lorraine O.: Toward a clearer understanding of the concept of nursing theory. *Nursing Research,* 20:428–435, September–October 1971 and the commentaries by Ellis, Rosemary, Powhatan Wooldrige, Jeanette R. Folta, and James Dickoff and Patricia James in the subsequent issue, *Nursing Research,* 20:493–502, November–December 1971.

For different view of theory or science in nursing see Rogers, Martha: *An Introduction to the Theoretical Basis of Nursing.* Philadelphia: F.A. Davis, 1970; Wooldridge, Powhatan, et al.: *Behavioral Science, Social Practice and the Nursing Profession.* Cleveland: Case Western Reserve University Press, 1968; Johnson, Dorothy: Theory in nursing: borrowed or unique. *Nursing Research,* 17:206–209, May–June 1968; Putnam, Phyllis: Conceptual approach to nursing theory. *Nursing Science,* 3:430–439, December 1965; Leininger, Madeleine, et al.: Conference on the nature of science in nursing. *Nursing Research,* 18:388–411, September–October 1969; Schlotfeldt, Rozella M., *et al.:* Symposium on approaches to the study of nursing questions and the development of nursing science. *Nursing Research,* 21:484–517, November–December 1972.

Jacox, See Note 4; and Johnson, Jean: Nursing research, vital for the profession. *American Nurse* (American Nurses Association newspaper), September 15, 1977, p. 15.

11. Goodrich, Annie W.: *The Ethical and Social Significance of Nursing.* New York: Macmillan, 1933, p. 14. Reprinted by Yale School of Nursing, 1973, on the occasion of the 50th anniversary of the School.

12. Mahaffey, Perry R.: Effects of hospitalization on children admitted for tonsillectomy and adenoidectomy. *Nursing Research,* 14:12–19, Winter 1965. Wolfer, John A. and Madelon A. Visintainer: Pediatric surgical patients' and parents' stress responses and adjustment. *Nursing Research,* 24:244–255, July–August 1975; Visintainer Madelon A. and John A. Wolfer: Psychological preparation for surgical pediatric patients: the effect on children's and parents' stress responses and adjustment. *Pediatrics,* 56:187–202, August 1975; Dumas, Rhetaugh G. and Robert C. Leonard: The effect of nursing on the incidence of postoperative vomiting: a clinical experiment. *Nursing Research,* 12:12–15, Winter 1963; Dumas, Rhetaugh G. and Barbara Anderson: Research in nursing practice: a review of five clinical experiments. *International Journal of Nursing Studies,* 9:137–150, August 1972.

Elms, Roslyn R. and Robert C. Leonard: Effects of nursing approaches during admission. *Nursing Research,* 15:39–48, Winter 1966. Johnson, Jean, E., et al.: Psychosocial factors in the welfare of surgical patients. *Nursing Research,* 19:18–29, January–February 1970. Pride, L. Frances: An adrenal stress index as a criterion measure for nursing. *Nursing Research,* 17:292–303, July–August 1968; Lindeman, Carol A. and Betty Van Aernam: Nursing intervention with the presurgical patient. *Nursing Research,* 20:319–332, July–August 1971. Tryon, Phyllis and Robert C. Leonard. Clinical test of patient-centered nursing. *Journal of Health and Human Behavior,* 7:183–192, Fall 1966.

13. Moss, Faye T. and Burton Meyer: Effects of nursing interaction upon pain relief in patients. *Nursing Research,* 15:303–306, Fall 1966. McBride, M. Angela: Nursing approach, pain, and relief: an exploratory experiment. *Nursing Research,* 16:337–341, Fall 1967. Diers, Donna, et al.: Effect of nursing interaction on patients in pain. *Nursing Research,* 21:419–428, September–October 1972.

14. Spitzer, Walter O., et al.: Nurse practitioners in primary care, III: the Southern Ontario randomized trial. *Canadian Medical Association Journal,* 108:1005–1016, April 21, 1973; Spitzer, Walter O., et al.: The Burlington randomized trial of the nurse practitioner. *New England Journal of Medicine,* 290:251–256, January 31, 1974; Sackett, David L., et al.:

The Burlington randomized trial of the nurse practitioner: health outcomes of patients. *Annals of Internal Medicine*, 80:137–142, February 1974.

15. Johnson, Jean E., et al.: Psychological preparation for an endoscopic examination. *Gastrointestinal Endoscopy*, 19:180–182, May 1973; Johnson, Jean E. and Howard Leventhal: Effects of accurate expectations and behavioral instructions on reactions during a noxious medical examination. *Journal of Personal and Social Psychology*, 29:710–718, May 1974; Johnson, Jean E., et al.: Sensory information, instruction in coping strategy and recovery from surgery. *Research in Nursing and Health*, 1:4–17, April 1978; Johnson, Jean E. *et al.* Altering Patient's responses to surgery: an extension and replication. *Research in Nursing and Health*, 1:111–121, October 1978.

16. Hodgman, Eileen Callahan: *The Nurse in a Community Action Agency*. New York: National League for Nursing (The League Exchange # 91), 1970.

17. Leventhal, Howard and Elizabeth S. Sharp: Facial expressions as indicators of distress. In Tomkins, Silvan and Carol Izard (eds.): *Affect, Cognition and Personality*, New York: Springer, 1965, pp. 296–318.

18. Glaser, Barney and Anselm Strauss: *Awareness of Dying*. Chicago: Aldine Publishing Company, 1966, especially Part II, pp. 29–118.

19. Kay, Marguerite: Disease concepts in the barrio today. *Communicating nursing research: collaboration and competition*. Marjorie V. Batey (ed.): Boulder, Colorado: WICHE, December 1973, pp. 185–194. Kay's article appears with a justified critique of the lack of information provided about how the categories were arrived at from the data as well as a remarkable critique by a minority respodent. See pp. 195–200 of the same volume.

20. Hodgman, Eileen Callahan: Gaining acceptance by ghetto teenagers. *American Journal of Nursing*, 69:1912–1917, September 1969.

21. Gebbie, Kristine M. (ed.): *Classification of Nursing Diagnoses: Summary of the Second National Conference*. St. Louis: National Group for Classifaction of Nursing Diagnoses, 1976, p. 45.

22. Wolfer, John A. and Carol E. Davis: Assessment of surgery patients' preoperative emotional conditions and postoperative welfare. *Nursing Research*, 19:402–414, September–October 1970.

23. Brown, Martha, et al.: Drug-drug interactions among residents in homes for the elderly. *Nursing Research*, 26:47–52, January–February 1977.

24. For a different point of view from sociology, see Gouldner, Alvin: Anti-minotaur: the myth of a value-free sociology. In Bennis, Warren, et al. (eds.): *The Planning of Change* (2nd edition). New York: Holt, Rinehart, & Winston, 1969, pp. 604–618; also, Greenwood, Ernest: The practice of science and the science of practice. In Bennis, Warren, et al. (eds.): *The Planning of Change* (1st edition). New York: Holt, Rinehart & Winston, 1962.

25. This discussion of the way in which knowledge in a practice profession is different from knowledge in basic or behavioral sciences is not at all intended to say that one is *better* than the other. Practice professions have the defined social charge of constantly improving their services. Until recently, social sciences seemed not to have the same kind of charge. Now, society is increasingly expecting that the public money poured into academic and social service institutions will have a pay-off in changes in *service*. Exciting programs in operations research, social change, clinical medicine, and interdisciplinary programs in law–journalism, economics–health care, or social science–human development show how traditional academic disciplines are changing. The points made here about prescriptive theory would apply to any field in which the need is for knowledge (theory) to shape or direct social change.

26. Dumas, Rhetaugh G. and Robert C. Leonard: Effect of nursing on the incidence of postoperative vomiting; for discussion of content of this study, see Wooldridge, Powhatan, Robert C. Leonard and James K. Skipper, Jr.: *Methods of Clinical Experimentation to Improve Patient Care*. St. Louis: C. V. Mosby, 1978.

27. Orlando, Ida Jean: *The Dynamic Nurse Patient Relationship.* New York: G.P. Putnam's Sons, 1961.

28. See especially the early part of the Dumas-Leonard article (Note 26 above), as well as Dumas, Rhetaugh G.: The effect of nursing care on the incidence of postoperative vomiting. Unpublished Master's report, Yale University School of Nursing, 1961.

29. Jacox, see Note 4 and Wade, see Note 9, especially.

There are hundreds of readings in the philosophy of science that deal with traditional ideas of theory. The interested reader might begin with Kaplan, Abraham: *The Conduct of Inquiry.* San Francisco: Chandler Publishing Company, 1964; Nagel, Ernest: *The Structure of Science.* New York: Harcourt, Brace, Jovanovich, 1961; Marx, M.H. (ed.): *Theories in Contemporary Psychology.* New York: Macmillan, 1963, especially Chapter I; Reichenbach, Hans: *The Rise of Scientific Philosophy.* Berkeley: University of California Press, 1966.

30. Dickoff and James, Theory of theories. (See Note 1.)

31. See Note 1.

32. Glaser and Strauss, see Note 18.

33. Kay, see Note 19.

34. Wilson, Holly Skodol: Limiting intrusion—social control of outsiders in a healing community. *Nursing Research,* 26:103–111, March–April 1977.

35. Hodgman, see Note 20. Also, Gebbie, Kristine M. and Mary Ann Lavin: *Classification of Nursing Diagnoses: Proceedings of the First National Conference.* St. Louis: National Clearinghouse for Nursing Diagnoses, (St. Louis: C.V. Mosby), 1973; also, Gebbie, Kristine M. and Mary Ann Lavin: Classifying nursing diagnosis. *American Journal of Nursing,* 74:250–254, February 1974.

36. For a lovely, small example, see Geach, Barbara and James Walker: Empathic resonance: a counter transference phenomenon. *American Journal of Nursing,* 74:1282–1285, July 1974.

This article is an unusually sensitive example of the very complicated kind of intellectual work in nursing, as well as a particularly satisfying example of theory construction grown out of analysis of nursing practice.

37. Janis, Irving: *Psychological Stress.* New York: John Wiley & Sons, 1958.

38. Glaser, Barney and Anselm Strauss: The social loss of dying patients. *American Journal of Nursing,* 64:119–121, June 1974.

39. Dickoff, James, et al.: Theory in a practice discipline, Part I: Practice oriented theory. *Nursing Research,* 17:415–435, see especially p. 421.

40. Northrup, F.S.C.: *The Logic of the Sciences and the Humanities.* New York: Meridian Books, The World Publishing Co., 1966, especially Chapter III, pp. 35–38.

41. Oleson, Virginia L. and Elvi W. Whittacker: *The Silent Dialogue.* San Francisco: Jossey-Bass, 1968.

42. Duff, Raymond and August Hollingshead: *Sickness and Society.* New York: Harper & Row, 1968. See also for methodological and content criticism Paul Beeson's review of this book in the *Yale Journal of Biology and Medicine,* 41:226–241, October 1968.

43. Leininger, Madeline: *Nursing and Anthropology: Two Worlds to Blend.* New York: John Wiley & Sons, 1970.

44. Glaser, Barney and Anselm Strauss: *The Discovery of Grounded Theory.* Chicago: Aldine Publishing Company, 1967, especially pp. 1–43.

45. See, for example, Lindeman, Carol A. and Betty van Aernam: Nursing intervention with the presurgical patient; Lindeman, Carol A.: Nursing intervention with the presurgical patient: the effect of group and individual preoperative teaching. *Nursing Research,* 21:196–209, May–June 1972; Lindeman, Carol A. and Steven L. Stetzer: Effect of

preoperative visits by operating room nurses. *Nursing Research*, 22:4–15, January–February 1973; Schmitt, Florence and Powhatan Wooldridge: Psychological preparation of surgical patients. *Nursing Research*, 22:108–116, March–April 1973; Dumas, Rhetaugh G. and Barbara Anderson: Research in nursing practice: a review of five clinical experiments.

46. See Note 12. See also Crowley, Dorothy: *Pain and Its Alleviation*. Los Angeles: UCLA School of Nursing, 1962; Johnson, Jean E. and V.H. Rice: Sensory and distress components of pain: implications for the study of clinical pain. *Nursing Research*, 23:203–209, May–June 1974.

47. Hollingshead, August and Fredric Redlich: *Social Class and Mental Illness*. New York: John Wiley & Sons, 1958; Meyers, Jerome and Lee Bean: *A Decade Later: A Follow-up of Social Class and Mental Illness*. New York: John Wiley & Sons, 1968.

48. The point that prescription involves more than a simple x-leads-to-y relationships needs emphasis. In Jacox's otherwise excellent article (see Note 4) prescription is treated as simply prediction with a goal in mind. The reader is urged to study carefully the Dickoff and James papers to appreciate the enormous complexity and subtlety of the notion of prescriptive theory, see Note 1.

49. Dickoff and James, Theory of theories, see Note 1. Some of the philosophers' papers have been collected in *Readings in Nursing Research*, Vol. I. New York: *AJN* Company, 1971.

50. Rosemary T. McCarthy made a valiant attempt to use the levels of inquiry framework for her own research. See A practice theory of nursing care. *Nursing Research*, 21:405–410, September–October 1972.

51. Levy, Barry S., et al.: Reducing neonatal mortality rate with nurse midwives. *American Journal of Obstetrics and Gynecology*, 109:50–57, January 1, 1971.

52. Dickoff, James and Patricia James, Theory of theories, see Note 1, p. 198.

53. Dickoff, James and Patricia James, Researching research's role in theory development, see Note 1, pp. 204–205.

54. See Brink, Pamela and Marilynn J. Wood: *Basic Steps in Planning Nursing Research*. North Scituate, Mass.: Duxbury Press, 1978, especially the Preface for a somewhat similar organization of research into levels. Brink and Wood do not quite make explicit the underlying continuum—kinds of theory—thus implying a rank order of their three levels. They do not include the fourth kind of theory—prescriptive—either. A good term paper could be written comparing Brink and Wood's scheme with the one presented here. See also Beckstrand, Jan: The notion of a practice theory and the relationship of scientific and ethical knowledge to practice. *Research in Nursing and Health*. 1:131–136, October 1978. This author argues that there is no such thing as "practice theory," that it is subsumed under either "scientific" theory or "ethics."

55. For example Wandelt, Mable: *Guide for the Beginning Researcher*. New York: Appleton-Century-Crofts, 1972.

56. Henderson, Virginia: *The Nature of Nursing*. New York: Macmillan, 1966, pp. 32–40. Wald, Florence S. and Robert C. Leonard: Toward nursing practice theory. *Nursing Research*, 13:309–314, Fall 1964; Simmons, Leo and Virginia Henderson: *Nursing Research*. New York: Appleton-Century-Crofts 1964, pp. 1–31; Leonard, Robert C.: Developing research in a practice oriented discipline. *American Journal of Nursing*, 67:1472–1475, July 1967; Dilworth, Ava: The need for patient oriented studies. *Nursing Research*, 5:134–135, February 1957; McManus, R. Louise: Nursing research—its evolution. *American Journal of Nursing*, 61:76–79, April 1961; Ellison, Margaret, et al.: Use of behavioral science in nursing: further comment. *Nursing Research*, 13:71–72, Winter 1964; Abdellah, Faye G.: Overview of nursing research, 1955–1968, Parts I, II, and III. *Nursing Research*, 19:16–17, 151–152, 239–252, January–February, March–April, and May–June 1970.

57. Dickoff, James, et al.: Theory in a practice discipline, Part I, p. 433.

58. *Ibid.*

3

The Research Process

INTRODUCTION

No matter what kind of study is called for by the research problem, all the elements of the research process will exist. They may be in different forms depending on the level of inquiry and other considerations, but every study will include every element. The elements of all studies are (1):

Statement of the Problem
Background—Conceptual Framework
Study Design
    Setting
    Sample
    Instruments/Measurements
    Data Collection
    Data Processing/Analysis
    Interpretation/Implementation

The purpose of this chapter is to clarify some terminology and cover some parts of the research process that need to be understood before the next chapters on study designs. Some of the elements in the research process are discussed in detail in later chapters, and only general comments are made here.

STATEMENT OF THE PROBLEM

Analysis of clinical problems to turn them into research problems was covered in Chapter 1. A statement of the problem is the result of analysis of the clinical discrepancy, a condensation of all the thinking that went into defining a discrepancy in clinical practice, stating the conditions and variables involved, and reducing the analysis of the problem to a few carefully constructed paragraphs. At the bare minimum, a statement of the problem should include how the problem came to be perceived as a problem, and what it is an instance of. The statement of the problem is, in effect, an introduction to the study, so it should convincingly lead the reader to a quick grasp of what the problem is and why it's a problem, that is, why it is something that if solved has the potential for improving clinical practice.

The statement of the problem should be as brief as possible; the longer the statement, the more likely it is that the problem isn't yet clear in the researcher's mind. It is not necessary to detail elaborately all the theories that might be involved, or all the ways of thinking about this one instance of larger problems. There will be plenty of opportunity for fleshing out the problem when it comes to the conceptual framework, theoretical background, rationale or literature review. All that is needed in a problem statement is the clearest possible, straightforward explication of what it was that prompted the researcher's attention to it, and of what this clinical problem is a small part.

Take a hypothetical example: a medical/surgical nurse is fed up with irrigating Foley catheters. It takes a lot of time, it can't be delegated to anyone else and she wonders whether it does any good anyhow. That's a perfectly decent beginning of a clinical problem. Suppose further that the nurse recognizes that doing Foley irrigations is an instance of a larger problem, that is, that nurses do a lot of procedures that seem to be done without thought, just following routine.

That may be quite enough to say as a statement of the problem (edited to be a bit more formal). The problem is there, the larger problem is stated and there is enough buried in the clinical example to lead to the literature review and develop the conceptual framework.

Another nurse might come to the same problem from the other end. She might have been brooding that nursing practice seems to contain a good many rituals, procedures done without thought. . . . Further thinking might lead to examples of such rituals, and Foley catheter irrigation might pop to her mind.

It doesn't much matter what order the problem statement uses, whether it moves from the clinical problem to the larger more abstract level, or from an abstraction to an example. Writing the statement of the problem the way it actually occurred to the researcher is often best, for it reveals an internal logic that will prove useful when it comes to developing the conceptual framework. It is likely to be more interesting to read a research proposal or report that grabs the reader's attention with a clinical example in the very beginning.

BACKGROUND

This part of the research process means building up the context in which the particular problem is seen—what the problem is an instance of. It is variously called "theoretical background," "rationale," "conceptual framework" and other terms. Whatever it is called, the activity involved in this step in the research process is a combination of literature review and simply *thinking.* Combined with the analysis and statement of the problem, this step is most critical in the research process, since every other aspect of the process derives from these two. This step is, therefore, probably the hardest mental work.

Batey writes in her survey of twenty-five years of *Nursing Research* that she found that the majority of the major inadequacies in published studies were in the conceptual phase of the study, rather than in the empirical or methodological phase (2). How the problem is characterized and what concepts and theories are pulled together to elaborate the problem, and the logic and consistency of the connections between ideas can make or break the study.

The word background is intended to convey the sense not only of the previous thinking and concepts that might be related to the problem at hand, but also of the background of clinical experience and wisdom behind the problem. It may be that a given problem might not have previous research behind it, or at least none that is immediately on target for the problem found. For example, despite a growing body of literature on rape, only recently have studies been done by women, and by health care workers, on rape and the care of rape victims. These later studies had to depend less on previous research and theory than on theories generated from the data themselves. More recent studies have emphasized rape as an act of violent assault, not simply a sexual attack, a perspective that opens up a different way of thinking about the problem of how the nurse can help rape victims.

Clinical wisdom and personal experience may provide ways to interpret concepts and findings from previous studies to build a fuller and more subtle theory. For example, a black nurse graduate student had considerable experience growing up in the South with faith healers, root doctors, voodoo and other related alternative forms of health care. She began to wonder whether some of the patients who seemed not to comply with traditional medical regimens prescribed for them in a northern city were instead relying on nontraditional remedies or practitioners. The literature was not very helpful, consisting as it did of some anthropological studies of faith healers, witch doctors, root healers and so forth. And the compliance literature was equivocal at best in determining patterns of complying with recommendations of traditional health practitioners. The nursing literature urged non-specifically that nurses take proper account of patients' cultural backgrounds and patterns of belief. And the literature on alternative forms of healing was mostly exhortative and inspirational. Here, the nurse had to depend on her own understanding and experience to devise a new way to think about the problem of patient compliance, one that included the notion that alternative forms of healing are not always in opposition to traditional forms, but that people might be selective in what kinds of problems they would bring to a healer and what kinds to a hospital clinic. Further, there might well be recommendations that doctors might make to patients that are contradicted by a local root doctor, or even more dangerous, some prescribed medications might be antagonistic to some herbal or other natural remedies.

As it happens, these examples would lead (and did) to factor-searching studies (3). Indeed, one of the reasons for conducting a study at the factor-isolating level of inquiry is that there is an absence of an existing conceptual framework, or even decent concepts to work with.

The purpose of the theoretical background is to provide the framework of ideas (theories, concepts) within which the study is to be conducted, and within which the results will be interpreted. The theories also show the place of the particular study in the line of inquiry, since research is a cumulative process, each study building on previous work, and each culminating in suggestions for future research.

Going from the clinical problem to the background in theories and then to the study design is an exercise both in induction and deduction. From the clinical problem, the researcher "induces" the related theory, as part of the analysis of the problem when the situation of which this problem is an instance is outlined. Then from the theories and previous research, the researcher deduces questions or hypotheses that will guide the study at hand.

The theories chosen (or found) depend to a large extent on the researcher's creativity in defining what the problem is an instance of. For example, a clinical problem about how to prepare women better for labor and delivery might be seen entirely within the context of theories about the childbearing cycle, adult development, physiological changes of pregnancy, and so on. But that same problem may also be seen as an instance of the larger problem of preparation for any new experience, and, therefore, literature on preparation in general—preparation for surgery, hospitalization, threatening treatments—might become available. Further, preparing women better might be viewed as a problem in information-giving, patient teaching, stress reduction, anxiety control or any number of other more or less psychological points of view. Thus, other sources of ideas—theories—are opened.

Similarly, a clinical problem about how to help women who have had mastectomies to adjust might begin as an instance of a problem in altered body image, but might also include theories about adult development, social stereotyping, family relationships, internal-external control, decision-making, "postdecisional regret" (4) or any number of other options.

Because the nature of nursing practice is that it lies at the conceptual crossroads of any number of other fields, from clinical medicine through the social sciences and humanities, clinical problems are usually capable of being characterized in almost an infinite number of ways. And no one way will be correct, or right. Conceptual frameworks may be more or less interesting, more or less logically derived, more or less internally consistent, more or less fully developed, but the actual choice (and it is a choice) of which theories to include, or which perspectives to take is an individual one. The major point here is that whatever conceptual background is built up, it be logically worked out, and lead naturally from the problem to the design.

Just because clinical problems can become so intricately complicated by competing theories, there is often the temptation to try to find absolutely every theory that might be related to a problem so as to build the biggest possible case for the importance of the problem and the study. This is likely to be wasted effort. Rather, the effort should be on developing as precisely as possible, the particular theory chosen to guide the particular study. Competing theories may be presented and criticized, and in any event, cannot be ignored. There should be evidence presented other than simply individual taste as to why a particular point of view is taken or a particular theory chosen over another available one.

A frequent error in clinical studies especially prevalent among those new to research, is picking a theory and adopting it wholeheartedly, without tracing it back to its beginnings and without carefully evaluating its fit to the problem at hand. For example, a good deal of laboratory research has developed theories about how information given to subjects to prepare them for a noxious laboratory procedure helps or hinders their coping. It is important to track these theories back to see what assumptions are included and what overall conceptual background was employed in inventing them, for example: what assumptions were made about how people cope, or about the nature of psychological threat. Further, one must examine carefully the circumstances under which the theory was developed—do they apply to the clinical problem? In the case of preparatory communication studies, it may be that they do not translate into clinical situations in which the threat is by definition inescapable (as in surgery) and in which it is clearly of a different order than a relatively less complex laboratory application of a tourniquet to an arm or showing a snake to a naive group.

Psychological theories are particularly tricky to use given the very wide range of theoretical perspectives that can be taken, from learning theories through cognitive theories through theories based on a psychoanalytic or psychodynamic model. But theory for a clinical study is incomplete without a fairly carefully done understanding of where it comes from and a decision that whatever the source, it is appropriate for the problem at hand.

It is often the case that the connections between theories needed by a particular study haven't yet been established. Again, because clinical nursing research crosses the boundaries between social science and clinical science, which do not communicate with one another a great deal yet, concepts from, say, psychology may not yet have their equivalent concept or measurement in, say, physiology. In the early days of clinical nursing research, physiological measures, such as blood pressures, pulse and respiration rates, were often used as measures of psychological stress (5), without full enough consideration of how the concepts in physiology related, or didn't, to psychological stress. The physiological measures were handy, and intuitively appropriate, but over the years, it became clear that there was no automatic one-to-one correspondence between, say, increases in blood pressure and increases in psychological stress. Lots of things make blood pressure go up besides stress, and psychological stress may affect lots of things other than blood pressure. In recent years as nurses have begun to know more about the autonomic nervous system and its indicators, and as the concept of stress has received considerable refinement, the studies have become more precise.

The state of the art in nursing research is such that at the moment, some theories that might be related to a given clinical problem are truly "mental inventions" but are not yet very fully developed beyond the idea stage. For example, while there have been several studies of the effect of primary nursing, with reasonably consistent results in improved patient welfare, the results themselves almost constitute the theory. So far there has not been very much abstract work done with the notion of primary nursing, nor with the underlying theories that might help explain why the results come out the way they do. Similarly, studies of the effectiveness of nurse practitioners in primary care show repeatedly that patients are at least as well off as under physician care, but again little theory has been developed to say why.

Thus, the theoretical background of a study has to provide some preliminary notions as to what may be operating in a given situation, so that when data come in, they can be explained.

The method for developing the theoretical background is the review of the literature.

REVIEW OF THE LITERATURE

There is no great secret about how to build up a reference collection, or how to review systematically the literature, though students are sometimes stumped when trying to figure out how to start. Just *start*, that's all. Find an article that has something to do with the general area one has picked for a problem, even if it's not precisely on target. Read that article's relevant bibliography and note the concepts involved.

Experience eventually teaches that it is wise to keep notes on everything one reads whether it's immediately relevant or not. Interesting ideas, criticisms of someone else's ideas, obscure references to be followed up on a day when one has time, new concepts or theories, new relationships between ideas—they will all find a time, and if one contemplates a career in nursing, one had better begin early to be systematic about recording references (6).

The statement of the problem will guide the literature search. It is often handy to go through the written statement of the problem, underlining the key words as they come along, then compile the list to be a beginning for a bibliographical search. Dempsey has outlined an exercise she uses for graduate and undergraduate students that gives good order to the process (7).

The concepts or words in the statement of the problem become the headings for searches through the published cumulative indices.

There are numerous indices to nursing literature available (8), as well as published abstracts of nursing and other literature (9), collections of studies (10), and after an initial period of foundering around, the problem becomes less one of finding something relevant, than figuring out when to stop.

A *Medline* search is a good tool, but most useful later in the literature search than earlier, when one wants to make sure one has a complete collection of relevant articles. The *Index Medicus* or *Excerpta Medica* are both good places to begin. *Dissertation Abstracts* has a section devoted to health-related dissertations, as well as indexed sections in major fields. *Psychological Abstracts, Child Development Abstracts,* the *Journal of Clinical Medicine* (which publishes internal medicine abstracts) and abstracting publications in other fields are very useful, since more content is contained in an abstract than in a bibliographic citation in an index. There are numerous regular series of abstracts in schizophrenia research, surgery, women's issues, drug addiction and almost any field one can think of. *Nursing Research* published abstracts of nursing-related work until Nov.–Dec. 1978, and all abstracts were indexed by author and content yearly in the annual index (the November-December issue). There is a *Hospital Literature Index* and a *Hospital Abstracts.* Abstracts of papers presented at professional meetings are often contained in the "proceedings" of the session, indexed under the name of the organization, for example, American Orthopsychiatric Association, Association of Children in Hospitals, American Public Health Association and so on.

The *Reader's Guide to Periodical Literature* may be more useful than one would think. Among other publications, it indexes *Science,* and very often in news magazines or other lay literature, reference is made to studies published in the professional literature which can then be tracked down. Card catalogues should not be forgotten, and one should pay attention to how any given book is cross-indexed because the subcategories may lead to other whole bodies of literature.

Textbooks, especially recent editions, are a fine place to start. In schools of nursing, faculty often have painfully built up card files and reprint files to which students may have access. A chat with a professor in whose area one's clinical problem is may be a way to start. Rapping with colleagues may provoke ideas.

The purpose of reviewing the literature is not to compile the longest possible list of citations to prove one's erudition. The purpose is to use the literature to develop logically the theory for a study, and to use it to provoke thinking about theory not yet developed by anyone else. Further, the literature has to be read selectively and critically, not mindlessly. Review articles when available are very good resources, since if done well, the article will have a critique of relevant studies in an area. But when a study looks relevant, one is bound to track down the original source; a review article is never a primary source. Whatever notes are taken about an article should contain enough information about what the study is about, where the major theories came from and what holes in the study might need patching to allow the article's inclusion in a thorough critical review.

While it should not be necessary to state, it is all too often the case that a researcher has not yet developed a personal system of collecting citations and references consistently. A great deal of later pain will be avoided if in the beginning one develops a system for recording references and making sure the complete bibliographical information is included. It can be irritating when one is writing the final draft of a study to discover that one forgot to copy down the page numbers of an article, or that one author's first name is missing from the citation.

It is also wise to begin to develop one's own indexing system to make order out of the references collected. How the system will develop will depend on the individual and what areas or topics are most often contained in an individual collection. The system need not be complicated, but has to have enough meaning to the person inventing it so that any reference can be retrieved later.

The literature should be reviewed not only for previous research on the topic chosen, but also for methodological ideas, instruments or measurements, other clinical examples and even statistical procedures. The literature is a goldmine of information and used efficiently will prevent a good deal of reinventing of the wheel.

Once references begin to be gathered, they tend to organize themselves almost without a great deal of effort. Sequences of studies begin to collect, common themes emerge, subheadings almost write themselves. But writing the literature review is not simply recording all the things one has read. The literature is to be used to stimulate thinking, not do the thinking by itself. Therefore, the best method to write (and therefore conceptualize) the literature is to do it in the order it happened, that is, in the order the investigator used to find the literature, not necessarily the chronological order of the citations. Nothing is more boring than reading list upon list of "so and so found," and then "so and so found something else," and it is not necessary to comment individually upon every single reference. The major themes and their adherents should be grouped, and whatever analytic comments are necessary made about that theme, then move on. And always, the literature review should be building toward some point, in this case, toward the research questions or hypotheses for the study.

It is a matter of institutional and individual style how the review of the literature is woven into the theoretical background and into the whole research proposal. As long as all the material is there, without redundancy, and with logic and clarity, the order and form it takes are not so important.

The literature review is never completely finished either. Even though one makes an artificial stop when the theoretical background is finally written and the research questions or hypotheses stated, the activity of continually reading the literature continues. It is a common, if painful, phenomenon that very often just as the study is ending, one comes across *the* seminal article or paper that should have been found earlier and wasn't. Or someone publishes a new work that would have been perfect as part of the theoretical background just as the final draft of one's study emerges from the typist. That's the nature of research as a human endeavor, however, since any topic and every study are simply pieces of a larger fabric of increasing knowledge for clinical judgment.

When the theoretical background is pulled together and the review of the literature incorporated with original thinking of the researcher, it constitutes a theory in itself. Indeed, in studies at higher levels of inquiry (association-testing and causal hypothesis-testing), that's what the studies do—test the theory in the form of hypotheses. In more exploratory studies, factor-searching and relation-searching, the theory is less well developed and is more like a perspective or point of view taken on the clinical situation than like a theory itself. That's why these kinds of studies are called for—because there are not available concepts or theories pertinent to the problem to be tested.

Finally, a word on terminology: a good deal has been written about what a "concept" is, a "construct," a "theory" (11). For our purposes, a concept is simply a word to which meaning has been attached through formal definition or common usage. In research, a concept usually means an abstraction, something not directly observable, like anxiety, stress, maternal bonding, attribution, nurse-patient relationships and so on. Physiological concepts are a bit more empirical: blood pressure (though not seen directly), catecholamine level, palmar skin activity, mobility and so on. A construct is just a fancier kind of concept, one which has in it several concepts, like social class (income and education), ego dystonic sensation, disturbance in parenting and so on. And theory, as defined in the last chapter, is simply a mental invention to some purpose, the purpose being description, explanation, prediction or prescription. Most of the theories one runs across in a review of the literature will be predictive or descriptive: the more a person balances the consequences of a decision, the less cognitive dissonance (postdecisional regret) he will have; the more externally controlled a person is, the more trust in his physician will be important in recovery from surgery; the bigger the newborn baby, the lesser are the chances of developmental disturbances; the more the nurse is attuned to the patient as a feeling, thinking and doing person, the more the patient is likely to experience relief from pain through the nurse-patient interaction. Each of these small theories has its own theoretical background, and was developed more or less logically and soundly. But all of them are theories, and could be part of studies and study designs.

Once the theoretical background is stated, ending with the research questions or hypothesis, the next step in the research process is to design the study.

STUDY DESIGN

Designing the study means stating the questions to be answered or the hypotheses to be tested, determining the level of inquiry, defining the variables, selecting a setting and sample, choosing measurements or instruments, designing a way to obtain the data and processing and analyzing the data.

Level of Inquiry

The level of inquiry is a shorthand way of stating what kind of research problem the one chosen is. What *is* this? problems are at the first level of inquiry; What will happen if . . . ? problems are at the third and so on, as described in the previous chapter. Forcing oneself to set down on paper the level of inquiry is a way to focus attention on the exact kind of problem one has, and thus the expectations of the design for the kind of information — theory — to solve it.

Research Questions and Hypotheses

By the end of the theoretical background development and literature review, there will be research questions to be answered or hypotheses to be tested. Depending on the level of inquiry, the research questions take different forms. For the first level of inquiry, the research questions almost literally take the form of What *is* this? with this named. "What are Soteria House's interactions with the world?" Wilson asked (12). "What is it like to die in hospitals today?" was Glaser and Strauss' question (13). For studies at this most basic level of inquiry, rarely is it possible to state more subtle questions.

Studies at the second level of inquiry, which also begin with research questions rather than hypotheses, translate, What's happening here? into questions about *relationships*. (These are factor-relating, or relation-searching studies, remember?) What factors are related to recovery from surgery? What is related to outcome of pregnancy? What is related to drug-drug interactions among elderly people in a nursing home? are examples of possible research questions at this level of inquiry.

Association-testing or causal hypothesis-testing studies begin with hypotheses, which are predictions of relationships among variables in contrast to research questions about relationships. Hypotheses are always stated in future tense: nursing interaction will produce reduced postoperative stress; ice to the perineum will reduce postpartum swelling; preparing parents for their child's surgery will reduce children's upsets might be examples of hypotheses for causal hypothesis-testing studies. Infant temperament will be related to mother's coping ability; need for personal space will be related to self-disclosure; social class will be related to specific patterns of mental illness distribution are examples of association-testing study hypotheses.

Note that every hypothesis states a prediction of a relationship. If no relationship is predicted, it is not an hypothesis. For example, a statement simply of the occurrence of something (social class differences will be found in this sample) is not a true hypothesis.

A good hypothesis has several characteristics. First, it is conceptually clear; that is, the terms used in the hypothesis are generally understandable. A quick survey of any research literature will show you how often this characteristic of a good hypothesis is violated. However, if studies are to be repeated to accumulate evidence of the generality of the findings, the hypothesis has to be stated in such a way that it is clear to other investigators. A second condition of a good hypothesis is that it has empirical references. In other words, the factors in an hypothesis must be measurable and related to observable phenomena. The third requirement of a good hypothesis is that it be derived from theory and/or research. This last requirement is not very hard to meet considering that an investigator will have analyzed a problem by the time she proposes the hypothesis and the relationship between the hypothesis and the theory is part of the analysis of the problem.

Hypotheses may simply predict relationships or they may predict the direction of a relationship. For example, There will be a relationship between patients' personality type and recovery from surgery, simply states a relationship. But, Patients with personality type . . . will experience fewer complications in recovery from surgery, predicts the direction of the relationship. Often, causal hypotheses state the predicted relationship in the form of a statement of *difference*. For instance, Pediatric patients who have nursing preparation for surgery will experience less postoperative difficulty than pediatric patients who do not experience preparation. Or, Patients cared for by a nurse practitioner will have higher rates of compliance with follow-up appointments than patients not seen by the nurse practitioner. In these cases, the relationship is between the group to which the patient is assigned (experimental or control) and the outcome, but it makes more sense to state the hypothesis as a prediction of difference.

Predicting the direction of a relationship has certain consequences for data analysis and interpretation of findings. Statistical inference from testing a "one-tailed" hypothesis—a prediction of direction—is different from inference from a "two-tailed" distribution, when no prediction of direction is made. The mathematical technicalities are beyond the scope of this book (see any standard statistics book), but it is important to realize early that the way the hypothesis is stated determines a good bit of what kind of statistical analysis and interpretation is possible.

Sometimes one will run across studies reported where the "null" form of the hypothesis is stated instead of the research hypothesis. That is, instead of predicting a relationship and perhaps the direction of it, the hypothesis states there will be no difference, or no effect of the independent variable. Batey points out that stating the hypothesis in the null form is not logical. "The function of research . . . is to test the substantive research hypothesis, not the statistical hypothesis. The use of null (statistical) hypotheses denies the . . . logical formulation." (14) The null hypothesis, as Batey hints, is a highly technical statistical device, used to put in words the statistical assumptions against which the empirical data collected will be compared. To test the probability of any particular research result, one has to have something to compare the results to. What inferential statistics provide are populations of possible results, called sampling distributions, which take into account all possible results one could get if there is indeed no relationship between the variables studied. One then compares the statistical finding (such as a difference between means, or some other mathematical measure) against this statistically "known" population of possibilities, and can figure out how likely it is that the finding obtained could have happened just by chance alone, rather than as a true effect of the experimental treatment or as a true correlational relationship between the variables studied. The statistical function of the null hypothesis is its only reason for existing—it generates the sampling distribution. But it should not be stated as the hypothesis to be tested since it is not directly tested at all, and indeed, isn't even very interesting in and of itself (except perhaps to a statistician). What is of interest is the research hypothesis, and the null hypothesis is just a device, a tool, to help interpret the findings.

Often even in studies at higher levels of inquiry where hypotheses are formally stated, research questions may also appear, but not as the primary focus of the study. Studies at lower levels of inquiry never contain hypotheses; otherwise they would not be at the lower level of inquiry. Hypotheses are appropriate when the study is a What will happen if . . . ? study, and only in those kinds of studies. However, sometimes after the main hypotheses are stated and tested, the researcher wants to take a more exploratory look at some variables without a formal hypothesis. Often these kinds of research questions relate to antecedent variables, things the patients or subjects carry into the situation with them. For example, in preparation for surgery studies, it may be of interest to pose additional research questions about the extent to which age, sex or previous hospital experience is related to how well the patient does, quite apart from the independent variable. It is occasionally these reseach questions that turn out to be more illuminating than the hypotheses tested, especially when there are "negative findings," that is, when things don't work out the way they were predicted. For example, Dumas' long series of preoperative preparation studies ended with the conclusion that at least as the nursing was defined in the last study (preparation a month before surgery), it didn't work (15). But then Dumas and others reanalyzed their data with certain research questions in mind, and found some correlations and differences among patients in type and amount of surgery, race and other variables that accounted for some of the negative findings (16). At the very least, these kinds of research questions may show the way for the next series of studies, and it is perfectly appropriate to include in an hypothesis-testing study, some subsidiary research questions.

Definition of Variables

The research questions or hypotheses will have stated what the major variables that will be included in the study are. Now, one has to provide definitions of them, and a special kind of definition, called "operational definition," has to be created (or otherwise provided) for every variable under consideration. Operational definitions specify the ways in which bits of the real world—data—will be taken as defining the concept, whatever it is. In other words, an operational definition describes the operations (measures, data collection) used to provide meaning to the concept.

Each concept in the research questions and hypotheses will have a conceptual definition and an operational definition. On the way to an operational definition, there are some intervening steps, spelled out below:

	EXAMPLES
Conceptual definition	"social class" = relative socioeconomic position (17)
Properties (characteristics)	education; occupation
Indicants	number of years of school; job title, each with assigned points
Operations	ask the respondent
Measurement	count the points assigned and add them up

The conceptual definition will follow from the theories used in stating the problem and developing the background. Conceptual definitions are in abstract terms and are often simply quoted from other work or from the dictionary. They are invented (or borrowed) for the purpose of the study; there is no one "right" conceptual definition *per se*, but each concept in the research question or hypothesis has to have its conceptual definition so that meaning of the study can be determined when the data are in.

The concept will then have one or more defining properties. In the case of the example above, "social class," as Hollingshead and Redlich evolved it, consisted of a combination of educational level and occupation (18). Other characteristics or properties of the concept social class could be chosen. For example, a special study of census data has developed the concept "socioeconomic status" to define population groups (19). The concept has the following properties: median family income; percent of population twenty-one years of age or less with less than twelve years of school; percent of employed males in unskilled, semiskilled and service occupations; percent of dwelling units with more than one person per room; percent of children under eighteen living with both parents.

The "indicants" are things that point to—indicate—other things; in this case, number of years of school indicates education, and job title is taken as the indicant for occupation. Then each indicant must have specified for it data which will be taken as evidence of the indicant. In the case of social class, the response of the individual to the questions, What is your job? and, How far did you go in school? are the actual operational definitions. The "operation" is question-asking and writing down the response. Finally, each operational definition has a measurement—rules for using data collected through the operational definition. Hollingshead and Redlich devised a point system for both occupations and educational levels which when summed, provided a rank ordered scale from social class I (highest score) through social class V (lowest score). Scores then, in their classes, are taken to mean social class, or relative social position.

Tedious as the process of arriving at operational definitions and measurements is, it is critical for a study to make sense, and for any claims of measurement validity to be made (see Chapter 9). Actually, one usually doesn't consciously go through all the steps from conceptual definition to properties, to indicants and down the line, but rather provides conceptual definitions and operational ones which are combinations of what is called here "operations" and "measurement" and lets it go at that.

Notice how, as one descends the definition ladder, the concept narrows. This is unavoidable and necessary, but is often frustrating to those new to research when they begin to see "surplus meaning" carved away from a pretty concept.

Take another example: "relief from pain (20)," from a study testing the effect of nursing interaction on relief from pain in postoperative patients. Here the conceptual definition might be something like decreased sensation of discomfort. The properties of the concept were physiological signs and verbal and nonverbal behavior of the patient. The indicants were blood pressure, pulse and respiration rates, observations of nonverbal behavior and patient reports. The operational definition included applying the sphygmomanometer to the patient in a lying-down position, pumping it to 200 mm. Hg, and releasing the pressure slowly, counting the first sound heard and the last; for nonverbal behavior, applying a checklist on which there were various possible behaviors—crying, sweating, coughing, smiling,—as well as notations of body position and movement; and for verbal behavior, the question, How are you feeling? or How are you feeling now? asked at the beginning and end of the interaction was used. And the measurements were the recorded blood pressure, pulse and respiration readings; the written description consisted of nonverbal behavior (submitted to judges and rated as indicating more or less comfort from beginning of interaction to end) and the actual words of the patient in response to the question (also submitted to judges).

In casual hypothesis-testing studies, providing operational definitions and measurements of the experimental variable, which is often "nursing care," is a particularly interesting problem in definition (21). Sometimes the nursing care is defined by someone's theory about nursing, in a general or broad way. Sometimes it is defined essentially as nursing process—identifying the problem, ministering, validating—and sometimes a kind of script is written which the nurse follows. Difficult though it may be, operational definitions of the independent variable in experimental studies still must be provided so that when data are analyzed, they can be interpreted in light of whatever the "treatment" was, and so that other investigators may have enough information to repeat or replicate the study.

In theory, all the variables upon which data will be collected in a study should have both conceptual and operational definitions formally attached to them. In practice, however, usually only the major variables in the hypotheses or research questions, and certain other variables that might not be intuitively meaningful, are formally given operational definitions. For example, demographic data collected normally in the course of nearly every study—age, sex, race, marital status and so on—often do not come from formal operational definitions. Other variables that are not the major ones in a study, but still deserve formal operational definitions, are those on which there is choice of measurement, those which require particular understanding of the field to grasp or those on which data will be collected, but collapsed. For instance, in a study of recovery from surgery, pain tolerance might not be a variable in a major hypothesis, but might be considered an antecedent variable of the patients themselves. Since there are no widely accepted standard measurements of pain tolerance, it would be important to say specifically how such data were collected—by self-report, for example, or by dolorimeter, or by some experimental procedure. Similarly, in studies of laboring women fetal heart rate might be a variable of interest, but not a central one. It would be important to state whether the fetal heart rate was collected by fetoscope (and/or how long the rate was counted) or by external monitor, since there may be differences in the reliability of the count. And, in another postoperative recovery study, type of surgery might be a variable of interest, but the intention will not be to classify every single type of surgical procedure by surgical categories. Rather, the data may be collapsed into major or minor categories, or some version of rank-ordered scale. Again, it would be important to specify out loud which datum (surgical procedure) is going to be taken as evidence of the operational definition and measurement (major, minor surgery).

Some interesting theoretical problems crop up in choosing operational definitions. As mentioned earlier, studies in medical/surgical nursing in the early days of clinical nursing research often took pulse rate and blood pressure as operational definitions of "stress" or "distress" when the logical theoretical connections between the physiological state measured by blood pressure and heart rate and the psychological state of stress were not made. Similarly, some psychological measures have been incorrectly applied when a researcher was not aware of the difference in psychology theory between measures of personality *trait* and personality *state* (the latter being more equivalent to "emotional state," time limited and situation specific, while trait measures supposedly tap enduring personality patterns or characteristics). "Trait" measures do not always work well in measuring transitory emotional states, though the data on this point are equivocal.

Sometimes clinical wisdom will avoid problems of invalid operational definitions. For example, using the amount of pain medication taken as a measurement of "pain" is questionable, since a case can be made that the amount of pain medication taken is a measure of staff behavior, not of the patient problem. Similarly, length of stay in the hospital may or may not be a good measure of recovery, since length of stay depends upon, among other things, the utilization review procedures in a given setting, and an individual physician's choice.

A useful test of operational definitions and measurements for clinical nursing research is whether they make clinical sense or not. And a useful test of measures borrowed from other research in other fields is to determine the conceptual background of the measure as described by the original author. If it comes from a theoretical perspective that is not the one chosen for a given study, the measure is unlikely to be useful. Or if the measure was intended for one purpose and is now being used for another, it is unlikely to show the results wanted. For example, our measurement for nurse-patient interaction, the Nurse Orientation System, is deliberately just what it says, a measure of how the nurse is oriented in her verbal expressions to the patient and the patient to the nurse (22). It is not a measure of empathy, of nurse-patient relationship or of Orlando's theory of nursing (23), though people have tried to use it that way with limited success. When in doubt about what an instrument is intended to measure, contact the original author. Wolfer has written a useful critique of some commonly used measures of patient welfare and recovery which elaborates these points (24).

When the problem is stated, the theory developed, hypotheses or research questions posed, study design chosen, level of inquiry stated and variables defined, it is time to choose a place and some people to participate in the research.

Choosing a Setting

The choice of the particular space-time setting in which to conduct research depends, as does everything else, on the problem selected for study. No matter what setting is chosen the relationship between the research and the setting and between the researcher and others around her/him become critical. Considerations other than convenience come into decisions about which settings to use.

In general, there are two types of settings—real and artificial. Real settings would include (for nursing research) any setting in which clinical nursing practice is being carried out. Artificial settings are usually laboratories of various kinds. The "realness" of a setting is determined by how representative it is of usual or normal practice settings. For example, a small unit set up as part of a medical research project for the treatment of patients with terminal cancer is a real setting, but it may not be representative of other wards or units in even the same hospital. The generality of the research will be affected by the representativeness of the setting.

Lab settings or other artificial settings have been used in psychological, sociological and some nursing research. Their major advantage is the amount of control the investigator can have over extraneous variables and the amount of manipulation of the physical and environmental conditions that is possible.

The major disadvantage of lab settings is, of course, that they do not resemble practice settings, and, therefore, the results from research may not necessarily say anything important about practice. Studies of nursing practice that take place in nursing practice settings have more applicability, generally, than do studies done in artificially contrived environments.

The choice of setting is based on several things. First, the proposed emphasis of the research must be considered. If the research is seen as eventually, if not immediately, contributing to changes in nursing practice, this suggests that the study best be carried out in practice. This assumes that the investigator has a conception of practice *as it is now*, and, therefore, can assess settings for how closely they come to either the real practice situation or the ideal practice situation. The goal of the particular study, or the stage of inquiry, is another factor to be considered. How close or how far away from solution or resolution of the problem is this study? How clear is the researcher about factors in the setting that might be important to either control or collect data on? Lab settings can often be used to isolate variables, test manipulations, refine techniques or procedures, evaluate measurements, as long as the ultimate testing takes place in practice.

In a setting, what is surveyed to decide what setting to use? Among other things, one might find out how nursing research, or any research, is perceived within the setting and by whom. Is the setting likely to be suportive or at least tolerant of the investigation? Is the setting likely to be catalytic or inhibitory to the conduct of the research, thereby possibly influencing the findings? Is the setting research-sophisticated (as many teaching hospitals are), and, therefore, are patients or personnel likely to be more cooperative, more likely to resist attempts to control their knowledge about the study? Is the setting economical to the research (convenient) and practical? Is convenience its only strong point? For example, graduate students doing research often have only one choice of setting—the one in which their school is. It may or may not theoretically be the best one available, but time and money considerations preclude long-distance separation of the student from the school.

Does the setting contain the sample needed? This may seem an obvious question, but many times a researcher chooses a setting on the basis of convenience and finds out that there aren't enough patients of the kind she needs to go around. In research and teaching hospitals, there may be many projects being conducted, and researchers want to protect their patients by not having them participate in more than one study. In addition, some hospital's emphases in treatment will eliminate some samples. For instance, an obstetric service may use a great deal of conduction anesthesia which may eliminate patients who wish natural childbirth. A more obvious sample would be some religious-affiliated hospitals whose policies preclude teaching about artificial birth control methods. Dynamically oriented psychiatric hospitals rarely let their patients regress very much, and, therefore, they would not be good places to collect data on extremely regressed patients.

All of the things listed should be considered in choosing a setting, even though the major consideration in the eventual choice is convenience. The setting should also be described in some detail in any report of research so that the reader or listener can judge how closely the setting resembles others, and, therefore, how relevant the findings would be for other settings.

Chances are, the more closely a study approximates practice in a given setting, the happier the personnel in the setting are going to be about cooperating with the study; and the better the relationships between each researcher and the setting, the easier it's going to be for future researchers to use the same setting. The researcher should remember that she has no intrinsic right of access to patients—she is given access by the hospital, agency, or unit in which the study will be performed. Therefore, respect and acknowledgment of the personnel whose unit it is contributes to everyone's mental health. Some ways to build good relationships with the setting include being as open as appropriate about what one is doing, sharing information with the personnel as it is important to them, feeding back the results of the study when it's finished, following the established lines of authority in obtaining permission to do the study, but most important conveying to the personnel the investigator's own reasoning behind why the study is interesting and important to nursing practice and what it might contribute to better patient care (25).

Carrying out a study in a particular setting may in itself contribute to better patient care both during the study period and afterward—the "Hawthorne effect"; the study itself has an effect on the phenomena being observed (26). For example, one small study on a chronic unit of a large neuropsychiatric hospital involved all the personnel and all the patients in various kinds of group activities and tested the effect of different kinds of patient-staff involvement. The researchers found that the interest in patient care generated by the study enhanced the effectiveness of all the patient-staff groups, no matter what the internal composition or intent of the group was. In addition, after the study was completed, the effect continued and personnel continued to be more involved with patients than they were before the study started (27).

Obtaining administrative clearance to conduct a study in a given clinical setting may turn out to be an interesting exercise in Who Has the Power. As a matter of principle, nurse researchers should have access to nursing service for administrative clearance to conduct *nursing* research. As a matter of courtesy, other professionals should be informed that the study is going on and is likely to have an impact on the work of others. If the study is truly a nursing study which approximates normal nursing practice, it should require no formal clearance by individual physicians, the medical staff committee or the hospital administrator. Unfortunately, the ideal state of affairs has yet to become universal.

In summary, the major consideration in choosing a setting is whether it has enough of the phenomenon being investigated, in other words, how appropriate the setting is to the conduct of research on a particular problem. Secondary considerations (which may become primary) include how accepting the setting is of clinical nursing research and how practical collecting data in the particular setting will be (in terms of time, distance, clearance, permissions and so on). Experience suggests that when the clinical problem is something seen as a problem by the staff as well as the researcher, and when proper account is taken of the reality of the clinical situation, relationships within a setting are supportive and helpful. The researcher also has an obligation, which should be part of one's negotiations with a setting, to report back on the findings from the study unless there is some burning reason why this should not be done (28). When the intent of research in nursing practice is to improve the practice and patient care, then the researcher has even more than the ordinary obligation to make public the findings, especially in the place in which they were generated.

Sampling

The next step in the research process is defining the sample to be collected and deciding on how it will be obtained.

"Sample" is usually taken to mean people, but a sample may or may not be people, depending on the study itself. For instance, a sample may consist of nurse-patient interactions (taken from the same people), or it may be episodes of care. It may be incidents of a particular kind (such as incidents of dying in hospitals). It may even be words or phrases, sentences or speechs if the study deals with analysis of verbal behavior of patients. In factor-searching studies, as we shall see in the next chapter, sample has even a different meaning.

But most conventionally, a sample means a group of people from whom data are collected. The principles of sampling discussed here apply to other kinds of samples.

The first thing to be done before a sample is chosen is to decide what criteria will make people eligible to be in the sample. These "sampling criteria" then become the "sampling frame"—the box built around the particular sample to separate it from all other people. Sampling criteria are generated for the most part by the analysis of the problem itself and by the variables chosen and operational definitions. Obviously, the first criterion has to be who has the thing under study. The sample members have to all possess the variables of interest. Superficially this seems simple, but the state of knowledge in clinical nursing being what it is now, the simple may quickly become complicated. For example, suppose one were interested in stress reduction in surgery patients. On the surface, it would seem that any patient undergoing surgery would be eligible for the sample. But a little armchair thinking might suggest that patients with emergency surgery are not likely to be the same (with respect to stress) as patients undergoing scheduled or elective surgery. Similarly, patients having cosmetic surgery may not have the same kind of stress experience as those having mutilative surgery. And patients having diagnostic surgery for cancer may be suspected to have a different stress conception than patients having corrective surgery (cholecystecomy, for example) in whom cancer is not a question. Patients having surgery on reproductive organs may not be the same as patients having thyroid surgery and so on.

Whether the sample members have the thing being studied is also called a "base rate" problem. The base rate is the normal rate of occurrence of a variable in the sample (or population) at hand—the prevalence, if you like. The base rate problem can be seen in two ways: 1. does the variable occur with enough frequency to collect a sample? 2. is there enough of the variable in a given sample to make it a useful sample?

For example, suppose one wanted to do a study on the effect of some new kind of nursing procedure for changing dressings on the incidence of wound infections. With antibiotics and improved sterile procedures in the operating room, wound infections may be so few and far between that it would be difficult to get a large enough sample in the time available. This doesn't mean the study should not be done, just that the researcher might have to adjust the amount of time necessary to gather enough cases.

Some variables simply do not occur very often, but when they do, the consequences are serious. For example, the nurses mentioned in Chapter 1 who wanted to figure out how to predict cardiac tamponade must realize that it will probably take years to collect a large enough sample to do the study they want to do, but that does not mean that cardiac tamponade is not a good thing to study, or to try to prevent.

When possible, it is wise to try to get some information about the base rate of a given variable in advance of designing a study. For things like cardiac tamponade, data are probably kept in the recovery room or coronary intensive care unit. For something like stitch infections, the infection control committee of the hospital may have some notion about frequency. Data on frequency of operative procedures are often kept in summary form by hospitals, and if not, they are retrievable from operating room schedules. Numbers of diagnostic procedures, such as pneumoencephalograms, CT scans and other high-technology tests, are often routinely kept. Obstetrical outcome data—numbers of prematures, stillbirths, multiple births—are frequently readily available from delivery room records, without having to check charts. Medical diagnoses, especially on ambulatory patients are less easy to find in summary form, which may be frustrating if one is interested in a study, say, on the effect of nurse practitioner practice with patients of a particular, and relatively infrequent, diagnosis. This information is sometimes already in the literature, even if it does not pertain directly to the setting one finds oneself in. Ambulatory diagnosis statistics, for example, have been published, and it is possible to extrapolate from the statistics to a local population at least for the most frequently occurring diagnoses. Nursing diagnoses are, as yet, almost never included in hospital statistics or even in public health agency information, and chart review is almost the only way to retrieve them.

Dumas' original study illustrates the second kind of base rate problem (29). Because the nurse-researcher was interested in seeing if preopera-tive nursing care could lower the rate of postoperative vomiting, she had to find a sample of patients with a relatively high rate of vomiting; otherwise, she could not expect to lower it. She had to collect some data, because none existed, to determine which surgical groups seemed to produce a relatively high vomiting rate (and which groups also did not routinely have nasogastric tubes), and eventually gynecological surgery patients were selected. In experimental studies in which the attempt is to test whether a certain kind of nursing care can lower, or ameliorate, certain untoward patient conditions, the base rate problem is especially serious. The seriousness of the problem increases with the vagueness or newness of the definition of nursing care. When a vague or global nursing treatment is being tested, there has to be quite a lot of the variable it's being tested on for it to make a difference. For example, if a new nursing treatment designed to lower patients' stress on admission to the hospital based on reassurance and providing information is being planned, one has to be sure there's quite a lot of stress there for it to be tested on. The treatment is simply too weak to make a measureable difference if there's not a lot of stress to be reduced. Therefore, for an early or beginning study on this topic, it would be well to choose a sample in which the overall level of stress is higher.

After choosing a sample which has enough of the characteristic being measured, the next important consideration is how representative the sample is of the larger population. Given that it is rarely possible to study the entire population, the purpose of picking a sample is so that conclusions generated by one sample may be applied to others—generalized. Studies at the third level of inquiry and above, association-testing and causal hypothesis-testing studies especially, are aimed at testing or verifying theory, and they require more attention to the representativeness of the sample than do studies at lower levels of inquiry which are hypothesis-generating, such as factor-searching and relation-searching studies.

To establish sampling criteria, the researcher uses whatever information is available on the base rate of the variables of interest to decide what kinds of criteria will make an individual eligible to be in the sample. Sampling criteria often include some age boundaries (for example, children zero to two only, or children only up to the age of ten), derived from the theoretical framework which might say that the variables of interest are likely to be different in older children, and, therefore, older children should be excluded. Sampling criteria are usually based on demographic or antecedent variables such as age, sex, marital status, diagnosis and so on, and obviously the sampling criteria have to be things that can be identified in advance of collecting data so that the researcher doesn't bother people to collect data from them if they will not eventually fit the criteria.

The sampling criteria will be derived from the statement of the problem and the theoretical background. But two frequently stated sampling criteria are that the individuals chosen must be able to read and speak English (and perhaps one other language in which the data collectors are fluent), and that the individuals not be participating in any other study (to respect the time and effort of the subjects or patients). Although not often stated as part of sampling criteria, it is absolutely imperative that the sample members must be able to participate fully in whatever the procedure is for obtaining informed consent which sometimes means that people who are retarded, or deaf, blind, mentally ill and so on may be excluded from some studies (see Chapter 11 for a fuller discussion of informed consent).

Some studies will require particular kinds of sampling criteria. For example, a study on the effect of nursing interaction on patients in pain when p.r.n. medication is to be given might specify that the patients must be eligible for a p.r.n. pain medication (that is, not have had one for the previous three—four hours). The effort in setting sampling criteria, especially for studies at higher levels of inquiry is to produce a sample that is relatively homogeneous with respect to the major variables in the study. The smaller the sample is going to be, for studies at higher levels of inquiry, the more homogeneous it should be. Otherwise, there will be so many things varying that the effect of the variable one wants to test may not show through, and interpretation of results will drive one to drink.

All studies have sampling criteria, even studies at lower levels of inquiry. But the sampling method used may differ for studies aimed at discovering theory (hypotheses) than for studies aimed at testing hypotheses and generalizing from the test to other samples.

How representative a sample is is tested technically by knowing the probability of occurrence of each sample unit in the population. Thus, there are a number of sampling methods known collectively as *probability* sampling where it is possible to calculate what the chances are of any given sampling unit—person—getting into the sample from the potential population of possible sampling units.

The major types of probability sampling are random sampling, stratified random sampling, and cluster or multistage sampling.

The principle of random sampling is easy to grasp: all it means is that the sampling units are picked in such a way that within the sampling frame, every potential sample member has an equal (and known) probability of being selected for the sample. Another way of saying the same thing is that whether an individual gets in the sample or doesn't has nothing to do with that individual's place on the variables of interest. Once the sampling criteria are set, then hypothetically all persons who meet those sampling criteria (in a given space and time boundary) have a known and equal chance of being in the sample. What determines whether a given individual ends up in the sample or not is a strictly procedural matter, having nothing to do with whether the individual has more of or less of the qualities that will eventually be measured.

There are several methods for picking a random sample. If it is possible to have the name of every person within the sampling frame, all of these names can be thrown into a hat and a percentage drawn. This is usually completely impossible, so there are various other ways to select samples. If all the possible units (regardless of *who* they are) are known, they can be numbered and the numbers selected from the total. One device used in such selection is a table of random numbers found in the back of almost any statistics book. This is a table in which numbers from 1 to 1,000 or 10,000 or 1,000,000 have been randomly arranged by a computer. If all the units in any particular population have been numbered, a table of random numbers can be used to select cases simply by reading down the columns of the table, starting anywhere, and picking the numbers of the cases.

Suppose the first block of numbers in a table of random numbers looks like this:

$$
\begin{array}{ccccc}
10 & 09 & 73 & 25 & 33 \\
37 & 54 & 20 & 48 & 05 \\
08 & 42 & 26 & 89 & 53 \\
99 & 01 & 90 & 25 & 29 \\
12 & 80 & 79 & 99 & 70 \\
\end{array}
$$

The sample size to be selected will be fifty people. Since fifty is a two-digit number, it is possible to use the rows and columns just as they are. It doesn't matter whether one reads the table across or down, just so the decision is made in advance of the study. Reading the table across, the first person selected would be number 10 (the tenth person in a list, or the tenth to be admitted to the hospital and so on); then the ninth person. The next number, 73, is larger than the fifty the sample needs so it can be skipped. The next people selected would be the twenty-fifth, thirty-third, thirty-seventh, twentieth and so forth. Notice that there are two 25s and two 99s in the table. When duplicate numbers come up they are just skipped and the next available number used.

If the sample size had been 100 instead of 50, the table would be read in columns or rows of three digits each. For example, the first person selected would be number 100, then (reading down) number 84 (since 375 is larger than the hundred needed) and so on.

One needs to be just a bit wary of lists of names because the underlying principle of listing may produce a list with systematic variations in it that will have to be considered. Alphabetical lists are supposedly the least "biased," but even then, depending on what is known about the population from which the list is generated, there may be problems. Lists may be incomplete, such as is the case in a telephone directory (where people with unlisted numbers and people without telephones are not included). Similarly, city directories or university directories may be out of date.

Lists of patients by hospital number (unit number) may be accurate as long as the system of assigning numbers is unsystematically related to anything else. For example, new babies may be assigned a new number in the sequence, and if one is going simply by unit numbers to pick a sample of adults, some babies are going to be included and will have to be edited out later. Billing lists may or may not be complete, depending on the institution's billing procedures. Lists of patients in visiting nursing agencies may be a problem if children in a family are listed only under the parents' name or number.

When the total number of entries in a list (or a population) is known, or when the total sample size to be drawn is, there are other methods of producing a "random" sample that are not truly random, but are systematic. For example, every fifth or twentieth, or thirty-third name or number can be picked from a list. If the total number of potential people in the sample is known, and one has decided on a total number wanted for the sample, then one can simply divide the total list by the sample number and take every n-th case. But suppose it was known that a certain clinic had, say, 500 patient records, and the researcher wanted a sample of 50. If the researcher takes every tenth record, everything is fine (sampling either alphabetically, if that's the way the records are arranged, or by consecutive number). But if the researcher started out taking every fifth number, the sample would be complete long before the population had run out, and people with names in the last part of the alphabet, or with unit numbers late in the sequence (perhaps new patients) would be underrepresented.

There are other approximations of these systematic random sampling methods used sometimes in clinical research. For example, all patients admitted to one room may be taken, and patients admitted to other rooms not selected. Or all patients in the hospital on Mondays and Thursdays may be sampled, and not any patients on the other days. These methods will produce a random sample only when there is no systematic pattern in room assignment, or admission in these examples.

Studies which use chart data retrospectively often make use of clinical knowledge to determine how the sample should be drawn. For instance, a study of obstetrical outcome might make sure that equal numbers of cases are drawn from each month of the year or each quarter, to take account of the fact that obstetrical residents rotate every summer, and it might be expected that new residents are less skilled than those who are finishing up their year. Or it might be the case (and is, as it happens) that the rate of delivery of babies varies across the year. (September is highest, in many facilities. Count back nine months and figure out why.) If so, then the researcher may want to take account of that and draw a sample of . . . percent of the deliveries per month, so that any high-delivery month will not be underrepresented.

When there is no systematic pattern to the underlying list from which the sample is drawn, a systematic, regular method of drawing a sample will be good approximation of a strictly random sample (30).

In some cases, a different kind of sample is used. *Stratified random* sampling makes use of the information that there are certain unequal groups within the population from which equal numbers are to be drawn. For instance, hospitals may have unequal numbers of medical and surgical beds. If equal numbers of medical and surgical patients are desired, the sample is stratified on the basis of service and two separate random samples are drawn as usual. Samples could also be stratified on the basis of race, social class, age or any number of other variables. The procedure for drawing the sample once the strata are identified is the same as that for random sampling.

While on the subject of lists, a few comments about how to obtain lists. It happens that many institutions do not have complete lists of patients over time. If master lists are not available from an admissions office, or a medical records office, there are other resources. For example, the billing office has complete lists of patients billed, which should be a complete list altogether (but isn't often, if it is known that some patients are seen and never entered into the system). Clinical microscopy laboratories, or bacteriology laboratories, have complete lists of the tests run, with patients' names and chart numbers. If one were interested, for example, in choosing a sample of patients with urinary tract infection from a general medical clinic population, one would ordinarily be faced with having to go through every single medical clinic chart to identify the UTI patients. However, it may be simpler to go through the bacteriology laboratory duplicate slips, kept in the lab, and identify those patients who had culture and sensitivity tests done and who were referred to the lab from the medical clinic. Sometimes special lists of patients are generated for other purposes, such as medical research. Individual physicians or a medical department may have complete lists of patients who have had particular experimental procedures, or who have conditions that were of special interest to medical research. Log books kept on nursing units, like delivery logs or operating room logs, may be a resource. If narcotics record books are kept, they may consititute a way to define a population of patients in pain, for example. Or the physical therapy department may have a list that can be used to detect orthopedic surgical patients of certain kinds.

Another type of probability sampling less frequently used in nursing research is *cluster* sampling, or *multistage* sampling. In this case, the units in the several stages are all selected randomly. For instance, one could randomly select from the entire United States a certain number of hospitals. Then from the hospitals, a certain number of wards could be selected, from the wards a certain number of patient units and from the units a certain number of patients. The selection of hospitals, wards, patient units and patients are all done randomly. The major disadvantage of this kind of sampling procedure is that all possible patients do not have an equal chance of being chosen, for if any hospital is eliminated, all its patients are, too. This has considerable implications for statistical procedures and generality of the findings.

Often in clinical nursing research, nonprobability sampling methods are used, for practical reasons. Because these methods produce samples that may or may not be representative, conclusions drawn from the studies are always somewhat more tentative. However, even probability samples drawn as rigorously as possible in one institution may or may not be generalized to other settings, if there is considerable difference among settings in the variables being tested. For instance, even probability samples drawn from medical centers or other teaching institutions may not be like samples from community hospitals or more rural settings in terms of patient diagnosis, severity of condition and so on.

Convenience or *accidental* sampling is a method most often used in clinical nursing research. Here, one takes all the sampling units one can get in the time allotted to get them, for example, all patients having gynecological surgery in October and November (the data collection period) of a given year. The assumption is that there is no particular reason for thinking these patients are any different from patients admitted at any other times of the year. But that assumption is just that, short of comparing the patients selected with records of patients taken at another time of year. (It happens, by the way, that there can be odd systematic variations in samples over given periods. School teachers, for instance, will schedule their elective surgery during academic vacations, so samples of gynecological patients, or patients with herniorrhaphies drawn in December and in the summer may contain more school teachers than usual. This may be important only if school teaching is related to other variables, such as social class, which it is. In this case, a sample with a good many school teachers in it will not necessarily enable one to generalize to samples with other kinds of patients, say unemployed people, especially when the study deals with nursing measures that might be differently experienced by people of different social class.)

Again, some clinical wisdom will help interpret findings from convenience samples when there is a suspicion that there may be systematic differences between the sample drawn and other possible samples. For instance, one study drew a convenience sample of all cases of distal limb fracture seen in a certain emergency room during July and August of a given year in order to compare the effectiveness of nurses as triage officers for fractures with physicians (31). It happens that new interns and residents join a service in July every year, so it became important to understand what the background of the two groups being compared was. The nurses, it turned out, were all experienced, none having less than twenty-seven months of ER under their belts. While data on the physicians were not presented, it can be assumed that just because it was July and August, more relatively inexperienced physicians consituted the comparison group. Here, the findings from the study may be compromised entirely by having essentially noncomparable groups.

Convenience samples are often the total timebound population—all cases of a particular kind in a given time. But they are still *samples* of the total theoretical population of *all* patients at *all* times.

Another method of nonprobability sampling used sometimes in relation-searching studies (see Chapter 5) is called *purposive* sampling. This method is never used in hypothesis-testing studies but may be appropriate in a more exploratory study when one wants to be sure that the entire range of a phenomenon under investigation is covered in the sample, and that the sample is going to be small enough so that one cannot assume that by chance alone all possible limits of the variable range will just happen. For example, suppose one were studying the pain experience. One might want to make sure that patients with all kinds of pain and all degrees of severity were included. To draw a purposive sample, the researcher identifies actual *individuals* who have more or less of the thing under study, in this case, pain. One might then go around to various nursing units and ask for actual names of patients with, say, migraine, or intractable pain from cancer; or patients with chest surgery, and patients with skin biopsies—any way of defining likely cases with different kinds of pain will be all right. The difference in this kind of sampling method is that instead of simply setting a sampling frame and taking everyone (or every n-th person) who fits the sampling criteria, in purposive sampling, the sampling frame is set, then actual individuals are picked *because* their position on the variable of interest is known. The claim cannot be made that samples drawn purposively are representative of anything in particular in the usual sense of generalizing to a population. But that's not why this method is used. Rather it is used when one wants to get a sample of people who "represent" the variable in question so that the findings from the study may encompass as much of the variable or phenomenon as possible. Since this method is used only in descriptive relation-searching studies when the outcome of the study is hypotheses for further study, generalization to other populations is not the purpose anyhow.

Another version of nonprobability sample is *quota* sampling, used perhaps in large interview studies. In this case, the sampling strata are identified and each interviewer is given a quota of each to be obtained. For example, interviewers may be told to talk with ten whites, ten blacks, and five orientals, but it is left to the interviewer to choose which people he interviews. Being human, he is likely to choose those people most convenient to him. Quota sampling is nonprobability sampling since it is not known what the probability of any person getting into the sample is. Data from such sampling requires statistical modifications and conclusions based on quota sampling are necessarily tentative.

Finally, there is something that might be called *nominated sampling*. Here, once having set the sampling frame, the researcher asks others for names of people who might be included (32). For example, a nurse might be interested in studying multiproblem families in a community agency. She might ask the local visiting nurses to tell her the names of families in their case loads that met the definition she had set. This method has obvious consequences for the generality of the findings, since it cannot be known whether each visiting nurse provided the researcher with a complete list or not. But a nominated sample may be the only kind that can be gathered when there is no objective way of picking the sampling units from existing lists, and when surveying thousands of family charts is not possible.

Sample Size

No easier criticism of any study can be made than to accuse it of having too small a sample. Debate rages in some academic circles about how large a sample size must be to be "large enough" to trust the findings. The larger the sample (assuming it was selected in some approximation of random) the more representative it will be, since it takes in more of the total population. There is not a one-to-one correspondence between rigor of sampling method and representativeness; a sample of one, no matter how randomly chosen, is unlikely to be representative. Similarly, a very large but sloppily selected sample may also not be representative of the population. So sample size and sampling method go hand-in-hand.

Another consideration in sample size is how big the phenomenon is that is being investigated, or how large the potential population is. For example, some things simply do not occur that often, like cardiac tamponade, or failure to thrive in infants, or toxemia of pregnancy or stillbirth. So a smaller sample of infrequently occurring events (smaller than a sample of more frequently occurring events) may just do. On the other hand, pain occurs a very great deal in hospitalized patients, so a larger sample of patients in pain may be required to claim representativeness of the population.

There are formulas that have been worked out by statisticians that can be used to estimate the needed size of a sample. (33). These formulas make use of "error estimation"—the degree of error in a statistical sense, that will be tolerated by the study. For example, the degree of error may be set in advance as 5 percent, meaning one wants to have confidence that 95 percent of the time, one's findings will be "true," all other things being equal. Plugging this level of confidence into a formula will produce an estimate of the size of the sample needed (since all statistical tests take into account the size of the sample).

But such rigorous estimation is not the rule in clinical research where factors of cost and practicality may outweigh even the most zealous desire for rigor. The three factors that most count in determining sample size are the degree of error to be tolerated, cost and the homogeneity of the sample (34). If the sample can be made to be homogeneous with respect to everything but the variable being tested, then small samples will suffice. The more homogeneous the sample (for hypothesis-testing studies) the better. Here homogeneity refers to the sample units being as much alike as possible along the dimensions of the background or antecedent variables—age, sex, social class, diagnosis or whatever. The more random variation there is in all the variables, including the one being tested, the more "noise" in the system there is, and the harder it will be to detect variation attributable to the thing one is interested in studying because so many other things are going on. Therefore, the larger the sample will have to be before a pattern of variation can emerge.

For instance, suppose a nurse were studying relief from pain through nursing. If the sample frame were very large and patients with incisional pain, intractable pain, chronic pain, as well as other pain were included, and if at the same time adult patients of all ages, both sexes, all diagnostic categories were included, the sample would have to be extremely large since so many other things could effect the results. But if the sampling frame were made smaller and only, say, postoperative patients without a diagnosis of cancer were included, then a smaller sample would probably suffice.

Besides fancy statistical formulas, there are other ways to guess at what size a sample might have to be. Various statistical procedures have lower limits (or upper limits) of numbers below which the results are no longer reliable. Knowing what kind of statistical treatment of the data will be used may give some guidelines for the sample size.

No matter what the desired sample size is, the real sample size will be smaller. Frustrating though it may be, the reality of clinical research is that some sample members will have to be dropped because they turn out not to meet the sample criteria, or patients will be discharged home before the researcher can get there to interview them, or charts will be missing or lost, or people will die, or surgery will be cancelled or some physician will refuse to let the researcher see his patients. Therefore, it is always wise to set a desired sample size, and at the same time, the minimal size sample that one can live with and hope for more.

Selecting Instruments/Measurements

The first criterion for selecting tools or instruments to measure the variables of interest is how well the measurements fit with the problem and with the theories involved. Other considerations about reliability, validity, appropriateness, sensitivity and precision are dealt with in a later chapter (see Chapter 9).

All measurements come with their own conceptual background, whether it is stated or not. Psychological tests, for example, often have whole manuals available detailing the background of the instrument and its conceptual framework. Other measurements, especially of physiological data have less background spelled out, though it exists intuitively. What is important in selecting measures, as a stage in the research process, is that the measures match the theoretical background of the problem, and that they match the problem itself.

Earlier in this chapter, some of the difficulties in matching measures with theory in the problem were discussed. For instance, a measure of personality trait will not serve to measure personality state, if that's what the problem is about, no matter how interesting the measure or how much fun it is to complete the forms. A measure of the gate control theory of pain will probably not be a good one for a study which takes a different theoretical approach to pain. Physiological measures may or may not be good measures of pyschological state, since all the connections between psychology and physiology have yet to be ironed out.

Similarly, some things that are intended to measure patient states or experiences turn out to be measures of something else. For example, measures of patient satisfaction may instead be measures of how much the patient trusts the interviewer and, therefore, is willing to tell the interviewer about (35). Amount of pain medication taken may be a measure of staff attention to patients, rather than a measure of pain itself (36). An index of foods eaten by prenatal patients may or may not be a good index of effective nutrition counseling, depending on what resources the patient has to get the kind of food needed. Length of labor may be a measure of patient anxiety, or it may not be, depending on whether there is cephalopelvic disproportion and whether certain kinds of regional anesthesia have been used. Rehospitalization for mental patients may or may not be a measure of the effectiveness of discharge planning, depending on other things like a patient's social resources. And so on and on.

Measures of the effectiveness of nurses in the expanded role are particularly interesting examples of the problem of what is being measured. When the expanded role expands into the traditional provinces of medicine, it is tempting to use as measures of the effect of nurse practitioners traditional measures of the effect of medical practice such as morbidity, mortality, control of symptoms and so on. But such measures will not tap the "nursing" component of nurse practitioner work, and, thus, they will measure only a small part of the effectiveness dimension.

The exercise of systematically providing an operational definition of each concept in a research problem helps to prevent a peculiar kind of error in selecting measures. Sometimes a thing is selected to be measured that is not really a measure of the effect but is part of the treatment itself. For example, in a study of nursing interaction effect on pain, part of the "nursing treatment" was to explore with the patient her/his pain and to offer alternatives to medication to deal with it. In this case, amount of pain medication taken cannot be used as a measure of the effect of nursing; it's part of the nursing itself, and while the data may provide a check on the independent variable (to see if the nurse did what she said she was going to do—offer alternatives), it is not a measure of the goodness of the treatment itself.

Careful clinical analysis of the problem and the constant application of clinical wisdom to all aspects of the research process is essential, not only to prevent the kinds of problems listed here, but to assure that the study when completed will have meaning to other clinicians.

Data Collection

A research plan has to include a specific plan for collecting data that will include how the subjects or patients will be informed and give their consent, who will collect the data, exactly how and when and where, and how the data will be written down or otherwise recorded. Special forms must be developed to record the data to assure that the same data will be collected on all patients in the same way. Even in factor-searching studies, special forms for writing down the data are developed, though they may be less systematic and more informal than the kinds of forms needed for hypothesis-testing studies.

Considerations in obtaining informed consent are dealt with in Chapter 11. Besides informed consent, however, patients or subjects must be assured the right to privacy and anonymity, the right to know that information collected from them will never be personally identifiable and will never be reported by name. The immediate implication is that in designing forms to collect data, the patient's name should never appear on the forms themselves. A code number, initials, the hospital number or any other device may be used, and a master list of names with code numbers kept in another place. Only the researcher should have access to the master list, and unless a long-term follow-up is planned, once the data are collected, the master list should be destroyed.

The data collection procedure should specify how names of subjects or patients will be obtained, from what source. It should note who, exactly, will collect the data (researcher? staff nurse? record clerk? research assistant?), and if the person is other than the researcher personally, how such people will be trained. What guidelines will be given them to make sure they all do it the same way, if multiple data collectors are being used?

Exactly how data will be collected must be thought through, in exquisite detail. If pulse and blood pressure are to be taken, for example, will they always be taken with the patient in a sitting position? In the left arm? The right? For one minute (pulse) or half a minute? If interviews are to be done, who will do them? Will the interviewer tape record responses or write down answers? Verbatim? Reconstructed from memory later? If self-reports of patients—written responses or checklists—will be used, will they be filled out in the presence of a data collector so interpretations can be made? Or left to be mailed back later? If chart data are to be used, how much of it will be written down "raw" and how much will be collapsed initially? For instance, if elevations in body temperature will be recorded, will it be done by writing down every temperature reading, or by simply counting the number of readings out of the total that were above 98.6 F.?

The reason all of these considerations must be thought through in advance is primarily to assure consistency in collecting data. But in addition, the details of data collection will become part of a report of a study, reported so that readers may decide how much faith to put into the study findings and so that other readers may have enough information to repeat the study, if they wish.

Sometime early in designing a study, some thought also has to be given to how much data to collect, not on the variables of interest themselves, but on other things. Always, data are collected on the characteristics of the sample so that the sample can be described later. But some thought given to other kinds of data that might be collected just in case they might be valuable in explaining the findings later will prevent a whole lot of later headaches. In clinical research the data collection period is the only encounter the researcher is going to have with the people and the problem, and it can never be duplicated. Therefore, it is wise to think in advance about the possible kinds of things that it might be well to keep track of for later reference. Among the things that might turn out to be relevant are such things as the physician's name, length of time in the hospital before surgery, patient occupation, unit of the hospital where the patient had a room, date, day of the week, time of day data collection happened, patient's race-nativity, family members available and untoward events that happened during data collection like a heat wave, an assassination, a holiday. Even when a retrospective chart review is the method of data collection, it is wise to make sure that as much data as can be justified are collected from the chart the first time around, because repeated trips to the record room are time-consuming and frustrating.

Major methods of data collection are covered in Chapter 10.

Data Processing/Analysis

How the data are to be handled once they are collected is also something to be spelled out in advance because how the data are to be analyzed may determine how they are to be collected. For example, some kinds of statistical procedures require raw data, so provision has to be made to collect them, even if they end up being collapsed later. If computer-assisted data analysis is to be used, a thorough run-through with a consultant who knows the actual computer system to be used and the programs will prevent many headaches later. For instance, some computer programs will not read zeros, but will read blanks, or vice versa, and such a tiny thing may turn out to be a very large problem if not anticipated. Some statistical tests in computer packages require equal numbers in all groups of data (equal numbers of experimental and control patients, for example) and that must be built into the design.

The fewer forms and pieces of paper the researcher has to handle, the less the chances of error in copying material, so it is wise to design data collection forms so that data can be immediately copied to machine read cards or format sheets without going through an intermediate step of coding or processing.

Qualitative data (narrative summaries, verbatim responses to interview questions and the like) may also be prepared initially for the kind of analysis that will later transpire. Sometimes carbon copies of interviews are a good idea if verbatim responses are going to be judged later—the carbon can then be cut apart without having to be recopied. Any device to make handling the data easier once they are collected should be invented in the beginning. Color coding of different parts of a questionnaire, special envelopes for putting EKG strips in, file folders for each set of data from each respondent, special papers or notebooks to keep data together—anything that will help make order out of the volume of data that will pour in will increase the researcher's mental health later.

Technical aspects of statistical analysis of data are beyond the scope of this book.

Insofar as possible, data analysis should be thought through in advance, and even dummy tables, or dummy data analysis forms, should be invented. Especially important in hypothesis-testing studies, and especially when there is more than one hypothesis, is to make a dummy table for each hypothesis, showing data to be entered in the table, and the table headings. Doing all of this in advance helps make sure that the logic of the study is consistent and that the researcher knows how to manage data once they are in.

Interpretation and Implementation

The final stages in the research process are to interpret—give meaning to—the data collected, and then to propose and hopefully take the next step to implement the improvements in practice suggested by the findings.

Interpreting the findings means referring back from the data collected to the theory and the research problem. Reporting research is not just a matter of giving the numbers and frequencies and statistical tests; rather, the empirical data are given meaning by reference back to what the ideas were that began the study. In this phase of the process, clinical judgment is as important as in any other phase, for some findings will be interesting only mathematically, and some will not be statistically valid but suggestive of important ideas. The state of the art of clinical research being what it is, some of the more interesting findings may be negative ones: a theory doesn't fit, a measure doesn't work, a treatment produces the opposite results from what is expected and so on. Because real-world research in real situations is never as well controlled and "pure" as laboratory research, interpretation of findings calls on the researcher's creativity and clinical sense.

In general, interpretation of findings can be separated into three relatively separate processes: discussion of findings, limitations and implications. Implementation may come later as a result of the mental work in the implications section.

In discussion of findings, the researcher deals first and most directly with the research questions or hypotheses as stated. The first job is to tell the reader what it is that was found, what the answers to the research questions were, or what the results of the hypothesis tests were. Then, one searches for qualifications, subtleties, nuances by paying attention to the background data on the sample, or perhaps other information that helps explain why the findings turned out the way they did. If the hypotheses are not supported, why not? Or if they are, are they still supported when the sample is broken down in different ways? For example, if the major finding for the hypothesis is that children recover better from surgery with a certain kind of nursing care preoperatively, does this finding also hold for children in different age groups? For children with different kinds of surgery? For children whose mothers roomed in or those who did not?

Relation-searching studies often end with answers to the research questions in the form of hypotheses for further testing. But if the researcher can offer some hints about how the study should be designed to test the hypotheses (what kind of sample might be chosen, or how data might be collected, or what measurements might be thought about) then they should be offered, after a thorough discussion of what the initial findings from the study are.

Limitations of the study should be stated as pointedly as the researcher's ego allows. Every study has its limitations and some are more serious than others. Sample size is an almost universal limitation in clinical research, but a small sample does not mean a study has no relevance at all. Reliability and validity of measures should be addressed head on, and any other aspects of the study that the researcher thinks might be improved next time around, or that should qualify the interpretation of data from the present study should be stated. But the researcher should also provide the best possible commonsense judgment of how important the limitations are, whether they really invalidate the study, or whether they are unavoidable complications that come from studying real-life problems. Stating limitations gives other researchers a standard against which to judge the study, as well as perhaps letting the next researcher avoid some pitfalls that are inevitable in the early studies in a building sequence.

Finally, the researcher should tease out of the discussion and the data implications for future research, for nursing practice, for nursing education or administration—whatever the source should be. The researcher is in the best position to begin to list implications because she/he is the one closest to the data and the one most invested in them.

In a practice profession, the researchers have an obligation that goes beyond simply reporting results and hinting at possible implications. Research in nursing practice has to be carried to the point of putting in place changes in that practice before it is completely done. The first step in implementation may simply be making the information gathered in a given study available to others through formal reporting or publication. When a research problem comes out of a clinical situation inspired by people who work there, there is a formal obligation to report back the results of the research, even when the results may not have solved the problem.

The improvement of practice will be advanced much faster when researchers and practitioners are the same people, or at the very least when they have constant communication, not just one-shot chats when a project is done in a clinical setting. Implementation is often a matter of organizational change, and that change cannot happen from outside, from the remote researcher dictating to uninvolved clinical people. When the research deals with real practice problems in a real situation, the process is speeded along somewhat, but until research and practice get much closer together than they are now, implementation will still be *ad hoc* and dependent on individual institutional commitment.

There is another way to think about implementation, however, addressed in some detail in Chapter 8.

THE RESEARCH PROPOSAL

The prospectus or research proposal is a plan for carrying out the study, and it includes all but the final stages of the research process outlined here (37). The outline used for a research proposal varies according to individual or institutional taste, but all the items must be covered: statement of problem, theoretical background, research questions or hypotheses, setting, sample, data collection, processing and analysis, limitations and procedures for protecting the rights of human subjects. The statement of problem and theoretical background will then become the first sections of the final research report, and if all details of the methods are spelled out in advance and followed, they can be lifted with just changes in verb tense to the final report.

Proposals are written not only to help the investigator carry out the study, but also are often submitted to research committees in the setting for approval, funding or advice. A thorough proposal allows the investigator to plan for and anticipate data collection procedures, analysis techniques, sampling problems and so on. Therefore, the proposal should contain enough explicit information so that those reading or judging it can determine how adequate the research plan is.

The proposal should contain first a statement of the problem that prompts the research. This statement is a condensation of the analysis of the problem and should include how the investigator came to believe this is a problem and how she/he sees the problem developing into a research project. The background section should also include an indication of previous work done in the area and why that work is not considered sufficient to have resolved the problem. The study design, sample, setting, measurements, data collection procedures and expected data analysis techniques should be covered in appropriate detail. All measurement tools, and data collection instruments should be determined in advance, and if possible, pretested.

A proposal usually includes a time schedule for the study so that the investigator can plan his time conveniently. If the study tests an hypothesis, there should be an indication of what will be taken as evidence that the hypothesis is supported and what it will mean if the hypothesis is supported or rejected. The briefer the proposal, the better, as long as all important material is covered.

The research proposal is considered to be a guideline for research. There will always be changes in the plan as the research is conducted and things not known before become obvious. It is important to look carefully at departures from the proposed attack on the problem and justify, at least to oneself, why they are necessary. And always, one must report deviations from the initial plan in the final report.

Sometimes one will find that the sampling criteria are too exclusive and that they are eliminating people who might well be included. It is legitimate to open up sampling criteria in a case like this as long as the basic principle of sampling is adhered to, and as long as the deviations do not make an entirely different sample result. Most often sampling criteria are opened up by increasing the age limits on the sample, or perhaps by including other diagnostic categories, in other words, simply extending the criteria already established.

Sometimes it will be discovered that certain measurements, especially interviews or questionnaires simply have some holes in them—questions that are not understood by respondents or redundancies. It is also legitimate in these situations to drop the offending question realizing that no data collected prior to dropping—on that particular question—can be used.

Sometimes a small variation in procedure has to be put into place because of an unanticipated clinical requirement. Some adjustment in measurement or data collection procedure is fine so long as the reliability of it is not compromised, and so that the data produced will still be useful.

Long-range studies involving a series of projects may proceed with only the initial study completely outlined, and the later studies to be built upon the first. When the first study is completed, however, subsequent studies have to have their own research proposal written.

The more the details of the study, including the anticipated results are thought and written out in advance, the easier will be the final phase of research—analyzing and interpreting the findings. The final phases are often the most fun because it is then that the researcher can let loose creative thoughts about what the data mean, and what implications can be drawn from the data. It is simply a kindness to oneself as a researcher, therefore, to provide the time and mental energy by taking care of as many details of the project in advance as possible, so that the later time can be as profitable as the subject demands.

Regardless of the level of inquiry or type of study, all of the aspects of the research process will have to be covered in a proposal, and all activities will be carried out as part of the design. The next five chapters (and part of a sixth) deal with how research is done for different kinds of problems, at different levels of inquiry, to produce different kinds of theory. The elements in the research process identified here are used as the outline for the chapters to follow.

NOTES

1. In their "8-4 research," Dickoff, James and Semradek suggest a different way of thinking about naming the parts of the research process that places emphasis on the place of the problem not only in instituting the research, but as an outcome of the particular research, and more important, as the "issue" (here, the situation of which the problem is an instance). See Dickoff, James, Patricia James and Joyce Semradek, 8-4 research: designing nursing research—eight points of encounter (Part II). *Nursing Research,* 24:164–176, May–June 1975, especially pp. 164–165.

2. Batey, Marjorie V.: Conceptualization: knowledge and logic guiding empirical research. *Nursing Research,* 26:324–329, September–October 1977. See also, Batey, Marjorie V.: Conceptualizing the research process. *Nursing Research,* 20:296–301, July–August 1971.

3. Ruggiero, Leona: Rape: the person, the event, the social field. Unpublished master's thesis, Yale University School of Nursing, 1977. Dixon, Beverly F.: A study of the use of root doctors as an alternative form of care. Unpublished master's thesis, Yale University School of Nursing, 1978.

4. Janis, Irving: Stages in the decision-making process. In Abelson, Robert P., et al. (eds.): *Theories of Cognitive Consistency: A Sourcebook.* Chicago: Rand-McNally, 1968, pp. 577-588. Janis, Irving and R. Mann: *Decision Making.* New York: Free Press, 1977.

5. Ellis, Rosemary: Fallibilities, fragments and frames: contemplation on 25 years of research in medical-surgical nursing. *Nursing Research,* 26:177–182, May–June 1977. See also, Wolfer, John A.: Definition and assessment of surgical patients' welfare and recovery. *Nursing Research,* 22:394–401, September–October 1973.

6. Taylor, Susan: How to search the literature. *American Journal of Nursing,* 74:1457–1459, August 1974.

7. Dempsey, Patricia: In "Letter to the Editor." *Nursing Research,* 26:390, September–October 1977.

8. Henderson, Virginia: *Nursing Studies Index* (for literature up to 1959), Vol. I–IV, Philadelphia: J.B. Lippincott Company, 1964–1972.

9. A useful list of reference sources in nursing is contained in Reference sources in nursing, *Nursing Outlook,* 20:338–343, May 1978. Many professional associations publish collections of abstracts annually, for example *Psychological Abstracts* (Washington D.C.: American Psychological Association). There are hundreds of compilations of research in various topic areas, usually catalogued as "recent research in . . ." or "summary of findings about . . ." The Department of Health, Education and Welfare lists numerous summary publications of recent research usually available from the particular Bureau (for example, Office of Maternal and Child Health of the Bureau of Community Health Services; Bureau of Health Manpower). DHEW summaries include completed research funded by the federal system and not necessarily published yet.

10. Collections of studies are published by the American Nurses Association in the annual series of nursing research conferences (Kansas City: A.N.A., series 1–12, 1965–1977) and by the Western Interstate Council for Higher Education in Nursing (WICHEN) as reports of their series, "Communicating Nursing Research", edited by Marjorie V. Batey (Boulder, Colorado: WICHEN, series 1–10, 1969–1978). The Division of Nursing, USPHS (Bureau of Health Resources Administration) publishes annually a list of current research supported by the Division, and back copies of previous years are available. (Research Grants Branch, Division of Nursing, DHEW, East-West Highway, Hyattsville, Maryland). Abstracts of master's thesis are often available from graduate programs with thesis requirements and several schools have collected their abstracts from previous years (the University of North Carolina, for example). Abstracts and lists of thesis titles are usually available by writing the librarian or dean of the school of nursing. Abstracts of Yale University School of Nursing master's theses are available by writing Mrs. Heide Miller, Librarian, 855 Howard Avenue, New Haven, Connecticut 06520, for a small fee.

11. Jacox, Ada: Theory construction in nursing—an overview. *Nursing Research,* 23:4–13, January–February 1974.

12. Wilson, Holly Skodol: Limiting intrusion—social control of outsiders in a healing community—an illustration of qualitative comparison analysis. *Nursing Research,* 26:103–111, March–April 1977.

13. Glaser, Barney and Anselm Strauss: *Awareness of Dying.* Chicago: Aldine, 1965.

14. Batey, *Conceptualization,* p. 329, see Note 2.

15. Dumas, Rhetaugh G. and Barbara Johnson: Research in nursing practice: a review of five clinical experiments. *International Journal of Nursing Studies,* 9:137–148, August 1972.

16. Johnson, Barbara, et al.: Research in nursing practice: the problem of uncontrolled situational variables. *Nursing Research,* 19:337–342, July–August 1970.

17. Hollingshead, August and Fredric Redlich: *Social Class and Mental Illness.* New York: John Wiley & Sons, 1958.

18. In Hollingshead and Redlich's early work, residence was also a variable. But it was too cumbersome and it correlated well with education and occupation. "Residence" meant that the city was analyzed to determine the "social class" of the area (block, census tract) using quality of housing, size of lot, single-dwelling units and so on. Every investigator who used this scale would have to analyze his own city.

19. Census Use Study: *Health Information Systems II,* Report # 12, Washington, D.C.: Bureau of the Census, 1971.

20. Diers, Donna, et al.: The effect of nursing interaction on patients in pain. *Nursing Research,* 21:419–428, September–October 1972.

21. Diers, Donna and Ruth L. Schmidt. Interaction analysis in nursing research. In Verhonick, Phyllis J. (ed.): *Nursing Research,* Boston: Little, Brown, 1977, pp. 77–132.

22. *Ibid.*

23. Orlando, Ida Jean: *The Dynamic Nurse Patient Relationship.* New York: G.P. Putnam's Sons, 1961.

24. Wolfer, see Note 5.

25. For what can happen when the setting is not respected, see Bermosk, Loretta and Raymond Corsini: *Critical Incidents in Nursing,* Philadelphia: W.B. Saunders, 1973, pp. 86–93. See also McBride, M. Angela, et al.: Nurse-researcher: the crucial hyphen. *American Journal of Nursing,* 70:1256–1260, June 1970; see also Hodgman, Eileen Callahan: Student research in service agencies. *Nursing Outlook.* 26:558–565, September, 1978.

26. The "Hawthorne effect" gets its name from experiments in industrial engineering conducted at the Western Electric plan near Chicago. Among the experiments was one testing the effect of different amounts of light on work productivity. The researchers found that no matter how little light was provided, productivity increased, apparently because the researchers were paying attention to the workers. See Simon, Julian L.: *Basic Research Methods in Social Sciences,* New York: Random House, 1969, pp. 97–98.

27. Harding, Roberta, Ned Tranel and Donna Diers: Unpublished paper.

28. The reporting requirement was spelled out nicely by a group of students of the class of 1968, at the Yale University School of Nursing. It is excerpted below:

The Discrepancy

Ideally, there should exist an ongoing, continuous, circular relationship (dialogue) between and among research, practice and theory:

1. The content and process of nursing research is derived from the problems *in* nursing practice and *with* theory.
2. The process and content of nursing practice and nursing research jointly contribute to theory—process and content.

In reality, there are breaks in the system. People are not talking to each other. As a result:

1. Nursing practice is deprived of input from research and theory development.
2. Nursing research is deprived of input from nursing practice and the validation phase of theory development.
3. Nursing theory is deprived of the benefits of joint contributions of nursing research and nursing practice.

And, the full potential force of practice-research-theory is not brought to bear on the process of improving practice.

Removing the Discrepancy

Although there are several possible approaches to removing the discrepancy, we are commited to begin communicating the process and content of nursing research to practitioners and other researchers. Approaching the problem by communing with the real world of practitioners, researchers, and students outside YSN fits the philosophy guiding selection of research problems, development of study designs/measurement tools, and conduct of the study/writing of the report (i.e., doing something that is intended to remove a discrepancy in the real world of nursing).

To facilitate the removal of the discrepancy, a committee was established. The committee formulated the following objectives for communicating nursing research:

TO PROMOTE THE COMMUNICATION OF NURSING RESEARCH

1. By facilitating an ongoing dialogue between and among nurse researchers and practitioners in all areas of nursing.

2. By assisting master's students to develop the skills needed to participate in and further the development of this dialogue.

It should be the student's responsibility, with appropriate consultation with her advisors, to identify the appropriate audience for her communication and to plan and arrange for a presentation.

Class of 1968	Elizabeth Chaney
	Andrea Joubert
	Mary Jane Kennedy
	Elaine McEwan
	Beth Strutzel

29. Dumas, Rhetaugh G. and Robert C. Leonard: The effect of nursing on the incidence of postoperative vomiting: a clinical experiment. *Nursing Research*, 12:12–15, Winter 1963.

30. In teaching hospitals, sampling can sometimes become very complicated, and the nurse's knowledge of the system critically important. For example, suppose the nurse knows that her institution is a regional center for high-risk pregnancy care. A random sample of charts of maternity patients will include a much larger number of patients with obstetrical complications than normally the case, with potential consequences for the generality of the findings. Or suppose the researcher knows of certain medical research projects going on, say in dermatology where some physicians are studying psoriasis and vitiligo. A sample of dermatology clinic charts will overrepresent this group.

The point here is only to alert the researcher to trust one's own information and knowledge of the system itself, in choosing a sample and in many other aspects of the research process.

31. Bliss, Ann, et al.: Emergency room nurse orders x-rays of distal limbs in orthopedic trauma: *Nursing Research*, 20:440–443, September–October 1971.

32. Daniel, Wayne W. and Beaufort Longest, Jr.: Statistical sampling and the nurse researcher. *Nursing Forum*, 16, (1):37–55, 1977. For an excellent discussion of sampling, see Slonim, M.J.: *Sampling*. New York: Simon & Schuster, 1960.

33. A very nice, brief treatment of the issue of sample size is Brown, Roscoe: Optimum sample size (research question and answer). *Nursing Research*, 25:62, January–February 1976.

34. Ibid.

35. Nehring, Virginia and Barbara Geach: Patients' evaluation of their care: why they don't complain. *Nursing Outlook*, 21:317–321, May 1963.

36. Johnson, see Note 16. The investigators discovered, for example, that black patients received demonstrably less pain medication than whites, which may be cultural, or an effect of racism.

37. For an excellent description of what should be contained in a research proposal to the federal government for funding, see Gortner, Susan: Research grant applications—what they are and should be. *Nursing Research*, 20:292–295, July–August 1971.

Granting agencies within the federal system provide outlines for writing research grant applications. Outlines (and entire application kits) may be obtained from the university grant and contract offices, or from specific research grants branch of the federal system to which the application will be sent. The outline for preparing the proposal is standard across all granting agencies, and includes as major headings:

Introduction and specific aims

Methods of procedure

Significance of this research

Facilities available

Collaborative arrangements

as well as sections on the investigator's own previous research background, previous research in the field, budget and other administrative forms.

4

Factor-Searching Studies

This chapter begins the discussion of study designs for problems at different levels of inquiry. Problems take different forms and require different kinds of knowledge to solve them, and thus different kinds of approaches to the problem—study designs—are called for.

Factor-searching studies are called for when the problem is to describe, or name the parts of, a given situation or event. Thus, the kind of theory produced in a factor-searching study is naming theory either in the form of narrative description, formal concepts with properties and formal definitions, or categories—a concept divided into its components, which are arranged in some kind of order and are all related to one underlying dimension.

"Factor" as used here pertains to an abstraction, not a fact, which is an empirical observation available to the five senses. The word is used in nonresearch contexts as well, with the same meaning: for example, What factors contributed to President Nixon's resignation? means more than just what the available facts were. It means what dimensions, or themes, or ways of thinking about events can be stated to characterize a great many complicated facts, opinions, suppositions and relationships. Similarly, in algebra, one "factors" (a verb) an equation, meaning one divides a whole into its parts, each one of which is a "factor." This second use gives the other shade of meaning to the word: the division of a whole into components.

Factor-searching studies literally look for ways to categorize, classify or conceptualize situations. They are used when the researcher wants to take a new look at an old situation, or when there is no useable information about a particular phenomenon available. Factor-searching studies are also called descriptive (1), exploratory (2) and formulative (3). The so-called case study of modern psychiatry and psychiatric nursing may qualify as factor-searching, if the investigator goes beyond mere reporting of the chronology of the therapy. The whole point of factor-searching is to devise or invent labels that taken together will usefully characterize the important aspects of a given

100

situation and the simple report of a single case without the requisite abstraction (intellectual work on the data) doesn't qualify.

Historical studies (narrative descriptions of events) may be factor-searching studies, and much of what is called ethnoscience is at this level of inquiry as well (4). In both these cases, the aim is description rather than hypothesis-testing, and often the data are put in the form of categories, or themes, after they are collected.

Some classical studies in sociology are wonderful examples of the kind of narrative descriptive study called here factor-searching. Whyte's *Street Corner Society,* for example, provides rich description and conceptualization of the social order in a street gang (5). A good deal of anthropological investigation might be classified as factor-searching—for example, Malinowski's classic study of the Trobriand islanders (6). Oleson and Whittacker's study of student nurses (7) or Schmahl's study of institutional change in a school of nursing are examples of factor-searching, descriptive, narrative studies (8). Mellow's thoughtful contribution to the understanding of psychiatric illness and nursing therapy is factor-searching (9).

In all these examples, the effort was to take a situation or event, and describe it through participant observation, or sometimes more formal data collection (questionnaires, interviews) so as to understand the situation better in conceptual terms. The concepts as they were invented are woven into the description, not separated out and formally provided with definitions of properties.

On the other hand, Glaser and Strauss have codified factor-searching as a method by bringing a different perspective on descriptive studies to the study of dying in hospitals (10). In their method—discovery of "grounded theory"—the steps in the research process are more formal and formalized, and the intent is to develop *concepts* (as opposed to narrative description) which are abstractions grounded in the data, but set off with specific definitions. The concepts can then be discussed by themselves so that their full meaning is understood by the reader. The Glaser and Strauss method intends to *conceptualize* a given event or situation, as opposed to *describing* it.

Finally, there are factor-searching studies intended from the beginning to produce sets of categories which, taken together, describe the entire situation. Naturally, these studies deal with rather smaller bits of reality than do the kinds of studies described above, since the event or situation to be described has to be small enough that one set of categories will encompass all of it (or at least that the categories will mutually exhaust the possible ways of describing the situation). Such categories, and the process of arriving at them, are also called taxonomy—naming—and there are thousands of examples. The periodic table of chemical elements is taxonomy, where the elements are arranged according to the structure of the atoms that make them up. Disease classification schemes are taxonomies (11). Classification of patients by amount of nursing care required, from self-care to total nursing care is a taxonomy. And the current nursing diagnosis project is a fine example of the work involved in inventing taxonomy, classifying and defining concepts (12). In the late 1960s a good deal of attention in nursing research went to the study of the nurse-patient relationship, particularly the verbal interaction of nurses and patients, and many ways of classifying what nurses and patients say to each other were invented (13). These too are taxonomies.

It is possible to devise categories without ever doing a study. The process is simply providing operational definitions for the concepts of interest, without reference to data. Factor-searching studies designed to produce categories out of the data are a different animal.

Factor-searching studies can be done also when the problem is to figure out why something works. For example, when early reports of experiments on the effects of nursing on patients began to be published in the early 1960s, there was a natural need to look more closely at the nursing care given to try to develop more precise ways of describing it, so that it could be taught and learned by others.

And, factor-searching studies may be done when the problem is essentially lack of a measurement for something. For example, when quality assurance became a factor in hospital accreditation and professional practice, there had to be invented ways to measure the quality of nursing. Here the research problem is What *is* this?—quality care?

Notice that all these examples are tied together by all being at the same level of inquiry, and all being What *is* this? problems. In factor-searching studies, there is no attempt to test the theory or concepts in the usual sense of experimental verification. Factor-searching studies may sometimes be the first step toward a measurement study, and the categories developed may later be tested for validity and reliability (see Chapter 9). But the purpose of a factor-searching study is simply (though it is not simple) to give names to aspects of a situation or event where there were no names before.

Factor-searching studies are the most basic that can be done. But one can move to a higher level of inquiry without first doing a formal factor-searching study to identify the dimensions of the situation. Conversely, just because a particular area has been investigated before, a "basic" study may still be warranted. There is hardly any area of science, including nursing, that couldn't profit from reconsideration of the nature of the variables involved, but at the same time if factors can be identified from other sources, a factor-searching study is a luxury.

The "method" for doing factor-searching studies is, in simplest terms, the psychological thinking process that is such a normal part of life that it is taken for granted put into systematic form (14). That process is discrimination, definition and classification and is done constantly, and often called "inference." One sees a woman patient in psychotherapy moving her wedding ring around her finger rapidly, and one doesn't think woman-patient-moving-ring-rapidly, one thinks anxiety, or hostility or something. That instant process of moving from the data to the concept is the essence of factor-searching as a process. The methods for factor-searching study simply bring that process, in all its steps, into the open so that others can make judgments about the validity of the concepts arrived at by knowing how they were arrived at.

Despite what looks like formlessness in a report of a factor-searching study, these kinds of studies have all the usual aspects of the research process, from a statement of the problem through data analysis and interpretation.

RESEARCH PROBLEMS

Problems for factor-searching studies are What *is* this? problems. Like problems for other kinds of studies, they can arise out of nursing practice, or out of the experiences of others recorded in the literature. Often, these kinds of research problems arise because no one has ever looked into a given area in depth before. At the time Glaser and Strauss began their monumental study of death and dying, no one had really looked at what it is to die in hospitals. Hodgman's study of nursing in a community action agency came about because, so far as was known, no nurse had ever entered this kind of nontraditional setting before nor described what it is to be there doing unorthodox nursing functions (15). As nurses have moved into the expanded role, it has become crucial to understand what that is like. Early studies in psychiatric nursing attempted to describe a kind of work now known as "nursing therapy (16)." Kay's study of disease concepts in the barrio came out of the health professional's need to understand better something about the patients or clients of her services (17). Wilson's study in a nontraditional healing community grew out of a conceptual model in sociology, but was aimed at understanding what it is for a radical institution to exist in a conservative community (18).

The kind of study design chosen must fit the way the problem is characterized. Most nursing problems could be usefully investigated at any level of inquiry, so the researcher has to justify why a particular kind of approach to the problem has been selected. In the case of studies of situations in which there have been no previous investigations, the rationale for a factor-searching study will be easy. (It would be harder, but possible, to justify a study at a higher level of inquiry.) In the case of a problem in an area where considerable information already exists, it should be explicit why the information doesn't fit, or is incomplete, or why the area deserves a new look. Very often such justification can simply be that a *nurse* has never looked at the area before, and the nursing perspective and philosophy may bring to the study a richness not available in existing studies by investigators more remote from the clinical impact.

The statement of the problem for a factor-searching study may simply be an explicit statement that the topic or area chosen is a significant one for nursing to investigate. The case for significance will be made by indicating how clinical judgment or patient care might be improved if the topic were studied and new information were forthcoming. Sometimes, when the topic had literally never been addressed before, it is not even possible to tell what this problem is an instance of, since the topic isn't even conceptualized to that degree yet. Perhaps the topic is something that is an instance of things nurses encounter in practice—not a very illuminating conceptual way of thinking about it.

Thus, the statement of the problem which begins a factor-searching study is delimiting a clinical topic, a focus, for the study to come. How specifically the topic is stated will depend on how the researcher came to notice it as a problem, but something more than just, I guess I'll study the nurse patient relationship is necessary. The statement of the problem and definition of the focus of the study have to be broad enough to allow the dimensions of the area to be discovered, but narrow enough to allow the researcher to decide how to collect data, how to find instances of the thing she/he is interested in.

These kinds of exploratory, descriptive studies may also begin with a kind of preset in assumptions which, if possible, should be stated out loud, early on. For example, it was a matter of some shock to Glaser and Strauss to discover not only that dying in hospitals had not been studied much, but that there was massive denial on the part of institutions that it even happened. Thus, they entered the study of death and dying already with some notion that dying was a taboo topic (19).

Similarly, Riley analyzes Whyte's *Street Corner Society* as having come from Whyte's desire to disprove the convenient generalization that there was no social order in economically deprived areas and that social disorganization prevailed (20). Hodgman embarked on her study of nursing in a community action agency out of concern that nursing was not reaching out enough into the community to find and deal with problems in their natural environment.

Since the most formal development of the method of descriptive study grew out of work in sociology (Glaser and Strauss), the available studies often have a more or less explicit sociological framework for the problem, with concepts like social control, tolerance for deviance, social organization and the like guiding even the way the problem is stated (21). There is no reason for thinking that only problems conceived of as sociological are suitable for this kind of descriptive research, however, but so few descriptive studies which have used explicitly the grounded theory methodology have been published that it is still too early to be entirely clear about what kinds of topics make for an effective use of the method (22).

Analysis of the clinical problem to make it into a research problem (see Chapter 1) usually reveals very early on that a factor-searching study is necessary. When the variables involved in the problem cannot be named, or when it is not possible to say what the problem is an instance of, then this kind of descriptive study may be called for.

BACKGROUND/CONCEPTUAL FRAMEWORK

Even though factor-searching studies grow out of the need to devise ways to characterize a given situation, they don't begin with a completely blank slate. The conceptual background may be more like a "perspective" on the problem than like the more deliberate analysis and synthesis of previous findings that characterizes studies at higher levels of inquiry.

For example, a sociological perspective automatically makes certain ways of viewing the situation predominate, as opposed to a psychological perspective. In the example of the nurse in the community action agency studied by Hodgman, it would have been possible to have taken any number of perspectives. The researcher could have viewed the situation sociologically and perhaps focused on role exchanges, intergroup relations or the relationship of the agency to other agencies. Or she could have taken a more psychological perspective and pursued the nurse's thoughts and feelings as a white middle-class professional entering a predominantly black, lower-class, lay organization. Instead, she took an eclectic approach and asked, "What happens when a nurse involves herself in a community action agency?" implying no particular point of view, and no preset categorization scheme.

Similarly, Mellow's original work with nursing therapy with psychiatric patients could have taken any number of more or less traditional conceptual approaches from theories in psychoanalysis about etiology of illness through learning theories, through role theories about the nature of nursing's work in psychiatry. Instead, she took an open, conceptual perspective and committed herself to collection of experiential data—on herself as therapist, on her observations of patient work.

Whatever the perspective or point of view taken, it should be spelled out as clearly as possible, and as explicitly as possible. This kind of study and this methodology is so new to nursing research, however, that this condition is rarely met and a great deal is left to the reader's imagination. Because nursing's point of view or perspective is so much broader than any one other conceptual field, nurses using this methodology have to make choices of perspectives that sociologists or others need not make, and have to make more explicit why any particular one is chosen.

To the extent possible, important assumptions that are behind the selection of the problem area should also be made explicit. In Wilson's study of Soteria House, a nontraditional psychiatric setting, an important assumption was that "preservation of autonomy is fundamental for the maintainance of conditions of structural and ideological freedom." (23) Here, this means that for a nontraditional setting to continue to exist, it has to be relatively free of external constraints and interference. This turns out to be a crucial assumption for her study which then deals with Soteria's attempts to keep the larger world at bay, or at least keep its peace with the surrounding professional and lay community.

In Hodgman's study, an important assumption might be that it is a professional obligation of nursing to find the needs of people, not just wait for people to come to traditional settings with their needs already identified. This assumption also became important to her study, which then focused on whether the nurse in a community action agency really did find needs; in other words, was there a role for a nurse in such a setting?

In the absence of a theoretical framework in the usual sense, the conceptual background for a factor-searching study may instead state general principles or even philosophies which provide a picture of the situation within which the problem is seen as a problem. As in studies at higher levels of inquiry, the purpose of even providing an explicit conceptual framework or background is so that the place of the problem at hand in the larger scheme of things is known, and so that, to the extent possible, the researcher's own theoretical or abstract way of conceiving of the problem is made available to others.

Factor-searching studies which are aimed at producing categories—divisions of a larger concept, such as quality of care, or nurse patient interaction—may have more traditional-looking background sections or conceptual frameworks. Here, since the major concept is already known (for example, quality of care), it is possible to provide some theoretical background for it, in contrast to studies in which the intent is to discover the concepts themselves. The literature may be surveyed, and there may even already exist ways of categorizing information pertinent to a given concept. Or it may be that the literature will be surveyed to analyze the various meanings that might be applied to the concept (not as categories, but as definitions). For example, in early phases of our study of nurse-patient interaction, it became clear that nurse patient interaction had several different meanings, ranging from nurses' attitudes toward the patient, through nonverbal behavior, through relationship, to verbal behavior (24). There were also by then several category systems already available, and each had to be analyzed to decide why it would not work for the purpose. Some were based in theories that did not apply to the clinical situation; some were too difficult to use and, therefore, unreliable; some were too oversimplified for use under a fairly complicated conception of interaction.

The background/conceptual framework part of the research process has the same purpose in factor-searching studies as in any other kind: to give an overview of what is known (in other theories, philosophies, previous research, or idiosyncratic assumptions) about the problem area. As in other studies, the conceptual framework will guide all other aspects of the research process. As far as possible, even when there has been no previous work on the topic, conscious mental work to give the background or rationale for the study must be done. If a certain perspective on the problem is taken, it should be made as clear as possible, and if certain important assumptions are made, they ought to be stated. It is difficult to make assumptions explicit, or make a perspective clear when it may be so intuitively logical to the researcher that she/he can't imagine it isn't obvious to others. One useful tactic is to state out loud the overall research question or topic area, then to ask oneself questions about it. For example, I guess I'll go study the dying patient situation, could be made clearer by some pointed questions to oneself: What do you mean—"situation?" Why do you call it that? What's a "situation?" What's a dying patient? All these questions could lead to rather more explicit sentences containing assumptions or sociological perspectives or whatever.

STUDY DESIGN

Factor-searching studies are at the first level of inquiry (factor-isolating theory). They begin with research questions rather than hypotheses but the questions are very general, and instead of naming variables or relationships, they may just name areas for inquiry (25).

In the community action agency study, for instance, the research question might have been, What happens when a nurse involves herself in a community action agency? with subsidiary questions like, What happens to the nurse? (What does she experience, think, feel?) What happens by the nurse? (What does she do?) What happens between the nurse and clients? and so on. These questions suggest sources of data but imply neither formal measurement nor predetermined variables. Similarly, in the dying patient study, subquestions might have been, What does the patient experience (think, feel)? What goes on around the patient, who participates, and what is said, done, thought, felt?

The way the research questions are posed implicitly directs the selection of a setting and sources of data. For example, since patients are dying in hospitals everywhere, almost any hospital would do as a setting. If the investigators wanted to look only at situations in which the patients' deaths were the predicted outcome for their hospitalization, as in the case of hospitals for the terminally ill, they would have to choose different settings. Most often the study begins in a convenient setting but may move to other places as the emergence of concepts of categories dictates. Similarly, if the intent is to look at the total experience of patients in this situation, one already knows that others will participate and the significant sources of data would include not only the patient, but his family and the hospital staff, as well as the observations of the investigators themselves.

It may be worthwhile repeating that while factor-searching studies are *the* most basic kind of study that can be done, they must proceed more formally than just starting with a vague idea about investigating some exciting new area and jumping in. Indeed, one of the points of considering factor-searching as systematic study—research—and, therefore, factor-isolating theory as knowledge is to distinguish it from nonsystematic, journalistic or reportorial description.

The method of factor-searching studies is to begin with as open a view as possible of the situation to be studied and immerse oneself thoroughly in the events rather than starting with preconceived ideas of what data are most likely to be important and thus missing the opportunity to enrich one's understanding by letting the data guide the conceptualization and the method, rather than the other way around.

In order to develop concepts or ways of characterizing the situation, one needs the richest possible data, data that will shed light on all possible variety of nuances, tints and shades of meaning of the evolving concepts. In contrast to other kinds of studies where the form of data collection is set in the beginning and cannot be changed in the middle of the study, factor-searching studies deliberately make use of "findings" as they are generated from the data, to lead to new sources of information. The data collection strategy does not change, but the kinds of information collected may.

Thus, factor-searching studies proceed in rough phases. Data, in the form of descriptions of events in the situation picked, are collected and recorded.

As the records accumulate, they are constantly surveyed for similarities, differences, themes, beginning concepts and records are made of these "analyses." The beginning analyses then point to new sources of information to be collected, and these are then also constantly reviewed. For example, in the Glaser and Strauss study, the data on the total experience of the dying patient began to suggest that one factor that seemed to characterize what was happening was the extent to which the patient and those around him were aware that he was dying. This beginning notion of "awareness" could then be tracked down by focusing in, for the next period of data collection observation, on how aware the patient and others were, what that meant to them, how it was seen and so on.

As concepts begin to be developed, the researcher searches for new and different situations in which the concept might occur in order to tease out all the subtleties of its meaning. This is a process called "theoretical sampling" (26)—looking for additional data in places or events dictated by the developing theory. For example, in rounding out the concept of social loss, Glaser and Strauss looked for different situations in which that phenomenon could possibly happen differently—the general medical ward versus the emergency room; the newborn intensive care unit versus a geriatric nursing home; the young, attractive patient versus an older patient and so on. Each new incident (in this case the incident defined as the dying patient) was then compared with every other incident in a method called "constant comparative analysis" with each comparison provoking new shades of meaning to the concept of social loss (27). These two processes continue until the concept is "saturated"—until new events or instances collected stop providing any new information.

Every concept discovered goes through this same process, and finally all the concepts are tied together with their definitions and perhaps with associated hypotheses into a coherent whole—a bit of factor-isolating theory. Throughout the data collection and analysis process, which occur simultaneously in this kind of study, the investigator builds in ways to assure that the data gathered are as objective and unbiased and reliable as possible.

The Glaser and Strauss method, summarized briefly here, is the model for factor-searching studies, followed in more or less rigorous a way no matter what the form of the theory to be developed is, that is, whether the theory will be in the form of descriptive definitions in narrative form, or in the form of taxonomical categories tied to one underlying dimension. Two points are implicit in the Glaser and Strauss model, however, and they should be made clear here. First, this kind of constant comparative analysis and theoretical sampling takes a very long time, especially when the area to be investigated is a large and untouched one, as in the case of the dying patient. While parts of the developing theory may come quickly and be isolated and defined rather early on, as in the case of the "awareness contexts," (28) a complete factor-isolating theory of the dying patient would be enormous and endless. The investigator must have the time available to collect data, code and analyze it, collect more, contemplate the direction of the theory development, collect more and so on. Unlike any other kind of a study where the end point of the various phases—data collection, data analysis—can be preset and one knows when they are done, factor-searching studies done in this model can go on and on. The "end" therefore is arbitrary, reached when the concepts and their properties have been saturated as much as possible, or when an artifical time boundary—the end of a grant period, or some other point—intervenes. Actually, no kind of study ever ends, in one sense, as there is always more to learn and understand on a given topic, and it is in the nature of science that understanding accumulates slowly, over long, long periods. But the end of one particular investigator's immersion in the data in a factor-searching study is difficult to set in advance.

The other buried point in this method is that it is probably best used when a team of investigators can be put together. The process of reviewing the field notes, developing concepts then returning for more data collection profits from discussion with others and from others' eyes on the data. It is particularly difficult for a single investigator to work her/his way through the mountain of material that collects all alone because when one has also collected the data oneself, it is hard to see the forest for the trees. It is possible for a single investigator to arrange with colleagues to act as consultants, reading the field notes as they accumulate, and discussing them to help draw out concepts, but this is a halfway measure at best. The critique of Kay's work on health-illness concepts in the barrio is a remarkably clear example of how a factor-isolating theory could have been improved if the viewpoint of the barrio could have been brought to bear on the study itself, with the addition of the research team of an investigator with the personal and cultural understanding the original investigator lacked (29).

Setting

As in any study, the principle behind choosing a place to collect the data is which place *has* it? In factor-searching studies, in which theory is being discovered or invented, the uniqueness of the setting may be more of an issue. If a study is to deal with description or conceptualization of a unique setting, the generality of the theory developed will be limited. For example, a descriptive study of patient experiences in a hospice (an inpatient facility for the terminally ill) might apply to other hospices, if there are others, but might not have general applicability to dying in other kinds of institutions. The problem of the uniqueness of the setting is important only if the descriptive research deals with the matters internal to, and uniquely characteristic of, that setting. In Wilson's study of Soteria House, for example, the setting might be considered unique, but since the study dealt with the relationships of that nontraditional setting to the outside world, it is simply an example of other nontraditional settings and their dealings with the world.

Studies aimed at developing categories usually need a "typical" setting, meaning that it is like most other settings in important ways. For instance, developing quality of care categories in specialized settings with a high staff-patient ratio, lots of equipment and money and relatively well patients would not produce categories that might be useful in a more typical institution. Similarly, developing categories to describe nurse-patient interaction using the interactions of clinical nurse specialists highly trained in interpersonal dynamics would not necessarily make the categories useful with more typical nurses.

At the beginning, the setting should be typical or else one runs the risk of developing theory which is unique to unique settings, when the purpose of theory development is to have it be as useful as possible, as general, to as many different settings as it can be.

Sample

The sampling principle in factor-searching studies is "richness," that is, how rich the data will be when supplied by the sample chosen. The sampling unit may or may not be individuals. In studies working from a sociological perspective, the sample is more likely to be incidents or events of a particular kind, which may involve more than one individual.

In the beginning of a factor-searching study there may be no true selection process at all; everything observed is recorded and the only selection is the natural one of the investigator's physical presence. Later, as concepts develop and theoretical sampling begins, purposeful choosing of which events to gather next is done.

Bits of reality are deliberately chosen for their potential to enrich the developing theory. In this kind of study, no proof is at stake, and since such studies are specifically done because the phenomena involved are not "known" or specified in advance, the usual notions of representativeness of the sample do not apply in the same way. That is, in studies at higher levels of inquiry where the intention is to be able to generalize the results of one study with one sample to larger populations, the sample has to be selected in such a way as to be representative of the larger group. But in factor-searching studies, the parameters of the phenomena are not even known—that's one purpose of such studies. Thus, the sample can only be representative in the sense that the events or instances collected and recorded attempt to cover the entire *range* of the phenomenon and the resulting concepts are as rich—full of meaning—as can be.

In studies at higher levels of inquiry, a sample is judged as adequate when it can be demonstrated to be selected according to methods that will make it representative of the distribution of attributes in the population. Samples for factor-searching studies (theoretical sampling) are considered adequate on the basis of how wisely and diversely the researcher has chosen his groups for "saturating" categories. Inadequate sampling is characterized by a theory that is thin and not well integrated, with many obvious unexplained exceptions (30).

But just as it is important in studies at higher levels of inquiry to report the sources of data so that other investigators can judge the likeness of their samples to the original, so in factor-searching studies it is important to record and report as much information about the events or sampling units as possible so that readers may judge for themselves whether the entire range of the phenomenon has been captured and whether the events that generated the concepts are typical. Thus, the participants in the events, the timing of them, the observable nature of them, the setting and so on all have to be taken into account and recorded.

The ideal in factor-searching studies is the Glaser and Strauss method of gathering data, beginning to construct concepts, sampling theoretically, gathering more data and so on until the concepts are fully saturated. When that method is not possible, usually because of time restrictions, one can approximate it with a smaller sample, that is, a more limited number of events or encounters. What one sacrifices is the richness and subtlety of the concepts, and any production of theory will probably have to be refined over and over subsequently in other studies. For example, in developing the Nurse Orientation System, a set of categories for classifying the verbal interaction of nurses and patients, the investigator had a limited time to collect the data to generate the categories. While the data were being examined as they were collected, and while some ideas for categories were emerging, it was not until the artificially limited time period was over that the categories were developed, and all from one set of data collected from one clinical setting (31). Over the next few years the categories had to be refined again and again, not in major ways but in increasing their precision and sensitivity, as other groups of data were collected.

The original set of data included conversations of nurses with chronically ill medical patients in a Veterans Administration Hospital. The nurses were permanent staff of the unit and not specially trained in interpersonal relations. When it came time to apply the developed categories to sets of data from highly trained psychiatric nurses, or data from patients with other than medical conditions, the categories had to be refined and made more inclusive. One early refinement, in fact, was to include in the category definitions and coding examples of data from women patients in order to supplement the male examples contained in the original data.

In summary, the sample in a factor-searching is that chunk of reality that is observed and recorded. The sampling unit in the beginning may be an observation, an event, an incident, a conversation with artificially defined boundaries such as time or setting. When concepts start to develop, theoretical sampling may be used, deliberately choosing new events or instances to observe and record because they have the potential of illuminating the developing concepts.

Instruments/Measurements

Rarely in factor-searching studies are formal instruments such as interviews, questionnaires, psychological tests used. Sometimes an open-ended interview may be used to structure responses or focus attention on some aspects of the problem, especially when the information cannot be obtained by participant or nonparticipant observation. For example, a study on rape might use a semistructured, focused interview with rape victims, to be sure that major dimensions of the event, the participants, the reactions of the victim and others are covered, since it is not possible for a researcher to be present during the event itself (which would be carrying participant observation a bit too far!).

Thus, there are rarely "instruments" or "measurements" in the usual sense of the word in these kinds of studies. Rather, data in the form of narrative notes and descriptions of events, conversations, observations are recorded systematically in "field notes," to be analyzed as they are recorded. Various mechanical devices may be used to help this process — tape recorders or dictaphones, for example.

The usual concerns about reliability and validity of the instruments used in a study do not apply in factor-searching studies. Rather, there is concern for the reliability of the *sources* of data and of the recorder (person or machine). That is, the concern is whether the sources of data represent well the developing concepts and whether the person recording the data gets it all down. The ultimate test of reliability in this sense is, as in sampling, whether the theory when developed is rich and full or thin and weak, whether it is all-encompassing of the concept or has large holes and unexplained ambiguities.

If the researcher is part of a team, or at least is subjecting the field notes to others' scrutiny periodically, lapses in recording or gaps in information can be detected. But there is no formal test for reliability of data in factor-searching studies, again because the purpose of the study is to develop theory, not to "prove" it.

Data Collection

Factor-searching studies may use a wide variety of observational techniques combined sometimes with interviews, or references to written reports of others (for example, chart data). Participant and nonparticipant observation are probably the primary data collection procedures.

Again, the notion of richness guides the data collection methods as well as the sampling method. Participant observation, where the investigator becomes part of the events themselves, provides some dimensions that can enrich the concepts, since information on the participants' own feelings become available. Glaser and Strauss used nonparticipant observation entirely, probably because as sociologists they could have no role in the clinical settings in which they collected data. In either case, data collection can be supplemented by interviews and references to information recorded by others (for example, chart data, minutes, reports). Informal, unstructured, focused interviews may be used to check on the accuracy of the observer's perceptions by asking the participants in a given event how they saw it. Audio- or video-taped events can be used as the primary source of information, though they may be somewhat thin if not supplemented by direct questioning or participation in the situations. In Kay's study of disease concepts, interviews were the only source of data collected, and, therefore, the theory developed from that source could only encompass what the respondents *said* they did, not what their actual behavior was, which limits the usefulness (and the accuracy) of the information.

Sometimes descriptive literature can be used as an additional source of information. For example, psychiatric theory development often uses reports patients themselves have written and published to shed additional light on material collected by therapist-investigators. A study of the dying patient done today would probably make reference to some of the very moving accounts written by people who were dying (32).

The most often used method of recording data is the field note. Here, notes are made during the events (if possible), then a full description of events is written later. In the beginning of a factor-searching study, the attempt is to get down on paper everything that was observed and/or felt. Later, as concepts begin to develop, the field notes can be refined to include only those aspects of the events that are being sampled at the time. The beginning process of isolating factors often produces small notions of themes or emerging concepts which then become something like a checklist, carried with the investigator so that one is reminded to look for and record special aspects of situations.

Modern dictating and audio recording make producing field notes much easier. Time must be planned in collecting data, however, to go to a quiet place and reconstruct the events on paper or verbally for transcription later. In one instance, an investigator equipped her car with a dictaphone and used her forty minute commute home to record the events of the previous hours. Obviously, the closer in time the recording is to the event, the less likely is information to be lost.

The notes taken during the events may follow any format, but certain identifying information should be recorded—the participants, the time, place, date of observation, circumstances and so on. In this kind of study as in any other, participants should never be named by their real names, but some kind of code developed to which only the investigator has access. Since the notes taken are an aid to reconstructing the observations chronologically, any form that works for a particular investigator is fine. Pertinent verbatim comments that help order the observation and recording the actual time at intervals are only two possible schemes.

Field notes can be written in any form, but one that seems to work well is to write the observations, or have them transcribed on only one vertical half of the paper, leaving the other half as a column for later writing in emerging themes or concepts. If interviews or direct tape recordings are used to supplement the field notes, they can be transcribed onto different colored paper. Glaser and Strauss advocate the writing of "analytic memos" at specified intervals throughout the data collection period—summaries of one's developing thoughts about the data, from which concepts begin to emerge, or directions for future data collection start to form (33). Discussions among the research team members, if there is a team, also become part of the data to flesh out the observations.

As one might suspect, field notes rapidly becomes voluminous. Thus, some kind of indexing system needs to be developed so that events of interest can be retrieved quickly. A master list of general topics, participants in the events, settings or even developing concepts can be used as an index with page numbers or dates or other identifying information recorded.

It is especially important in factor-searching studies to preserve the flavor or quality of the data as much as possible, since one test of how useful the theory will be is how "sensitizing" or evocative—convincing—it is (34). A conversational, anecdotal style of writing or dictating is most useful.

Data collection, processing and analysis occur simultaneously in these kinds of studies. One cannot help having abstract thoughts about the events being observed or recorded, and these thoughts become beginning concepts. Therefore, it is entirely appropriate to include in the recording of data the I wonder if this means . . . ideas that naturally come to mind. Indeed, these may lead one into theoretical sampling, or at least into looking more closely at some aspects of the next set of observations. Also, one cannot help making connections between the observations of one day and previous ones and these can be noted while one is dictating or writing: This reminds me of. . . .

The importance of having time to get away from the data to think about them cannot be overemphasized. Contemplative time is important in any kind of study, but in factor-searching studies the contemplation, or conceptualization, *is* the method of theory development and has to be provided for.

Since data collection aims for richness, another source of data is the investigator and her/his own perceptions, thoughts, feelings, as long as such information is treated as *data* to be compared with and analyzed with other data, rather than as definitive in itself. The creative use of personal insights can greatly enrich a factor-searching study, but only as long as proper precautions are taken to balance those kinds of data with other data which might disconfirm one's own impressions (35). The principle of rigorously subjecting one's own observations to the test of others is no less held in these kinds of studies than studies at higher levels of inquiry—it is just done less formally. In predictive studies, for example, the hypothesis is the investigator's perception, to be tested by conventions developed in research methods. In factor-searching studies the perceptions are raw data, to be compared and contrasted with other raw data, with the same open mindedness as hypotheses are tested.

Data collection is said to end when the factors or categories are "saturated," that is, when new data no longer reveal new dimensions (36). However, given the volume of information that becomes available and the literally infinite possibilities for developing new concepts, data collection usually ends because of time limits imposed outside the study. The investigator then does as much as can be done to develop theory to characterize the situation, knowing full well that any kind of reality is capable of being characterized in numberless ways and in many degrees of specificity. Any set of concepts or categories will tap only a few dimensions of any situation, just as any hypothesis tested and supported encompasses a tiny bit of reality. Thus, the slow progress of science or theory development.

Data Processing/Analysis

In factor-searching studies, data processing is the noting of themes, beginning concepts, ideas stimulated by the data and the isolating of the events or instances that provoke or amplify the thought. Usually notes of such thoughts are made in the column next to the raw data, then summarized or gathered together at intervals and separated from the raw data on different pages. The "processing" of data takes place in the investigator's head literally, but the results of that process are recorded as well as the data themselves so that later others can understand where the concepts came from.

In studies at higher levels of inquiry, data processing means getting the raw data in shape to be analyzed, usually by mathematical means. In factor-searching studies, some of that processing goes on as the data are collected. To the extent possible, especially in the beginning of data collection, every attempt should be made to record as fully as possible everything in a given situation. Later, as concepts evolve and theoretical sampling takes place, the focus is narrowed, but full description is still necessary as the force of the study shifts from breadth of observation to depth. Throughout, a self-conscious monitoring of one's own thinking process is maintained and recorded in order to keep the raw data that provokes concepts and the concepts themselves as close together as can be.

Data analysis goes on concurrently with data collection and processing in a factor-searching study. But when the time comes to write up the study is when the finishing touches to data analysis are put on. Then, the developing concepts are defined, illustrations given, the concepts are threaded together in some meaningful pattern and properties of the concepts are provided. The mental process here is trying to see different instances of events as related, and linking these instances with bigger (more abstract) and bigger concepts—names which fit all the events within that abstraction. One tries to reduce the volumes of data collected into a meaningful handful of named concepts.

(One student once wryly remarked that for her this process was the exercise of devising bigger and bigger concepts that encompassed more and more of the data so that when she finished, she felt her entire study could be contained in just its title!)

Wilson's article is a fine illustration of both the method and the way of reporting factor-searching studies (37). She reduced a very large amount of data to one large concept: limiting intrusion (of the outside into Soteria

. House), with three defining properties—minimizing approachability, deflecting and disengaging. The major concept and its properties are formally defined, and illustrations given to show the shades of meaning and subtleties of the concepts.

Some factor-searching studies will present the data not in formal concepts, but in a running narrative description, perhaps organized around important phases, or themes. Here the "phase" or the "theme" becomes the concept, and other than being less formally derived, the process of data analysis is the same as in the grounded theory approach.

Still other factor-searching studies will analyze data to arrive at a set of categories, all related to one underlying concept. Sometimes categories are part of other studies, sometimes their production is the aim of one single study.

These kinds of categories are distinguished from more general groups of concepts by the fact that they are all related to one underlying dimension, and taken as a whole encompass all there is of that dimension. Glaser and Strauss' "awareness contexts" are one form of categories. They identify one dimension—awareness of the patient's terminality—and two conditions—the patient's awareness and that of others—put together to form classes of "awareness." In the first category, the patient knows he is dying and so do others—"open awareness." In the second, the patient knows, but others do not—"mutual pretense." In the third, others know but the patient does not—"suspicious awareness"—and in the fourth, no one knows—"closed awareness." (38) By definition, when one puts together two dichotomies (patient knows or doesn't, others know or don't), the four resulting categories exhaust the possibilities.

This example also illustrates the other principles that guide the kind of factor-searching called "category construction." The first principle is that the categories taken together are jointly exhaustive—everything has a place. The second is that they are mutually exclusive—everything has only one place. Then categories must be a "significant division of the whole" meaning that the distinctions among categories should be neither too broad nor too trivial for the purposes of the study. The final principle is that the categories be unidimensional—that is, all related to only one underlying dimension.

Some studies begin with the notion of developing categories along only one dimension. In some cases the dimension itself is chosen in advance and the force of the study is to invent the properties or categories of that dimension. Hollingshead's "Two Factor Index of Social Position" is the result of such a study (39).

The Nurse Orientation System for content analysis of verbal interaction of nurses and patients uses as its underlying dimension the concept orientation—the verbal stance one actor takes toward the other, how one views the other. This concept was generated from data which consisted of tape recordings of verbal interactions, supplemented by notes and informal interviews. The orientation dimension is then divided into its subject—orientation to the patient, to the nurse, to others or to objects which exhaust the possibilities.

Then within each of these properties, interaction can be categorized as orientation to the person as a feeling person, a thinking person or a being-doing person (see Figure 4-1). These categories exhaust the realm of orientations, yet every unit of verbal interaction can be placed in one category.

Figure 4-1. *Nurse Orientation System* (40)

CATEGORY NUMBER	CATEGORY
0	*Object Orientation*
	Patient Orientation
1	Feeling
2	Knowing-thinking-evaluating
3	Being-doing
	Nurse Orientation
4	Feeling
5	Knowing-thinking-evaluating
6	Being-doing
	Other Orientation
7	Feeling
8	Knowing-thinking-evaluating
9	Being-doing

In category construction, the "constant comparison" comes not so much from comparing event with event (in this case category with category), but in devising a beginning set of categories and applying them to some data, often the same data used to generate the categories, then seeing how they "fit." Applying categories to data means seeing if it is possible to divide up the data and put units of it into the first-draft categories. This procedure is repeated usually many times until a set of categories evolves which does encompass all the data meaningfully. Often the first tentative set of categories is just a list of all the possible labels for the data the investigator can imagine. Some of them will turn out to be too trivial or too general, or will not fit the data. Those that don't fit are discarded, those that are too small can sometimes be combined, those that are too general can be subdivided. Reworking the categories over and over constitutes the major portion of data analysis for this kind of factor-searching study.

Factor-searching studies rarely employ inferential statistics (indeed, given the way the data are collected, inferences to even known statistical populations are inappropriate, though they have been known to be attempted). Even descriptive statistics are rarely used except perhaps to describe the sample or the number of events categorized. "Qualitative analysis" is the appropriate term for data analysis in factor-searching (41).

INTERPRETATION

In studies at higher levels of inquiry, interpretation of data is done after data are analyzed mathematically, in an attempt to figure out what the data mean. In factor-searching studies, the step of data interpretation goes on simultaneously with data collection and analysis, so that the final phase in the research is less "interpretation" than it is reporting. By the time one gets to the writing-up stage, it should be quite clear what the data mean, and the concepts, description or categories should be clear in one's mind. If one has used the method of field notes and analytic memos then a good deal of the final report writing will come from the analytic memos themselves. If one is aiming for a narrative descriptive report, some reorganizing of the information may be needed to tease out the themes or phases. By the end of the data analysis for a study intended to produce categories, the categories will be listed and defined and coding instructions for their use provided.

Factor-searching studies belong to the "context of discovery" rather than the "context of verification." (42) There are no tests of hypotheses here, no statistical proof involved. Rather, they are intended to develop theory, and a particular kind of theory at that. The product of a factor-searching study, therefore, is a bit of theory, in the form of conceptual description or in the form of a set of categories related to one underlying dimension. For the former, the report of the study takes the form of a narrative, often a lengthy one, liberally using examples from the data to illustrate concepts or their properties. The latter kind of study ends with the categories and their definitions reported together with illustrative examples and, sometimes, beginning assessments of the reliability and validity of the categories developed.

Glaser and Strauss suggest that a good factor-searching study is one in which the concepts are saturated and sensitizing, and the theory integrated (43). The test of how well a study at this level of inquiry was done is a pragmatic one—credibility. Is the theory developed believable? Or, in the case of categories, are they indeed mutually exclusive, exhaustive, unidimensional and a significant definition of the whole? Factor-searching studies aim to develop naming theory and how good the names are depends mostly on what use is made of the concepts or categories and whether they stand rigorous tests of empirical utility, as well as formal tests of prediction.

Developing categories in a factor-searching study may be the first step in a measurement study (see Chapter 9), the next steps being to test the reliability and validity of the categories developed. Narrative descriptive studies, or studies which devise concepts, may or may not be carried on to tests at higher levels of inquiry. Even though these studies are called exploratory, or descriptive, the results may indeed explain sufficiently some set of events so that no further formal testing of the concepts or predictions is called for. For example, the concept of social loss of the dying patient may explain why some dying patients are treated differently than others (are ignored, or attended to) sufficiently so that the notion of social loss may be immediately incorporated into nursing practice to improve patient care. That is a head nurse might adopt social loss as a concept to help her when she counsels nursing staff caring for dying patients in order to help them understand their feelings about different patients. Or the concepts of awareness contexts may also be useful in practice without any further testing in order to help clarify different behaviors of dying patients with family or staff. Simply providing names for phenomena is in itself explanatory theory, and may be as useful *for its purpose* as the more conventional notion of experimental scientific theory. If what the practice situation needs is simply a way to conceptualize events, naming theory will do. If the practice situation (the clinical problem) requires tested predictions, naming theory will not completely serve the purpose, but it was never intended to.

Factor-searching studies may also end with formal hypotheses that might lend themselves to further testing. If so, the researcher has the obligation to outline the hypothesis, as a piece of theory, and include any ideas for how it could be tested, including suggestions for sampling, setting, measurement or whatever else might be useful.

Because factor-searching studies accumulate vast quantities of information, secondary analysis of data may go on for a long time after an artificial end to the study, and the production of the primary report.

In summary, factor-searching studies are called for when the clinical problem is how to understand a set of events or phenomena. In this kind of study, encounters with the real world (data) are used to generate the theory, rather than being used to test theory, as is the case with studies at higher levels of inquiry. Studies begin with an area or topic of investigation, and with broad research questions about What *is* this? Data are collected through observation, questioning, interviewing or access to recorded material in charts, papers, minutes or reports. Data are analyzed as they are collected, by constantly comparing like instances with one another until a name for the class of instances is produced. Theoretical sampling may be used to find other instances of a given concept. Factor-searching studies may produce narrative descriptions, usually organized around themes or chronological phases, concepts formally defined with properties, or categories of one single concept, all related to one another in some kind of ordered system. The kind of theory produced is called factor-isolating or naming theory, and it may itself be explanatory or fit into prescriptions for practice or it may lead to further testing.

Factor-searching studies are the most basic kind of study that can be done, but not the least sophisticated, and certainly not the easiest. The mental work involved in inventing theory from data is extremely taxing, especially if done alone without a team of colleagues with whom to share the experience. Such studies are not best done if the researcher is impatient with abstraction, or wishes more concrete, instant results, for the study demands contemplation and highly complicated conceptual work (44). The reward is in seeing developed a new way of thinking about an important clinical problem, with perhaps some suggestions for how this new thinking can be used to change nursing practice and patient care for the better.

NOTES

1. As in Goode, William and Paul Hatt: *Methods of Social Research*. New York: McGraw-Hill, 1952.

2. Abdellah, Faye G. and Eugene Levine: *Better Patient Care Through Nursing Research*. New York: Macmillan, 1965; Fox, David J.: *Fundamentals of Nursing Research* (2nd edition). New York: Appleton-Century-Crofts 1970; Wandelt, Mabel: *Guide for the Beginning Researcher*. New York: Appleton-Century-Crofts, 1970.

3. Selltiz, Claire, et al.: *Research Methods in Social Relations*. New York: Holt, Rinehart & Winston, 1960.

4. See Christy, Teresa E.: The methodology of historical research. *Nursing Research*, 2:189–192, May–June 1975 for a brief overview. On ethnoscience, see Bush, Mary T., et al.: The meaning of mental health: a report of two ethnoscientific studies. *Nursing Research*, 24:103–138, March–April 1975 for a good, brief explanation of method, illustrated with data. See also Leininger, Madeline: *Nursing and Anthropology: Two Worlds to Blend*. New York: John Wiley & Sons, 1973; Ragucci, Antoinette: Ethnographic approach and nursing research. *Nursing Research*, 21:485–490, November–December 1972.

5. White, William Foote: *Street Corner Society: The Social Structure of an Italian Slum*. Chicago: University of Chicago Press, 1943.

6. Malinowski, Bronislaw: *Crime and Custom in Savage Society*. New York: Harcourt, Brace, Jovanovich, 1926.

   Both Whyte and Malinowski are excerpted and discussed in Riley, Matilda White: *Sociological Research* (Vol. I). New York: Harcourt, Brace, Jovanovich, 1963.

7. Oleson, Virginia L. and Elvi W. Whittacker: *The Silent Dialogue*. San Francisco: Jossey-Bass, 1968.

8. Schmahl, Jane A.: *Experiment in Change*. New York: Macmillan, 1966.

9. Mellow, June: Nursing therapy in the acute and post-acute phases: an atypical case. *Three Reports of Nurse Patient Interaction in Psychiatric Nursing*. New York: NLN Exchange, 1959; Mellow, June: Research in nursing therapy. In *The Improvement of Nursing Through Research*. Washington, D.C.: Catholic University Press, 1958; Mellow, June: The evolution of nursing therapy and its implications for education. Unpublished Ed.D. dissertation, Boston University, 1964. See also, Colliton, Margaret A.: The history of nursing therapy: a reactionnaire to the work of June Mellow. *Perspectives in Psychiatric Care*, 3(2):10–19, 1965.

10. Glaser, Barney and Anselm Strauss: *Discovery of Grounded Theory*. Chicago: Aldine Publishing Company, 1967; Glaser, Barney and Anselm Strauss: *Awareness of Dying*. Chicago: Aldine Publishing Company, 1966. See also, Quint, Jeanne C.: *The Nurse and the Dying Patient*. New York: Macmillan, 1967. Also, Glaser, Barney and Anselm Strauss: *A Time for Dying*. Chicago: Aldine Publishing Company, 1968.

   Some reviewers have not granted credibility either to Glaser and Strauss' methods or to their findings. Leonard Reissman said that after reading *Awareness of Dying*, he agreed with physicians that sociologists (as Glaser and Strauss are) have nothing to offer physicians. Reissman also attacks the methods. See Leonard Reissman's review of Barney Glaser and Anselm Strauss' *Awareness of Dying* in *Annals of the American Academy of Political and Social Science*, 366:202–203, July 1966. Contrast this review with Elizabeth Strutzel's review of *Discovery of Grounded Theory* in *Nursing Research*, 17:364–365, July–August 1968.

   See also Quint, Jeanne C.: Awareness of death and the nurse's composure. *Nursing Research*, 15:49–55, Winter 1966. Glaser, Barney and Anselm Strauss: The purpose and credibility of qualitative research. *Nursing Research*, 15:56–61, Winter 1966; Glaser,

Barney and Anselm Strauss: Discovery of substantive theory: a basic strategy underlying qualitative research. *American Behavioral Scientist*, February 1965, pp. 5–12; Glaser, Barney: The constant comparative method of qualitative analysis. *Social Problems*, 12:436–445, Spring 1965. These authors have written voluminously on their findings, in the medical, nursing, sociological and hospital literature. Readers are encouraged to seek out other references, since their ideas and their data are so rich.

11. The process of defining and redefining disease classification schemes occupies the entire lives of a good many people. The general history of disease classification schemes is presented in Gebbie, Kristine M. and Mary Ann Lavin: *Classification of Nursing Diagnoses: Summary of the First National Conference*. St. Louis: C.V. Mosby, 1973, especially the section, "Principles of Classification," pp. 7–20. One of the more intricate problems in disease classification (other than nursing diagnosis) is psychiatric disease nomenclature. The *Diagnostic and Statistical Manuals* of the American Psychiatric Association (which are patterned after the International Classification of Disease Process) are a particularly interesting example. See especially the Forwards and Introductions of the existing manuals (DSM I, II, III), Washington, D.C: American Psychiatric Association, latest revision, 1977.

12. Gebbie and Lavin, see Note 11. See also Gebbie, Kristine M.: *Classification of Nursing Diagnoses: Summary of the Second National Conference*. St. Louis: National Group for Classification of Nursing Diagnoses, 1976; also, Gebbie, Kristine M. and Mary Ann Lavin: Classifying nursing diagnosis. *American Journal of Nursing*, 74:250–254, February 1974.

    For a brief but cogent article on taxonomy as theory, see McKay, Rose: What is the relationship between the development and utilization of a taxonomy and nursing theory? *Nursing Research*, 26:222–224, May–June 1977.

13. The sequence of studies is listed and discussed in Diers, Donna and Robert C. Leonard: Interaction analysis in nursing research. *Nursing Research*, 15:225–228, Summer 1966. See also Diers, Donna and Ruth L. Schmidt: Interaction analysis in nursing research. In Verhonick, Phyllis J. (ed.): *Nursing Research* (Vol. II). Boston: Little, Brown, 1977, pp. 77–132. For some reason, interaction studies have not been in fashion in recent years. One of the most recent, after a lapse of some years is Altschul, Annie: *Patient-Nurse Interaction: A Study of Interaction Patterns in Acute Psychiatric Wards*. University of Edinburgh, Department of Nursing Studies, Monograph #3. Edinburgh: Churchill Livingston, 1972.

14. Bruner, Jerome: *A Study of Thinking*. New York: Science Editions Inc., 1965.

15. Hodgman, Eileen Callahan: *Nursing in a Community Action Agency*. New York: National League for Nursing (League Exchange #91), 1970.

16. Mellow, see Note 9.

17. Kay, Marguerite: Disease concepts in the barrio today. In Batey, Marjorie V. (ed.): *Communicating Nursing Research: Collaboration and Competition*. Boulder, Colorado: WICHE, December 1973, pp. 185–194.

    Two other factor-searching studies using only interviews were relatively more successful in comprehensiveness of categories derived, probably because the problems tackled were smaller. See Hampe, Sandra: Needs of the grieving spouse in a hospital setting. *Nursing Research*, 24:113–120, March–April 1974 and Leavitt, Maribelle: The discharge crisis: the experience of families of psychiatric patients. *Nursing Research*, 24:33–40, January–February 1975. See also Burgess, Ann and Lynda Holmstrom: Crisis and counseling requests of rape victims. *Nursing Research*, 23:196–202, May-June 1974.

18. Wilson, Holly Skodol: Limiting intrusion—social control of outsiders in a healing community. An illustration of qualitative comparative analysis. *Nursing Research*, 26:103–111, March–April 1977.

19. Glaser and Strauss, *Awareness of Dying*, see Note 10, especially pp. 3–15.

This phenomenon (denial of death by health professionals) is documented in numerous places, among them Kübler-Ross, Elisabeth: *On Death and Dying.* New York: Macmillan, 1969.

20. See discussion by Riley of Whyte's work (see Note 5), especially pp. 57–75.

21. See Wilson, Note 18; Quint, Note 10; see also: Strauss, Anselm, et al.: Pain: an organization-work-interactional perspective. *Nursing Outlook,* 22:560–566, September 1974; Fagerhaugh, Shizuko U.: Pain expression and control on a burn care unit. *Nursing Outlook,* 22:645–650, October 1974; Wiener, Carolyn L.: Pain assessment on an orthopedic ward. *Nursing Outlook,* 23:508–516, August 1975.

   The latter three articles do not describe the methodology for the studies (which are all related) but give an excellent picture of theory development and reporting at this level of inquiry.

22. It is characteristic of factor-searching studies (except perhaps those where measurement categories are the end product) that they are more suitable for book publication than for articles, which may explain why there are so few in the literature as yet. Factor-searching studies are very complicated to report, and since the data are so enormous, take a good deal of scarce journal space. Even in a most recent report of such a study (Wilson, see Note 18) reports only a part of her findings in a journal article.

23. Wilson, see Note 18, p. 103.

24. Diers and Leonard, see Note 13.

25. Glaser and Strauss use the word "hypothesis" in a somewhat loose way, and roughly equivalent, sometimes to "guess," at other times clearly meant as a specific statement of relationship. For this book, "hypothesis" has the latter meaning—a technical statement of defined relationship between two or more variables; a prediction of relationship or cause and effect. Thus the statement here that factor-searching studies do not begin with hypotheses, but rather with research questions may be read to be in conflict with Glaser and Strauss' method. On the whole, I would rather use technical terminology, even when it has a non-technical meaning, rigorously.

26. Glaser and Strauss, *Grounded Theory,* see Note 10, especially pp. 45–77.

27. Glaser and Strauss, *Grounded Theory,* see Note 10; Wilson, see Note 18.

28. Glaser and Strauss, *Awareness of Dying,* see Note 10, especially pp. 1–100.

29. Martinez, Aurora: Minority response to Disease concepts in the barrio today. In Batey, Marjorie V. (ed.): *Communicating Nursing Research,* pp. 197–200.

30. Wilson, see Note 18, quoting Mullen, P.D. and Richard Reynolds: The potential of comparative analysis for health education research. Paper submitted for the Dorothy Hyswander International Symposium, September 27–28, 1974.

31. Diers and Schmidt, see Note 13.

32. Stewart, Alsop: *Stay of Execution.* Philadelphia: J.B. Lippincott Company, 1974 is only one example, but a particularly moving one.

33. See Wilson, Note 18.

34. Glaser and Strauss, *Grounded Theory,* see Note 10.

35. See Wilson, Note 18, for an excellent description of how this works.

36. See Note 34.

37. Wilson, see Note 18, especially p. 103.

38. Glaser and Strauss, *Awareness of Dying,* see Note 10, especially pp. 29–115.

39. Hollingshead, August and Fredric Redlich: *Social Class and Mental Illness.* New York: John Wiley & Sons, 1958.

40. From Donna Diers: The nurse orientation system: a method for analyzing nurse-patient interactions. Unpublished master's report, Yale School of Nursing, 1964. Revised, January, 1966. See also, Studies of nurse-patient interaction. USPHS grant NU00179, Bureau of Health Manpower, Division of Nursing; see Note 12.

    This is only the outline of the categories—coding instructions including complete definitions of the categories are necessary to use the NOS.

41. Glaser and Strauss, Purpose and credibility of qualitative research, see Note 10.

42. Glaser and Strauss, *Grounded Theory*, see Note 10.

43. Glaser and Strauss, *Grounded Theory*, see Note 10.

44. Glaser and Strauss intimate that their method can only be used by sociologists, or at least that sociological training in non-participant field work is essential. (See Purpose and credibility of qualitative research, Note 10). This statement was made early on in the development of the method, and by now several nonsociologists have used it, and several participant observers so I suspect that opinion would not now be held. It seems reasonable that the method can be used in the study of nonsociological phenomena (indeed it has been), and that methods other than nonparticipant observation may be used. Experience with student studies suggests that the method outlined by Glaser and Strauss in *Grounded Theory*, see Note 10, is comprehensible, and applicable to a wide variety of situations. Recent studies (as yet unpublished) have used this approach for two studies of cotherapy in psychiatric nursing, for a study of rape, for a study of nontraditional healers and so on.

5

Relation-Searching Studies

INTRODUCTION

Relation-searching studies are called for when the names of the factors (variables) are known, or selected, but the researcher hasn't the faintest idea how they might be related to each other, or to one other common factor. These studies are still exploratory, or descriptive, in contrast to hypothesis-testing, because while the factors can be named, the state of theory development is such that it is not possible to make formal predictions about relationships or effects.

Relation-searching studies are concerned with developing theory rather than with testing it. The kind of theory to be developed is factor-relating theory (or situation-depicting), so these studies are at the second level of inquiry. The theory behind them is developed at least to the point that the variables can be named and operational definitions for them provided, but the relationships among variables cannot yet be derived.

Relation-searching studies are done when a situation is new, or at least new to nursing; or when previous studies have not examined the same sets of variables, though the topic area may have been investigated; or when there is a search to see whether a relationship found in one context will also be found in others when the original theory did not necessarily predict that it would.

In the literature, there is some confusion between this kind of study and the kind addressed in the next chapter—association-testing. Relation-searching studies do not have hypotheses, while association-testing studies do. In general, the theory which guides a relation-searching study is less fully developed, more tentative. It may well be that the topic has not been investigated before at all, so that new measurements or operational definitions are called for. Since the purpose of relation-searching studies is not to generalize the findings to other populations or samples, but simply to describe the relationships found, sampling criteria are different. And data analysis may include a number of techniques for searching out relationships,

124

and interpretation of the results will be in the form of hypotheses for further testing, rather than necessarily substantive tests of relationships.

As a general rule, if the theory permits stating formal hypotheses, a relation-searching study should not be done. Rather, an association-testing or causal hypothesis-testing study is a more direct attack on the problem, and represents a somewhat larger step on the road to prescriptive theory development than does an exploratory, relation-searching study. Using a relation-searching study design when an hypothesis-testing design could be used is not very efficient, though it may represent less intellectual risk-taking.

RESEARCH PROBLEMS

Problems for relation-searching studies are What's happening here? kinds of problems. Like other problems, they may come from clinical observations or perceptions of discrepancies, or from previous work by others.

Whole groups of relation-searching studies have come from various nurses' desire to figure out what kinds of variables in patient background, physical condition and so on, may be associated with problems that the nurse has to deal with. For example, a nurse might wonder what factors are related to the occurrence of decubitus ulcers in hospitalized patients (1). Another nurse, faced with having to do health teaching with women patients, might wonder what kinds of things seem to be associated with the incidence of *Candida albicans* in her patients (2). A medical/surgical nurse wondered what variables were related to the amount of tracheobronchial secretions she was forever having to suction in patients with tracheostomies (3). Despite a fair number of experimental studies testing the effect of nursing on postoperative patients, a pair of investigators wondered if nursing couldn't be used more efficiently if it could determine what things were associated with smoothness (or lack thereof) of postoperative recovery (4).

Another group of research questions which have led to relation-searching studies have dealt with nursing needs of particular groups of patients, for example, the elderly living in congregate housing (5). Here, the relationship that is being sought is between the characterization of the patients (elderly) and their nursing needs, with some additional searches for relationships among variables within the major classification, such as whether men and women have different needs, or whether married or single people do and so on.

Still other kinds of relation-searching problems spring from the need simply to describe a new situation. For example, a quite useful study of the kinds of patient conditions dealt with by nurse practitioner students led to some powerful suggestions for different ways to classify patient condition that made more sense for this kind of practice (6). Here, the relationship was between kinds of nurse practitioners (nurse midwife, family nurse practitioner), and the kinds of conditions or problems seen. Other studies have looked at the kinds of things bereaved people might think important in the care of their loved ones, with relationships sought according to whether the bereaved person was male or female, and what religion she/he was (7).

Other studies have looked for different perceptions of being transferred during hospitalization (8), or subjective perceptions of coronary care (9) or noise levels in acute care settings (10), all to define different conditions under which different perceptions (noise or whatever) occur.

Then there are relation-searching studies in which theories developed from other situations are examined in a new context to see if the theory "fits," and if new relationships can be teased out. Several such studies have used the notion of life crisis (amount of life change) to see if it will predict other things such as problems of pregnancy (11). In addition to using the theory in a new situation, these studies often incorporate a new piece of theory into a situation to help develop more subtle hypotheses or relationships. For example, Nuckolls took the life crisis work of Holmes and Rahe which had, to that point, hypothesized only direct linear relationships (the more life crisis, the more illness) and added a notion of psychosocial assets as mediating the effect of life crisis or life change (12). Here a new variable is examined in an old situation in order to see if it relates both to life crisis and to an outcome variable, in this case problems of pregnancy, and as it happens, the findings suggest the hypothesis that if people have social assets to depend on (family, friends and other assets), the amount of life crisis will not necessarily predict illness. But if people do not have high social assets, life crisis is more directly related to problems of pregnancy.

Finally, there are research problems in which the relationship being searched for is not even specified in advance, but the researcher plunges into the situation to try to discover if there are any relationships among the variables of interest. For example, a pediatric nurse felt she needed to know more about how children perceive their bodies, so as to know how to gear her health teaching or counseling. So she did a study to see what children knew about or understood about the insides of their bodies, then related this to the age of the child and to the child's sex (13). Another investigator wondered what kinds of health teaching information hospitalized patients get, then looked for clues about how they get it, from whom, what kind of information it is and when it is received (14). And other nurses felt that nursing is left to deal with the dependence or independence of patients during hospitalization and surgery without knowing much about what that is, or how it changes, so they related dependence-independence to stages of hospitalization (15).

In all these examples, the general form of the research problem is What's happening here? translated in technical terms to What factors are related to what? In general, the purpose behind all these studies is to understand better a situation so as to know how to intervene in it, or how to form one's prescriptions for care more accurately or acutely. Thus, one sees a good number of relation-searching studies aimed at discovering new information about patients in various situations on the theory that the more nurses know about patients and how they experience things, the better able we will be to care for them.

Even though there well may be applicable theory, either from previous studies of the same problem or studies of related problems in other areas, the theory is not yet in shape to make formal predictions, though it is well enough developed to provide operational definitions and general guidelines for the investigation. The creativity in relation-searching studies is in seeing a problem area as a brand new one, or in bringing to it new eyes and new ideas to make richer the existing knowledge—and in taking the risk of delving into an untouched area.

Note that in all the examples here, the variables are already named, in contrast to factor-searching studies where even the variables are not known. Recovery from surgery, dependence, life crisis, social assets, prognosis of pregnancy, patient condition, decubitus ulcer are all names of variables or factors, and for each one in the study, an operational definition and measurement have to be created, invented, borrowed, found or otherwise provided. There is another subtle difference between relation-searching studies and the factor-searching ones discussed in the last chapter. Here, implicit in the problem is the fact that there will ultimately be *comparisons* among cases, for example, older versus younger children, major versus minor surgery, married versus single elderly people or people with high social assets versus people with low assets. In factor-searching studies, no comparisons are implicit in the way the problem is defined because not even enough about it is known to know what to compare (16). This point is important throughout study design because when comparisons are going to be made, the same data must be collected on every case; otherwise, it is not possible to make comparisons. As we saw in the last chapter, data collection could be altered, and entirely different or new data collected when a category or concept dictated it. In relation-searching studies (and any other kind where comparisons will be made), exactly the same information must be retrieved from each sample unit.

BACKGROUND/CONCEPTUAL FRAMEWORK

In contrast to factor-searching studies where so little is known in advance that the conceptual framework may be more a perspective on the problem area than anything else, in relation-searching studies, there is some available background information from the literature or experience, but it isn't enough to allow formal predictions. For example, previous studies may have shown that life crisis or quantity of significant life change was associated with illness onset, but no one has looked at life change in a nonillness, but crisis situation, such as pregnancy. Or, investigators may not have associated social assets as "protective," that is, as mediating the linear relationship between life crisis and disease (17).

Or, despite volumes of research on psychological states, no one has examined how psychological states, such as fear and anxiety, relate to real-life situations, such as recovery from surgery. Further, no one has tried to determine the relative incidence or base rate of untoward preoperative and postoperative emotional and physiological states (which would be necessary to design studies to try to relieve untoward states) (18).

Or, in spite of several studies on decubitus ulcer formation, only increased pressure over prolonged periods was consistently related to skin breakdown, while other factors—nutrition, anemia, shearing force, heat, moisture, friction, infection and the like—had been suggested, but not documented. In addition, an investigator might have her own ideas about other things that might be associated with decubitus ulcer formation (19).

Sometimes, the information available from previous studies and the theory developed from previous research just don't fit the way an investigator has experienced the problem. For example, studies may have shown that children were not very informed about what the inside of their body was like, or where certain organs were located, but the pediatric nurse might believe from her own experience that children are really better informed than previous studies would suggest. A new study might be called for using a more sensitive technique to determine children's perceptions, and relate the perceptions to age of the child and other variables (20).

Clinical experience may lead an investigator to extend the information available in the literature to include other variables not studied, ones that might be derived from nursing knowledge. For example, it may well be known (from research in microbiology) that *Candida albicans* is related to drug addiction and diabetes, but a nurse might deduce also that there is the possibility that constant wearing of pantyhose might be related to *Candida* incidence (21). Or, the literature might suggest that urinary tract infection follows Foley catheter use frequently, but a nurse might wonder if it makes a difference whether the catheter is inserted on the ward or in the operating room (22).

The conceptual background for a relation-searching study is an attempt to pull together the available information to show the relationship of the problem to other, like problems (what the problem is an instance of). The effort is to build a conceptual case for why there is even any reason to suspect the factors chosen *might* be related. Sometimes that case will simply turn on logic. Even in the absence of previous theoretical work or research, does it make common sense that, for example, preoperative fear level might be related to postoperative recovery? Or that steroid therapy might be related to development of decubitus ulcers? Or that having family and friends around might make a difference in the way life change is experienced?

Sometimes the conceptual background is simply an extension of previous work, such as when relationships among variables have been found in one population, and the present study will see if the relationships will appear in a different population.

The conceptual framework includes in it the abstract definitions of the variables to be used. Unlike factor-searching studies in which it is not possible to provide such definitions, since that's the purpose of doing the study, in relation-searching studies, the theoretical background behind the major variables has to be stated. In the case of physiological variables such as infection rate, or secretion, or decubitus ulcers, or *Candida albicans*, the definitions are fairly simply produced. (Operational definitions may be more difficult.) In the case of psychosocial variables, it should be clear how the investigator is using the terminology, since there are sometimes competing ways of defining things like anxiety or fear or even life crisis.

Since relation-searching studies are aimed at discovering theory where there was none before, the conceptual framework is necessarily less complete than it has to be for hypothesis-testing studies. At the very least, the available literature should be reviewed to point out what is known in the area, and, therefore, what yet needs to be known. If new concepts are being added to existing knowledge, and if they come from clinical experience, they too must be defined, and the reasons why they are included, stated. Very often that statement is simply a matter of intuition coming from clinical wisdom, and no further justification is needed.

Part of the conceptual background will be why the problem is a problem for nursing, and why it is necessary to investigate it at all. Thinking this through is a bit more complicated than simply thinking that nursing needs all the knowledge it can get, and, therefore, nearly anything is legitimate to study. Some relation-searching problems are clearly attempts to figure out when, how and with whom to prescribe nursing activities in order to change a situation for the better. Some problems are more preventative—how can something we don't want to happen be stopped? Some are apparently aimed at increasing the precision of prescriptions by understanding better some aspects of patiency as in the study about children's perceptions of their bodies, or a study of social assets in life crisis. The value of the information obtained in any study depends on how the problem is characterized, since that will determine how the data are collected, so time spent in figuring out so what (So what if we find out. . . ?) is time well spent.

STUDY DESIGN

Relation-searching studies are at the second level of inquiry, factor-relating (or situation-depicting).

The time framework for relation-searching studies may be prospective, retrospective, or it may dip into the empirical situation at one particular point in time. A study of factors associated with decubitus ulcer formation was prospective (23). Certain patients were followed for two weeks to see if they developed decubitus ulcers and to find out what variables were associated with that development. A study of factors related to recovery from surgery was also prospective (24). Patients were selected before surgery, and certain measurements and tests were given before and after the operation.

Some phenomena demand a prospective approach. For example, a study of life crisis and pregnancy might require that the measurement of life crisis be taken at some arbitrary point in pregnancy (say seven months), with the measure of the outcome of pregnancy being taken two months later. Or a study of dependence-independence of hospitalized patients might examine this variable over time, to relate it to different phases in hospitalization.

The advantages of using a prospective design are two: new data that would not ordinarily be available from charts or other records can be collected; and, as a general rule, prospective studies are considered more rigorous (discussed in more detail in the next chapter).

When it is not possible to do a prospective study, retrospective studies can be done, using existing records such as charts or other sources of data. For example, it would be inefficient to follow a large group of pregnant women to determine what factors are associated with stillbirth, since it is known that the incidence of stillbirth is quite small. It is easier to study this problem retrospectively, pulling the charts of those women who had still-births to compare them with a sample of women who did not.

Other studies may examine all the variables occurring at one particular time; for example, a study of factors associated with tracheobronchial secretions might collect data on secretion, as well as all the other variables of interest, all at one time.

Research Questions

Relation-searching studies begin with research questions rather than hypotheses. The questions all take the general form, What's happening here? made specific for the problem at hand.

Castle and Osterhout's study of urinary tract catheterization and infection provides some very nicely stated research questions:

1. . . . *Who* is catheterized? Under what *circumstances?* For *how long?* and *by whom?* (Emphasis in original.)
2. . . . Which patients are already infected at the time of catheterization, and which patients become reinfected with different organisms following one or more catheterizations?
3. Which of the descriptive variables concerning the method and management of catheterization, if any, are associated with the incidence of urinary tract infections, and what are the relative risks of infections due to these associated variables? (25)

These questions spell out quite clearly what the variables are to be investigated, by classes, rather than each one specifically. For example, research question 1 implies categories of variables about patients, about time, about the care giver and about certain "circumstances," in this case, whether the catheter was inserted on the ward or in the operating room.

Sometimes research questions are even more general, stated as, What factors are associated with. . . ? (for example, with tracheobronchial secretions, with postoperative recovery). In most cases, the more specific the questions can be, the more useful they will be in guiding the investigation, and the more likely it will be that the relationship between the questions and the conceptual background will be clear. Sometimes, when the study is tackling a new area, the research question does not even specify potential associations, but simply states, for example, What are children's perceptions of their body parts? Or, What are patients' subjective impressions of the coronary care unit? Or, What kinds of patient conditions do nurse practitioner students see most commonly? On the whole, it is wise to make research questions somewhat more specific than these examples and to make explicit whatever kinds of associations will be sought. It is quite common in relation-searching studies that an area is selected for study, a very general research question is posed, data are collected on anything that looks interesting within the area, and after the data are in, decisions are made about what variables to try to relate to what. For a study at this level of inquiry, that is acceptable, but when the potential associations can be stated in advance, they should be. Even though relation-searching studies are still exploratory, that's no excuse for just messing around in the data. The more the study can be guided by prior thought, if not by explicit theory, the better the study will be and the larger the increment of theory construction.

The excitment of relation-searching studies can come in trying to think through all the possible variables that might be associated with each other, or with one single criterion variable. For example, the study of children's perceptions of their bodies could have been enriched by thinking in advance about all the things that might be related to how children think about the inside of themselves. For example, age of the children, and sex were two variables included in the study. But how about birth order? Education of the parents? Occupation of the parents? Intelligence of child? Certain kinds of life experiences of the child, such as previous surgery? Forcing oneself to state research questions as specifically as possible forces one to think consciously about potential relationships where stating a general research question and then plunging into the problem does not.

Setting

As in all other kinds of studies, the first criterion on which to select a setting is whether it contains the variables of interest. Then, is it possible to collect the data in the setting chosen? General considerations in choosing a setting and in researcher relationships within one were covered in Chapter 3, and they do not differ for relation-searching studies.

Sample

Since the purpose of relation-searching studies is not to generalize to other samples, the sampling method may or may not attempt to be representative of some larger theoretical population. Most often, relation-searching studies use convenience sampling, taking the first one hundred cases of urinary tract infection with catheterization, or the first ninety cases of general abdominal surgery, or as many pregnant women as one can find from a given clinic in the time one has to find them.

When it is possible to select a sample randomly, it is a good idea even for studies at this level of inquiry. The criticism of other kinds of sampling is always that it cannot be known how representative the sample is of the population. While the results of relation-searching studies may not be intended to apply to larger populations (be generalized), theory developed from samples chosen rigorously may be more useful than theory developed from unique samples in special settings or small samples of any kind.

Often, relation-searching studies contain a large number of variables, all to be related to one another, or to one other criterion variable. When this is the case, the sample size has to be larger than the number of variables, otherwise, one will run out of cases to compare when cross-tabulating variables on each other. There is no magic number that makes a sample size "adequate." The larger the number of variables, the larger the sample must be in order to detect any relationships that might be there.

The principle guiding the selection of a sample of patients or observations in relation-searching studies is how much can be learned (about the relevant factors) from them. In order to compare cases and specify relationships, there must also be variation in the sample of things to be compared. Put another way, the sample is heterogeneous. For example, if the study is about the relationship between age and recovery from surgery, one would have to have within the sample a distribution of ages. If only people of the same age were included, no statements about the relationship could be made.

There are several ways to be sure that the sample will contain variation. If the dimensions of the factors are known (for example, people's ages can differ), sampling units can be selected according to their place on the continuum. Such sampling is called *purposive* —deliberately selecting people on the basis of some *a priori* characteristic.

When it is possible to think in advance of a variable that is particularly crucial to the problem, then purposive sampling may be used to make sure that in a small sample, the entire range of variables can be encompassed. For instance, if one wanted to study life crisis among the elderly, and a small sample had to be used, one might deliberately look for people on different points in the life crisis continuum, for example, recently retired people versus those still working; widows or widowers versus those with living spouses; people with families versus those without and so on. (Death of a spouse, change in work, family change are all items on the life change scale.) To sample purposively, one has to know not only what the potential range of the variable is, but one has to have a way to locate individuals who occupy particular points on that continuum. When it is possible to do so, purposive sampling can be a powerful tactic, as long as it is realized that conclusions from a sample selected purposively are chancy at best. But as a tool for theory construction, it can be quite useful to know for sure that the sample contains a wide range of variation on the variables of interest.

Given a large enough sample selected at convenience or randomly (and again there is no magic number), one can expect that the entire range of the phenomena will be included just by chance alone, unless the setting from which the sample was gathered is unusual. For example, in a study about children's perceptions of their bodies, data gathered from a school for exceptional children would not necessarily contain the whole range of children's perceptions.

Sometimes relation-searching studies begin with convenience sampling and change to purposive sampling after a while to be sure that there will be variation. If after a few cases it seems that the age of the patients is relatively constant, the researcher may skip the next few people of the same age and wait for someone older or younger to appear. Similarly, the researcher may be interested in a combination of characteristics. For example, age, previous hospital experience and diagnosis might be the three factors considered important. The researcher might begin with convenience sampling, then select deliberately to fill all possible combinations of people with the three variables—for example, young age, no experience, medical case; young age, some experience, medical; young age, no experience, surgical; young age, some experience, surgical; older age, no experience, medical and so on. Such purposive sampling can become time-consuming if there are a number of factors in various combinations. Even with only three factors in this example, there are six possible combinations if each factor has ony two categories (old-young, for example). To obtain a sample large enough so that all the people in one category combination can be compared with all those in another combination would be quite time-consuming. Even with only ten people in each possible combination, the total sample size would be sixty, which is not very large.

Another way to increase the heterogeneity of the sample is to select the very typical case and the very atypical case. This assumes, of course, that some of the major factors that make a case typical or atypical are known. Yet another way is to select cases from the extremes of a continuum. For example, talkativeness may range from muteness to extreme verbosity. The researcher might select a sample of people from both ends of the scale—extremely taciturn and extremely verbose—in order to compare them with respect to other factors.

These kinds of sampling are also known as "known groups." Some research problems will call for samples of known groups, when the criterion variable (the outcome) comes only in the form of presence or absence. For example, the study of factors associated with stillbirth would demand selection of a sample of women who had stillborns and a sample who did not, since stillbirth is a variable that only has two possibilities—either it's there or it isn't. And, of course, one cannot study the relationship of factors to stillbirth if one looks only at a sample of women who had stillborns; one could never conclude that whatever associations were found wouldn't also be found in a sample of women with live births.

As in other kinds of studies, data on the sample characteristics are reported in detail, as are details on how the sample was gathered. Very often, sample characteristics are themselves the variables of interest (age, sex, marital status, social class and the like) so sample descriptions are not reported separately, but as part of the data analysis. Enough information about the sample has to be provided the reader so that the reader can judge how applicable the findings from the study might be to other samples and how relevant the theory developed from the study is.

Instruments/Measurements

Relation-searching studies may use any of a number of different kinds of instruments or measurements to give operational definition to the factors of interest. Interviews, questionnaires, paper-and-pencil tests, self-reports, scales, observations, physiological measures, nurse ratings, checklists—any instrument that fits the variable may be chosen. Often relation-searching studies will use a variety of techniques and instruments, since it may not be known which tactic will work best. A study of preoperative emotional state and postoperative recovery, for example, used several different measures of fear and anxiety and one aim of the study was to figure out which way(s) worked best (26).

Operational definitions, selection of instruments and measurements, follow directly from the research question and the problem. And every variable on which data are to be collected must have its own operational definition and a set of rules which guide how the data are to be coded, what evidence will be taken as indicating the presence or absence of a given variable, or a certain place on a continuum.

Since relation-searching studies may be called for when certain variables haven't been investigated before, these studies often include brand new instruments, invented for the study and never tested before. When this is the case, considerable time goes into constructing the instrument to be as sure as possible that it fits the concept, that it is practical, that it will produce enough data and enough variation and that it can be reliably used.

Comparisons among and between cases are going to be made in relation-searching studies, so the data from case to case have to be equivalent. Reliability of instruments and measurements then becomes an issue. Reliability is the extent to which repeated measures of the same thing, or measures by two different data collectors of the same thing at the same time, will produce exactly the same information. Therefore, any instruments used should have detailed instructions for their use so that everyone collecting data will do it in the same way.

Validity—the extent to which the measure measures what it's supposed to measure—is often simply assumed in relation-searching studies when a **new** measure has been invented. When an instrument has been used previously, information about its validity should be supplied. Reliability and validity and other measurement criteria are discussed in detail in Chapter 9.

When a study deals with the association of factors to one single criterion variable, the definition of that variable is critical. For example, if the study deals with factors associated with skin breakdown, that must be defined precisely: ". . . an area over which the skin has broken (is discontinuous), which has not shown signs of healing in one week as measured by decrease in diameter of the lesion." (27) Or, a study of factors associated with urinary tract infection defines infection: ">100,000 organisms per ml. in a carefully collected midstream specimen, >100,000 organisms per ml. in a carefully aspirated catheter specimen; ≥10 white blood cells per high power field in a uncentrifuged clean collected specimen; >100,000 organisms per ml. of a different pathogen than that in a previous culture." (28)

All details of coding or scoring raw data have to be decided in advance (though when the data are in, they may be collapsed or combined).

Data Collection

Data collection always aspires to be objective. In relation-searching studies, equivalent data are collected on all cases, meaning that the same data are collected in the same way from all sample units. Equivalence is assured by using written protocols or procedures, interviews, checklists and the like, and by strict adherence to these guidelines established in advance.

It is useful to plan in advance what categories of the factors will eventually be used in data analysis, though it is wise to collect data raw (uncollapsed) so that different kinds of categorization may be possible later. For instance, if age will be a factor, it is a good idea to collect actual ages of patients, even if later the ages will be grouped—twenty–thirty, thirty–forty and so on. Data are lost when collapsing is done, and since relation-searching studies are attempts to develop theory, the data should be as rich as possible to begin with. Later decisions may be made about how to reduce the data to some manageable amount, but the raw data will always be there.

Very often in relation-searching studies, even though the factors are all named in advance, subcategories or properties of factors may not be known. Interviews will sometimes contain open-ended questions to be categorized later. Just because relation-searching studies are at a higher level of inquiry than factor-searching studies, there is often a tiny factor-searching study built into relation-searching, and into studies at other levels of inquiry as well. The difference in process is that constant comparative analysis is rarely used to develop categories from anecdotal or other qualitative data in relation-searching studies; rather, all the data are collected, then the categories are developed from the data later, rather than as the data are being collected.

As in any other kind of study, informed consent and assurance of the confidentiality of information are mandatory.

Data Processing/Analysis

The three steps in any data processing are description, classification and enumeration. Description is already done as part of selecting the operational definitions for the factors. The particular data that will be taken as evidence of the existence of a category or factor are determined in advance. Classification may be done in advance, too, as in the case of using categories already developed. Classification as a part of data processing then simply means putting the case into the category in which it fits. Enumeration means counting up the number of things or people in the given categories, for example, frequencies, percentages.

Data processing reduces the amount of data to the point where it can be handled. Therefore, it is important to be aware of the number of reductions that are made in processing the data. The further the reductions from the original observation, the less relevant the findings will be. For example, suppose blood pressure readings had been taken on a number of patients admitted to a hospital. In processing the data, the readings might be rank ordered, then divided in the middle to form two categories—high blood pressure and low blood pressure. Suppose, in addition, that tape recordings of the conversation of the patient had been made at the same time the blood pressure readings were taken. One might simply count up the number of sentences spoken during that time, again rank order them, and come up with two categories—high verbal and low verbal. These kinds of procedures are fairly typical, though a little overstated here. The amount of data is greatly decreased by doing this. The more collapsing that is done, the more "real" data are lost. A person with a blood pressure reading of 140 may then be in the same category as a person with a blood pressure reading of 180, which may obscure important differences between them. Knowing what collapsing data does to the original observations will help determine the data processing procedures.

How and when such procedures are used is determined in part by the statement of the problem, in part by the precision of the measurements and in large part by clinical wisdom. If the statement of the problem has led to suggested relationships between large categories of information such as high verbal and low verbal, in the example above, it makes sense to analyze the data this way, knowing that medium verbal will be left out.

It is possible to obtain quite precise, but clinically meaningless, information if precise measurement tools are available. Clinical wisdom will lead to combining categories, or grouping data more meaningfully. For example, actual minutes of the various stages of labor can be calculated and counted, but minutes are probably too fine a measure for first stage labor (but not for second stage). Similarly, blood pressure in mm. Hg is standard, but the difference of 1 mm. Hg when the systolic reading is 120 versus 121 is probably meaningless, whereas grouping blood pressures into intervals of 5 mm. Hg may make more sense. On the other hand, centimeters or fractions of them may be crucial in a study about decubitus ulcers, and no attempt would be made to collapse the information or group it.

There are several kinds of relationships that can be discovered in relation-searching studies. Two factors may simply occur together; when one is present another is also present—they occur at the same time. Or factors may vary together, as one changes, the other(s) do too. One factor may cause another factor to change or to occur; one factor may inhibit another factor's occurrence or its change; factors may vary together without any statement being made about whether one causes the other; one factor may act as a catalyst to another factor, that is, although it does not cause it, it increases its action; or one factor may deter another.

The aim of data analysis in relation-searching studies is literally to figure out what the relationships among factors or variables are, if any. This usually means relating every factor to every other one in such a way that a conceptual chain of variables emerges. Depending on how the research questions are stated, the process may be modified and become more descriptive, as in the case of the study of urinary tract infection following Foley catheterization mentioned earlier. Here, certain relationships of particular interest were listed in the research questions—for example, "under what circumstances does urinary tract infection occur?" (29). Comparisons of frequency of UTI in women who had been catheterized on the ward versus in the operating room answers the question.

Data analysis consists of comparing cases to relate factors. The number of cases (or the exact reading) in a particular category of one factor is compared with the number in another category of the same factor. The statistical techniques of multiple regression, analysis of covariance and other tests lend themselves naturally to determining the probability that the relationships found occurred by chance or not. While these tests are beyond the scope of this book, the logic behind them and the general method can be illustrated by a kind of categorical analysis called "path analysis." (30) Here, the "path" among the variables is charted so that at the end, a theory can be constructed that hypothesizes relationships of particular kinds between and among the variables tested.

For illustration, take a study of what factors are related to the way women perform (how they cope) in second stage labor (delivery of the baby) (31). Here, the nurse had observed that women seem to perform differently and wondered what, in attitude, fear, first stage labor experience and other variables, were related to second stage performance. She felt that if the relationships could be teased out, nurses might be able to decide how and when to intervene with mothers in labor to help them cope better during delivery.

For purposes of this illustration, only four variables will be tackled: parity, planning of pregnancy, fear and attitude. Data on planning and fear level were obtained in a postpartum interview; data on attitude were derived from scores on a test of maternal attitude toward pregnancy. Each variable was collapsed into two categories: planned or unplanned pregnancy, optimal fear or not (based on theory), positive versus negative attitude and primiparity versus multiparity.

First, the relationships between each variable and the criterion variable—performance during second stage labor—were tested. Then, each variable was examined for its relationship to every other one, and finally three variables at a time were tested to see what pattern emerged. In the case of the variables used here for illustration, after the initial test had shown a relationship between planning, attitude, fear and performance during second stage, and there were some hints of relationship among them (and others as well), three variables were examined together, with one (in this case planning) serving as the test factor. The purpose was to see whether the relationship between attitude and fear would change if another variable—planning—were controlled.

Two tables were made, one of the relationship between attitude and fear in those women who planned the pregnancy, and one between the same two variables with those women who did not plan.

Table 5-1 (32). *Attitude and Fear Under Differential Conditions of Planning Pregnancy*

		PLANNED FEAR LEVEL				NOT PLANNED FEAR LEVEL	
		Optimal	Not Optimal			Optimal	Not Optimal
Attitude	High	70%	29%	Attitude	High	50%	50%
	Low	50%	50%		Low	43%	57%

When the relationship between attitude and fear (initially a weak one) was examined under different conditions of planning, the relationship disappeared. That is, there were no (or slight) differences in the percentages of cases that fell in contiguous cells of the tables under either condition of planning. The biggest difference was among women who planned their pregnancy and who had positive attitudes; they tended to have the optimal level of fear more often. All the other percentages in the tables are essentially equal, meaning there is no general relationship between the variables of fear and attitude, when planning of pregnancy is controlled, only a specific relationship when pregnancy is planned.

Then, different conditions of parity were introduced, to produce another table of relationship between attitude and fear (Table 5-2):

It appears that in primiparas, a positive attitude makes no difference in fear level, but primiparas with a negative attitude achieve optimal levels of fear more often. The relationship is stronger in multiparas, where positive attitude leads to optimal fear and negative attitude to nonoptimal fear levels, rather a more straightforward relationship. This means that parity is a variable that helps specify the relationship between knowledge and attitude,

Table 5-2. *Attitude and Fear Under Differential Conditions of Parity*

		MULTIPARAS FEAR LEVEL				PRIMIPARAS FEAR LEVEL	
		Optimal	Not Optimal			Optimal	Not Optimal
Attitude	High	67%	33%	Attitude	High	50%	50%
	Low	33%	67%		Low	67%	33%

that is, that it helps make clearer the relationship. (Planning and parity had already been examined and no relationship found.)

The next step would be to add another variable to the chain, say, knowledge about pregnancy, to see if under different conditions of knowledge, the relationship between fear and attitude stays the same or changes. If it stays the same, knowledge is not a specifying variable; if it changes, knowledge is a condition that affects both fear and attitude, and needs to be taken into account in developing a theoretical chain of variables.

All other variables that have earlier been shown to be related to performance would then be added to the equation until, after many, many of these tables, a theory can be built up to describe the connections among factors, under different conditions of each factor. In the example used here, the final theory suggested that planned pregnancy leads to increased knowledge, knowledge leads to optimal fear, optimal fear leads to positive attitude and positive attitude leads to increased performance. The time sequence suggested comes not from the path analysis itself, but from the nurse-researcher's own sense of what makes sense in the chain of factors. Indeed, picking which factors to use in path analysis is partly a clinical decision on which will be most meaningful.

This kind of procedure is specific to situations in which variables can be collapsed into dichotomies. The logic of taking two variables first, then adding a third, then a fourth and so on is essentially identical with the logic behind statistical procedures for variables not collapsed into dichotomies. In the case of variables measured on continuous scales, first every variable is correlated with every other one, then variables are taken together, with new variables being added to the maneuver at each step until a collection of variables accounts for as much of the relationship as possible. Computer programs make the process relatively painless, more so than the example given here which is done by hand and is very tedious.

As a general rule, data analysis in relation-searching studies should be carried to the point of multiple comparisons. Hypotheses derived from relation-searching studies are more likely to be useful if they can include as many variables as possible. Similarly, descriptive findings by themselves are more valuable when interrelationships among factors have been teased out than when each factor is simply related to every other one without elaboration. In the example of performance in second stage labor used here, the putative theory developed by arriving at a chain of relationships from parity through planning of pregnancy, knowledge, fear and attitude is more useful in advancing the cause of clinical knowledge than simple findings that planning, parity, knowledge are all related to performance by themselves. Similarly, a conclusion like "a profile of a patient likely to develop [decubitus ulcers]: a thin, febrile male with an infection who may be receiving cortico-steroid therapy" (33) is more instructive than statements about the frequency of decubitus ulcers in men and women, those with infections and not, those receiving steroids and not and so on, each taken singly. The whole point of relation-searching studies is to develop theory and the better stated and more encompassing the theory can be, the larger a step forward it is.

INTERPRETATION

The question to be asked of theory developed from relation-searching studies is how credible is it? Does the theory make sense? Does it seem adequate to explain the factors involved and their relationships? Does it leave unexplained cases?

Interpretation of data at this level of inquiry is necessarily tentative. Methods of measurement may be less than precise, samples may be small, statistical findings may be more suggestive than anything. The interpretations of data should be in the form of hypotheses for further investigation (as well as descriptions of what was found). Sometimes the suggestions for future research will lead to measurement studies, or back into factor-searching if the data lead one to conclude that further work on the topic must await better conceptualization of the variables.

Sometimes the results of a relation-searching study will suggest that next time around different variables should be included. The very exercise of encountering the real world in a relation-searching study may lead to reconceiving the problem with different, or additional, factors discovered not so much through the formal research, but through the informal process of collecting data and thinking it through. For example, in the second stage labor study, the researcher simply noticed that during delivery, when nurses or anesthetists gave their directions to "push" or not simply, directly and consistently to the patient, she was able to perform better. The activities of caregivers had been recorded, but were not the major focus of the study. At the end, one suggested direction for future research was for further study of this observation, perhaps in an experimental design where different forms of support during delivery could be tested.

Relation-searching studies often amass amazing amounts of data to be reported, and it is all too often the case that reports end with research jargon exposition instead of plain English. There is a significant correlation between fear level and performance during second stage labor is not nearly as helpful as, Women with moderate amounts of fear performed better, or whatever the English translation is. One purpose of any research effort is to stimulate other research efforts, and one way to do that is by making the findings make sense not just to the research-sophisticated reader, but to the interested nurse. Another purpose of any research effort is to improve practice, and part of the researcher's responsibility is to put the information gained into a form that can be used by one's colleagues in practice.

While the ideal state may be that relation-searching studies, and their suggested hypotheses at the end, be carried formally further to the point of confirmation of the hypothesis, it is simply a fact that "findings," even tentative ones, will be used without further confirmation, so great is nursing's need for knowledge to improve care. Therefore, when possible, the findings should be put into useable form. The "patient profile"of the decubitus ulcer study is one way to do it. When the data allow (as is sometimes the case in multiple regression analysis), results can be worded almost as a formula: If a woman without preexisting urinary tract infection has a catheter inserted preoperatively on the ward, she has a 33 percent chance of getting an infection.

As in any study, the first mission in interpreting data is to figure out, and then state, what the data mean. In addition, explicit suggestions for future research should be made, in the form of hypotheses, if that's what are suggested, or in the form of ideas for measurement studies or statements of the need for factor-searching to identify additional variables. Suggestions for improving the knowledge by tightening up on the methods of study should also be stated as directly as possible.

Because relation-searching studies are done when it is not possible to develop and test hypotheses or when a topic area is new or not investigated, the researcher can become quite excited by findings that open up new insights into an unknown topic. It requires some exercise of discipline not to go beyond the data in interpreting them, that is, not to make sweeping generalizations of findings that do not respect the limitations of the study itself. It is particularly hard to resist the temptation to attribute cause-and-effect relationships when they have not been tested at all (see Chapter 7). It is not at all wrong to suggest causal relationships as hypotheses for further study. And common sense will lead to some quasi-causal statements, simply because some variables occur before others, and, therefore, could naturally be treated as causing the variation in others that happen later. For example, planning of pregnancy probably happens before knowledge and attitude toward delivery (though a case could be made that attitude might lead to planning) so it is natural to develop the chain of variables in a certain order. But causal relationships, or even associational ones, are not *tested* in a relation-searching study.

As in factor-searching studies, the challenge in relation-searching is to make sense of the new information in a way that leads to further questions. The discovery of theory can be as compelling an experience as testing it (see the next three chapters). Generating new hypotheses, new ways to look at old phenomena or even new phenomena just discovered represents an important stage not only in the levels of inquiry as discussed in this book, but in the state of development of knowledge for a practice profession. The elegance of the method of discovery in clinical research lies not in the techniques of research so much, but in the "issues tackled, the questions raised, and the hypotheses proposed." (34)

NOTES

1. Williams, Ann: Study of factors contributing to skin breakdown. *Nursing Research*, 21:238–243, May–June 1972.

2. Daus, Anita and E.S.E. Hafez: Candida albicans in women. *Nursing Research*, 24:430–433, November–December 1975. See also letter to the editor by Joann McCloskey, *Nursing Research*, 25:141, March–April 1976 and the authors' response.

3. Ambron, Sylvia A.: Clinical signs associated with amount of tracheobronchial secretions. *Nursing Research*, 25:121–216, March–April 1976.

4. Wolfer, John A. and Carol E. Davis: Assessment of surgical patients' preoperative emotional condition and postoperative welfare. *Nursing Research*, 19:402–414, September–October 1970.

5. Hain, Sr. Mary Jeanne: Health needs of the elderly. *Nursing Research*, 25:433–438, November–December 1976.

6. Chen, Shu-Pi, et al.: Documented clinical experiences of primary care nurse students. *Nursing Research*, 26:342–348, September–October 1977: Chen, Shu-Pi, et al.: Patient encounters by primary care students. *Research in Nursing and Health*, 1:18–28, April, 1978.

7. Freihofer, Patricia and Geraldene Felton: Nursing behaviors in bereavement: an exploratory study. *Nursing Research*, 25:332–337, September–October 1976. This study has excellent examples of research questions.

8. Smith, Mary Colette: Patient responses to being transferred during hospitalization. *Nursing Research*, 25:192–196, May–June 1976. This study is an interesting example of how a patient problem perceived by a nurse turns out not to be a problem to patients after all.

9. Geertsen, H. Reed, et al.: Subjective aspects of coronary care. *Nursing Research*, 25:211–215, May–June 1976.

10. Woods, Nancy Fugate: Noise stimuli in the acute care area. *Nursing Research*, 23:144–150, March–April 1974.

11. Nuckolls, Katherine B., et al.: Psychosocial assets, life crisis and the prognosis of pregnancy. *American Journal of Epidemiology*, 95(5):431–441, 1972; see also, Peszecker, Betty and Jo McNeil: Relationship among health habits, social assets, psychologic wellbeing, life change and alterations in health status. *Nursing Research*, 24:442–447, November–December 1975.

12. See Nuckolls, Note 11. The work of Holmes and Rahe in life stress and illness is voluminous. Early reports, which stimulated a great deal of other work are Holmes, T.H., et al.: Experimental study of prognosis. *Journal of Psychosomatic Research*, 5(4):235–252, 1961; also, Rahe, R.H., et al.: Social stress and illness onset. *Journal of Psychosomatic Research*, 8(1):35–44, 1964.

13. Porter, Carol S.: Grade school children's perceptions of their internal body parts. *Nursing Research*, 23:384–391, September–October 1974.

14. Pender, Nola J.: Patient identification of health information received during hospitalization. *Nursing Research*, 23:262–267, May–June 1974.

15. Derdiarian, Anayis and Dorothy Clough: Patients' dependence and independence levels on the pre-hospitalization-post-hospitalization continuum. *Nursing Research*, 25:27–34, January–February 1976.

16. The reader should be aware of the difference between "comparison" as used here and terminology used in Chapter 4—"constant comparative analysis." The latter would seem to imply the kind of case-to-case comparisons being discussed here, but it really is a different kind of animal altogether. Constant comparative analysis is a conceptual, rather than empirical activity where events are "compared" not in order to find sameness, but to find the subtle differences that will enrich the meaning of the developing concept. For this kind of analytic activity, equivalent data from event to event are not only necessary, they may be counterindicated, when the purpose is to flesh out a concept, provide it with different properties, define it fully. This is quite a different process from empirical comparison, as it is presented in this chapter, where the intent is to see how many like (or different) instances can be obtained so that empirically derived patterns of relationships can be established, knowing that the data on each instance (case) were collected in the same way, with the same instruments, so that the data are equivalent.

17. Nuckolls, see Note 11.

18. Wolfer and Davis, see Note 4.

19. Williams, see Note 1.

20. Porter, see Note 13.

21. Daus and Hefez, see Note 2.

22. Castle, Mary and Suydam Osterhaut: Urinary catheterization and associated infection. *Nursing Research*, 23:170–174, March–April 1974.

23. Williams, see Note 1.

24. Wolfer and Davis, see Note 4.

25. Castle and Osterhout, see Note 22, p. 170.

26. Wolfer and Davis, see Note 4.

27. Williams, see Note 1, p. 328.

28. Castle and Osterhout, see Note 22, p. 171.

29. *Ibid.*

30. See Lazarsfeld, Paul and Morris Rosenberg: *The Language of Social Research.* New York: Free Press of Glencoe, 1955, pp. 111–166. This kind of "multivariate analysis" is not to be confused with statistical multivariate (factorial or multiple regression) analysis. Path analysis was invented for use with dichotomous data before the advanced kinds of statistical packages for multivariate analysis were available.

31. Kopp (Daniels), Lois: An exploratory study of the responses of mothers to support during the second stage of labor. Unpublished master's thesis, Yale University School of Nursing, 1967, especially pp. 73–75. I apologize for using an unpublished report for this rather lengthy discussion of path analysis, but it makes the point so well. It would be unusual to see in the nursing literature a full description of this kind of process since it occurs only in exploratory studies which are less likely to reach the publication stage in any event. The kind of detail necessary to understand the example simply demanded this particular citation.

32. In the original, the sample size was only 20, making percentages quite questionable. But for purposes of this illustration, they were useful.

33. Williams, see Note 1, p. 328.

34. Spitzer, Walter O.: Canadian studies of primary care delivery by nurse practitioners. In Williams, Carolyn and Joyce Semradek (eds): *Resolving Dilemmas in Practice Research: Decisions for Practice.* Chapel Hill: University of North Carolina School of Nursing, 1976, pp. 20–47. Spitzer distinguishes three "streams" in biomedical research: laboratory research, clinical research and health care research, in chronological order. In laboratory research, he says, "excellence is demonstrated by the hypotheses" (p. 21), and in health care research "the challenges are methodological (p. 22)."

6

Association-Testing Studies

INTRODUCTION

Studies at the third level of inquiry include association-testing studies (covered in this chapter) and causal hypothesis-testing studies (next chapter). Though the study designs are markedly different, both kinds of studies are at the third level of inquiry, aimed at developing predictive theory, through stating formal predictions of relationships, then designing a rigorous test of the predictions. In contrast to the kinds of studies discussed in the previous two chapters, in which discovery of theory was the end point, studies at the third level of inquiry are aimed at testing theory, or verification. Association-testing studies differ from causal hypothesis-testing studies by virtue of the difference in the formally stated, predicted relationship. Association-testing studies deal with topics, problems, research areas in which cause-and-effect statements are not directly tested. Instead, statements of relationship, or association between or among variables are tested. Because no tests of causation are going to be made, study designs for association-testing studies are different from designs for testing causal hypotheses.

Association-testing studies are also called "explanatory" in some literature (1), "correlational," or "survey design" (2) and are distinguished from exploratory studies on the one hand, and experimental studies on the other. Association-testing studies presume earlier factor- and relation-searching, if not formally in prior studies, then informally through the literature. Whereas relation-searching studies end with theory developed in the form of hypotheses for future testing, association-testing studies begin at that point, with stated hypotheses and formal procedures for testing them.

"Association" is a particular kind of a relationship among factors. Associations or correlations mean that factors occur together or vary together, but no attempt is made to say that one causes another. Associations can be positive—the factors vary together in the same direction; as one increases, the other does—or negative—the factors vary together but in different direc-

144

tion; as one increases, the other decreases. Hypotheses about associations come from previous research and/or from clinical hunches.

Unlike causal hypothesis-testing studies, in which the natural situation is deliberately manipulated to test the effect of one independent variable, association-testing studies depend on the natural variation already present in the situation. No attempt is made to change the natural situation; rather data are collected on whatever is going on, and the effort is to determine whether the predictions made in advance about what might be related to what will indeed be supported. Association-testing studies are at a higher level of inquiry than relation-searching or factor-searching studies because the factors are already named and defined, and the theory is developed to the point where predictions can be derived.

In the published literature, there are numerous studies that sit on the line between relation-searching and association-testing. The position taken here is that not only is this confusing, but to use a study design specific for one purpose (say relation-searching) to accomplish another (testing an association) is methodologically unsound. The power of association-testing comes from deriving hypotheses from theory, then designing tests of them that will later allow claims of tested relationship, with evidence about how probable it is that the relationship found is "real." Relation-searching studies, without hypotheses and with a true exploratory framework, do not allow such claims, nor were they intended to.

For some reason, the number of association-testing studies about problems in patient care is relatively small. There are large numbers of association-testing studies about nurses and other nonpatient-oriented problems (3). In clinical research, there is usually the overwhelming urge (as there should be) to study problems that will eventually lead to causal hypotheses and statements, rather than to be satisfied with establishing correlations among variables. Thus, as we will see in the next chapter, there are now a fairly large number of experimental studies in clinical practice in the literature which deal with the effects of different kinds of nursing practices on patients. Association-testing studies are not a poor substitute for causal hypothesis-testing studies; instead, they are specific to a particular kind of research problem in which the interest is in natural variation and the desire is to link up variables by formal statements of relationship.

RESEARCH PROBLEMS

Problems for association-testing studies are variants of What will happen if . . . ? stated more accurately as What happens if . . . ? "What happens to diabetics who are 'internally controlled,' will they learn differently and control their illness differently?" (4) "What happens to people who behave in certain ways in the recovery room, will they have different postoperative courses?" (5) "When patients have fevers, do they experience time differently than when they do not?" (6) "Do children of handicapped parents feel differently about their own bodies than children of non-handicapped parents?" (7)

Note that in all these examples, the interest is in *difference* or comparison. And note also, that in contrast to research problems for relation-searching studies, the problem itself implies more theoretical background, and less need to simply leap in and explore. Instead of asking What's happening here? research problems for association-testing studies assume that something *is* happening here, and particular somethings at that. Previous research and theory lead one to suspect—guess—or in technical terms, hypothesize, the particular variations in contrast to relation-searching studies where one is even guessing that anything is happening.

Problems for association-testing studies arise when the interest is in testing whether a guessed-at relationship is really there, with no intention to establish cause and effect, or in situations in which it is not possible to test directly cause and effect because the situation cannot be manipulated by introducing the cause to examine the effect. For example, one cannot make some parents handicapped and some not in order to compare them, but one can take methodological advantage of the fact that some parents *are* handicapped, and some are not. Similarly, one cannot assign particular personality types to individuals *a priori*, but one can depend on the fact that in a given sample of people, personality type will vary naturally.

It is no accident that the association-testing study design was developed most fully in sociology, where it is not possible to control the natural variation of phenomena of interest to sociologists, and where the variables themselves are social conditions. For instance, the variable social class cannot be introduced or manipulated, but sociologists can look at the natural variation in social class and predict relationships to other variables, such as mental illness (8).

Research problems for association-testing studies come from a wish to know more about a given situation and to know more specifically about certain aspects of the situation. Rather than taking a shotgun exploratory approach to a new situation, as would be the case with a relation-searching study problem, the situation is conceived of in such a way that particular variables are singled out to be of interest. Previous research and theory lead one to select particular variables rather than simply trying to find out if anything is related to anything else.

BACKGROUND/CONCEPTUAL FRAMEWORK

The review of the literature will have led the researcher to the conclusion that there is reason to believe that some association exists between or among certain variables. This does not necessarily mean that there is *more* literature on a given topic, than is available for topics at lower levels of inquiry, though there may be. Rather, the concepts have definitions and the theory has evolved to the point where explicit predictions are possible. The predictions are derived from the theoretical background and the connections between the hypotheses and the theory are made clear. The more explicit those connections and the clearer their derivation, the easier will be the job of interpreting data once they are collected.

Since association-testing studies are theory-testing, the use of theory both in defining the hypotheses and in interpreting data are different at this level of inquiry. Theory is more than merely a point of view or perspective (as in factor-searching studies), and more than merely an outline of possibilities (as in relation-searching). In prediction-testing studies, theory should make the logical case for the predicted relationship to be tested, and it should be easy to see how the researcher got to the hypothesis from the theoretical background.

This does not mean necessarily that there will have been previous investigations of the exact topic at hand. Theory developed in one area may be used to apply to another, to see if it will work, or fit, or predict as successfully in a new area of application as it did before. For example, one theory about the relationship of life change had built up tested associations between life change and illness onset. But the next study could take that theory and hypothesize that life change might also be associated with nonillness situations, such as aging (9). Or theory that predicts that people of certain personality types behave differently could be used to hypothesize that personality type will be associated with a particular kind of behavior, that is, recovery from surgery, as seen in the recovery room behavior (10).

The present state of clinical knowledge means that very often association-testing studies use theory developed in other situations and apply it to new ones, namely to clinical situations. Theories from psychology or psychiatry, as in the case of the life change work or personality types, or theories developed in other disciplines are tested to see if they will hold up under real-life conditions with clinical problems. The new application of theory is in the service of understanding more about how patients (or potential patients) experience situations or events in the health care system so as to know better when or how to intervene to prevent or alter untoward patient experiences.

The job of the clinical researcher is to make a case for why the theory developed in another context ought to work in the present clinical problem. This means that the problem itself has to be conceived of as an instance of the problem addressed by the theory. For example, the problem of how much diabetics know about their disease and how well they can control it has to be seen as an instance of "locus of control"—the extent to which people believe they control their own existence, versus being controlled by forces outside themselves (11). Or aging has to be seen as an instance of the larger notion of life change and life stress (12).

As discussed earlier (in Chapter 1), almost any clinical problem could be investigated at almost any level of inquiry. What makes a problem an association-testing study problem is the extent to which it is possible to see the relationship of the problem to existing conceptual material, and, thus, derive from theory specific, noncausal hypotheses to be tested.

STUDY DESIGN

Association-testing studies are at the third level of inquiry—situation-relating, or predictive.

In association-testing studies there is no attempt to deliberately change reality other than stopping the action to measure at a particular point. There are several types of study designs that are used in association-testing studies: cross-sectional, retrospective, prospective and mixed.

In the *cross-sectional* type of association-testing study, the action is stopped and measurements of both variables in the hypothesis are taken. For instance, an hypothesis about the relationship between the educational level of women and the number of misconceptions they have about labor and delivery could be tested by selecting a sample and measuring the women on both variables at the same time.

The cross-sectional design is familiar from opinion polls taken on national samples. In this case, respondents are asked not only their preferences or opinions, but also something about themselves—age, ethnic background and so on. Then correlations between preferences and other variables can be done.

In a *retrospective* design, one factor occurs before the other one, though both measurements may be taken at the same time. For example, suppose a nurse was interested in the relationship between APGAR scores on babies at one and five minutes and the length of the mothers' labors. Obviously, labor occurs before birth. The investigator might record the APGAR scores and then look back at the chart to determine the length of labor. Some epidemiological studies employ this design, for example, in looking for patterns in the lives of people who have died of leukemia. The diagnosis of leukemia is made first, then earlier health records are surveyed.

The *prospective* design is the third kind of design available in the association-testing study. This is more easily understood as a follow-up study. For example, suppose a nurse was interested in how the newborn infant's APGAR rating is related to the infant's physical condition on the first pediatric checkup. The investigator might first collect data on the APGAR ratings on the sample of infants, wait six weeks and then obtain the measurement of the infant's condition at that time. The example of the study concerned with the relationship between personality characteristics and recovery from surgery is also a prospective design. In this case, the measurement of personality factors was done preoperatively and then related to measurements of postoperative recovery taken in the recovery room and on the ward.

The fourth kind of design combines two of the other designs and is called a *mixed* design. Cross-sectional designs may be combined with either retrospective or prospective, and the latter two may be used at the same time. For example, a nurse might investigate the relationship between certain experiences in the recovery room and postoperative conditions. The cross-sectional part of the design would be done in the recovery room, perhaps looking at the relationship between sleep and rest and physiological factors. Then other measurements of recovery could be taken later and related to the earlier findings.

Association-testing studies take advantage of natural variation in situations without attempting deliberately to introduce variation into the situation, since it is known that the natural situation contains certain variations of its own. For instance, not all people share the same social class ranking, nor do all mental patients have the same diagnosis. Therefore, data can be collected on these two variables and then related to test the hypothesis that a particular social class is related to a particular kind of mental illness. Similarly, all people do not share the same personality characteristics, nor are they likely to recover in the same way from surgery. Therefore, these natural variations can be examined and their relationship tested.

Retrospective studies are "up until today." Prospective means "today on," cross-sectional studies mean "today," and mixed studies are combinations.

Retrospective designs depend on the data already available (or on recall of events that happened before today) and, thus, are somewhat weaker as designs. With prospective designs using available data, the researcher is limited to only those variables on which data already exist, which may or may not include all the potentially interesting ones. For example, medical records are a notoriously poor source of data for studies relating nursing diagnosis to other conditions because nursing diagnosis is rarely recorded. Psychosocial data on patients may also not be routinely recorded, when it might be of significant interest. Retrospective studies using recalled information obviously depend on the completeness of recall, a fairly unreliable thing to depend on.

Retrospective studies also may suffer the criticism of "affirming the consequent," in logical terms (13). Because retrospective studies begin with the outcome, then look back to see what is related to it, unwarranted conclusions may be drawn simply because the outcome is already known, and the research is limited to data already available. For example, a study of recovery room behavior might include people who were chosen in advance because they behaved in certain ways, then their charts would be examined to test hypotheses about what variables are associated with recovery room behavior. It might be concluded that, say, ethnic group is associated with certain kinds of recovery room behavior, when had the study been designed prospectively and new data collected, it might turn out that instead of ethnic group, it is personality type, or preparation for surgery or something else that is operating. Early studies of life change and illness onset were almost entirely retrospective, with a sample of ill people being chosen, then a record being made of the life changes that had occurred during the previous two years. Later, these studies became prospective—a sample of people were chosen and, asked to keep a record of their life changes over a period of time, then the frequency of illness was counted and the association with life change tested (14). The prospective study is a stronger test of association because it opens up the possibility of finding instances in which the outcome variable (illness onset, in this case) does not follow from life change, leading to development of a new theory that might specify the conditions under which life change and illness onset are directly related, and those in which they are not (15).

Hypotheses

Association-testing studies begin with formally stated predictions of relationships or correlations. The hypotheses are derived from the theoretical background and previous research, but have the force of extending the line of inquiry into a new area, a new instance, including new variables, or otherwise refining the state of knowledge.

The power of association-testing study comes from distilling theory to the point of making an explicit prediction rather than simply exploring to see what if any variables might be related to each other. To state an hypothesis is to put one's logic and theoretical work on the line.

Hypotheses are always statements of relationship: "Internally controlled diabetics will know more about their disease and therefore demonstrate more control over it." (16) Most often, association-testing study hypotheses predict not only that there will be a relationship, but what shape it will take, as in the example above. Such hypotheses are called "directional," since they state the direction of the expected relationship, in the case above, that the more the person is internally controlled, the more information and control he will have over his disease. (A nondirectional hypothesis would simply state that there will be a relationship between locus of control and disease knowledge.) The more explicit and directional an hypothesis can be, the larger the increment of information gained by testing it.

One sometimes sees hypotheses stated in the null form in the literature: "There will be no significant difference in the rank ordering of life events by the elderly and by the normative population." (17) As discussed in Chapter 3, the null hypothesis or prediction of no difference, no relationship or no effect, is useful only as an English translation of the statistical treatment of the data. It is sometimes argued that stating hypotheses in the null form is by definition "more objective." (18) This is specious reasoning, which assumes that stating an explicit expectation of relationship is somehow biased, when it is not at all. Deriving an hypothesis from theory is not bias in the sense of idiosyncratic value or preference; it is *reasoning* and, therefore, to be taken advantage of, not to be eliminated. It is the research hypothesis, not the null hypothesis that is really of interest; the researcher wants to know if internal control is related to diabetics' knowledge, not if it isn't. It may turn out in the end that there is no relationship, in which case the research hypothesis can be rejected, which makes more intuitive sense than stating a null hypothesis of no relationship, finding indeed there is none, then accepting the null hypothesis.

Hypotheses must be stated as simply and directly and clearly as possible. Terms in the hypothesis must be defined both conceptually and operationally, preferably not in the hypothesis itself. Sometimes one will see hypotheses with the operational definition built in: Life change, as measured by the Schedule of Recent Experiences (which is what the life change measurement is called) will be associated. . . . There is nothing really wrong with including the operational definition in the hypothesis itself unless it makes for cumbersome reading or confuses the hypothesis.

Studies may contain more than one hypothesis, depending on how the problem is construed and what variables are of interest. Sometimes additional research questions are stated, to supplement the hypotheses, though they are not the major focus of the study.

Independent and Dependent Variables

The terms "independent" and "dependent" when applied to variables are often used in association-testing studies. They are better understood and more appropriate in causal hypothesis-testing studies where the independent variable is the one introduced or manipulated, the one on which the variation in the dependent variable depends. Dependent variable tends to mean an outcome variable, while independent variables are the ones one wishes to relate to the outcome. Independent variables occur in time before the thing is measured as a dependent variable, as personality type is there before recovery room behavior, and locus of control is something that exists within an individual before diabetic knowledge. In association-testing studies that are cross-sectional, and when there is no attempt at all to imput causation, the use of the terminology of independent and dependent variables is simply confusing since it implies a casual relationship when there well may not even be a suspected one.

Setting

Selecting a setting to conduct a study is, as always, a matter of finding a place that has the population in it who have the variables under study. Considerations in selecting a setting for association-testing studies are no different from selecting a setting in any other kind of study.

Sample

In sharp contrast to exploratory, theory-generating studies, studies at the third level of inquiry are aimed at testing theory, and so samples need to be *representative* so that conclusions drawn from the study may apply to larger populations. Thus, more attention is paid to sampling in association-testing studies, and no maneuvers, such as purposive sampling used to increase the heterogeneity and richness of the sample, are tolerated. Association-testing studies take account of the normal, natural variation in the things under study, assuming that if the sample is selected in such a way that who gets into the sample is determined by some approximation of randomness, there will be sufficient variation in the factors studied to draw conclusions about relationships.

Samples for association-testing studies are heterogeneous with respect to the variables in the hypothesis. Unless there is variation, no relationship can be established. If the whole sample consisted of diabetics who were quite able to control their disease, no relationships could be established between disease control and other variables because people who were not able to control their disease would be excluded. Therefore, sampling criteria are defined in such a way as to be as inclusive as possible, as far as the problem statement will allow. For example, in a study of diabetics, including all adult-onset diabetics would be wise, but not juvenile diabetics since that may be a different kind of disease. In addition, since locus of control is supposedly a personality trait of adults, adolescents or children would normally be excluded anyhow.

The sampling principle in association-testing studies is *representativeness*. In real life, however, rarely are samples truly selected randomly. Instead, convenience samples are often used, under the assumption that there is no particular difference in the sample that happens to be convenient (the first n diabetics to appear, or a particular group of elderly people) and any other possible sample. What is important in selecting a sample is that how any one person gets into the sample is determined by something other than the individual's particular place on the variables of interest. Once sampling criteria are established for the entire group, who gets in the sample should be simply a matter of who turns up in the setting during the time allotted to data collection (if the sample is not to be drawn strictly randomly).

Generalization from samples of convenience is necessarily more tentative than from truly random samples, and there are only two ways to assure that convenience samples are representative. The first is by comparing the sample characteristics to other known samples, if they exist (for example to other diabetic clinics, or other elderly housing projects). The other way is through replication—repeating the study either again in the same setting or in a different one—then comparing samples. Neither tactic is used very frequently. Rather, data on the sample characteristics and on the setting, to the extent that might be related to the sample characteristics, are presented and it is left to the reader to decide how applicable the findings are to samples she/he has at hand.

There is a sampling method used in epidemiological research called "cohort studies" that is sometimes used in either prospective or retrospective association-testing studies (19). A cohort is a sample, simply stated. Cohort studies are those which pick several samples, or cohorts, each different in terms of some important variables. For example, a study might pick age cohorts—groups of people in different age groups, and the study might even pick the people from different settings. Or a study might pick a cohort of patients seen in a certain setting in 1970–72, another cohort seen in the same place in 1974–76, and so on, to look at a predicted association over time when there is reason to think time might be a factor, and when simply selecting charts from the record room back over the years is inefficient.

Instruments/Measurements

Association-testing studies depend on the natural variations in the factors under study. Statements about association require that other possible sources of variation besides the natural ones be controlled or ruled out. This means that the methods used to collect data must be reliable and objective, and that other sources of error in the instruments themselves, the data collector and so on, are closely checked. One wants to be able to conclude that there is a real relationship between one variable and another, not that an interviewer forgot to ask certain questions or that a measurement was unreliable.

All variables in the hypothesis have formal operational definitions and measurements, with clear and explicit indication of the type of data that will be taken as evidence of the variables of interest. Often, measurements already used and tested will be used in association-testing studies, since the theory will have been developed to the point where measurements actually exist. If previously used measurements are to be used, information on the reliability and validity of the measures will be presented so that the reader can judge the credibility of conclusions reached from their use.

If new instruments are invented for the particular study, more than just cursory evidence of the goodness of the measures is necessary. At the very least, this may mean a pretest of the instruments before the actual study begins, or perhaps recourse to a panel of judges or to literature which establishes that the content of the instrument is correct. The kinks in the instruments should be worked out before the study begins.

One general problem in choosing and using data collection instruments is the amount of inference required to classify the phenomenon. If observers are required, for instance, to classify women in labor as very uncomfortable, moderately uncomfortable or a little uncomfortable, they will have difficulty figuring out where the dividing lines are. In addition, observers will not be able to agree on the classification of particular mothers when such general categories are used. Therefore, categories should either be defined very specifically, or other more precise indicators should be chosen—motor activity, blood pressure, verbal reports of discomfort and so on. Reducing the amount of inference required will generally increase the reliability of any data collection procedure.

There is a particular problem in association-testing studies called the "halo effect." While not exclusive to this kind of study, it is a particular issue when one is trying to establish relationships between variables as hypothesis-testing. The halo effect occurs when the judgment or reading on one variable overlaps with the reading on another. For example, suppose a sociologist were studying the relationship between religiosity and church attendance. Suppose further that he sent his graduate students out to observe who went to church, then later selected a sample of townspeople to interview for their religious-ness. If the observer notes that a certain individual goes to church, and then interviews that person, it is possible that an unconscious bias could make the interviewer rate the person as more religious than the person really is, simply because he knows the individual goes to church. Thus, the halo effect can be a bias in data collection, cured in this case by using different data collectors for the two variables in the hypothesis.

But the halo effect can also be a conceptual difficulty, as when the operational definition of one variable in the hypothesis overlaps with the other variable. Measurement of life stress and illness onset provides an interesting example. The measurement of life change requires respondents to check whether in the past two years (or another period) they have experienced any of the items on the life change scale. The scale includes such items as death of a spouse (the highest ranked item), change of residence, change in job, loss of job, sex difficulties, change in health of family members, change in financial state, beginning or ending school, revision of personal habits, change in sleeping habits or eating habits and so on. If the measurement of life change is not restricted to the period *before* illness onset, then the illness itself could be not an effect of life change (which is what the hypothesis implies), but could *be* life change at least as this scale measures it. That is, illness might include the items of life change, rather than being a consequence of life change. In such a case, there is literally no test of the hypothesis because the halo from measurement of one variable encompasses the other and they become in effect the same thing (20).

In any hypothesis-testing study, the researcher wants not to have to worry that the variation found comes from something other than the real hypothesized relationship. Therefore, more attention is paid to operational definitions, and their relationship to the theory to be tested, and more effort is put into assuring that data collected will indeed be comparable from case to case.

Data Collection

Even more than in relation-searching studies, data collection in hypothesis-testing studies needs to be objective, unbiased and consistent. In addition to the usual methods for assuring objectivity and lack of bias, in hypothesis-testing studies there is the particular concern that simply knowing the hypothesis may influence the findings and should be guarded against. One method to help ensure against this kind of bias is to keep those who act as observers or those who score or code data "blind" to the purpose of the study and the hypothesis.

It is assumed that if the people are unaware of the intent of the study, there will be less effort on their part to unconsciously bias the data in the direction of the hypothesis. If observers are being paid to collect a certain amount of data, they are more likely to try to make their data come out the way they know their boss wants it to. Similarly, if classmates or students are coerced into collecting data, loyalty to the investigator may unconsciously prejudice it in some consistent way. The reverse is also true—data collectors who do not feel a commitment to the study may do a less than adequate job and even perhaps falsify data (21). Keeping observers blind and at the same time giving them a real sense of participation is a tricky interpersonal problem.

Checks on the accuracy of data can be built into data collection. For instance, questionnaires or interview schedules often contain the same question asked in different ways to estimate the respondent's consistency. The respondent's accuracy can be checked by including information that can be obtained from other sources. For example, an interview might include questions about how long the patient has been in the hospital, what was on his tray for dinner last night and so on, all of which can be checked through chart or diet records.

The details of checking reliability and validity of indicators are covered in a later chapter. It should be mentioned here, however, that the evidence concerning the extent to which observations can be agreed upon, and the extent to which data really does reflect the factors involved should be collected and presented in any study at the verification stage. All details about data collection, including the times of observations, length of data collection period, time of year, kind of equipment, training of observers and the like, are taken into account in determining how well an hypothesis was tested.

In many cases, it is inconvenient or impossible for the investigator to hire or coerce other people into collecting the data and she must do it herself. We have no reason to doubt any individual investigator's integrity, and no investigator has to prove that she didn't fake the data. But, if studies are to be replicated, all the details of how the data were collected should be supplied to other investigators who may then wish to tighten up the data collection procedures. The most important factor that will help an investigator collect meaningful data is probably sustained curiosity and interest, not so much in "proving" the hypothesis as in discovering the kind of information that can best serve to build nursing theory and improve patient care.

Data Processing/Analysis

Most of the data in association-testing studies is precoded in advance of data collection. It is possible to do a great deal of precoding, since categories or measurements from earlier factor or relation-searching studies are taken into account in the analysis of the problem. In addition, tools for collecting data are clearly defined. Data processing, then, generally means enumerating the data already described and classified and treating the enumerated data with appropriate statistics. It should be emphasized that the plans for data processing should be made well in advance of data collection, not only to economize on time, but also to prevent the bias that can occur when one knows how the data turned out and tries to develop categories *ex post facto*. The details of statistical treatment of data should also be ironed out well in advance of data analysis for the same reasons. In addition, different statistical procedures require different kinds of data, and it is frustrating indeed to have collected huge amounts of data inappropriately for the kind of analysis to be done.

There may be also a certain amount of unprecoded data in association-testing studies, since one wants to leave a little room for developing new hunches. Such data is treated like any other qualitative data, as described in earlier chapters.

Since the predicted findings will have been stated in the hypotheses, data analysis begins with tests to see whether what was predicted really happened. The interest is in both the direction of the relationship between factors, and the strength of the relationship. "Direction" means whether the factors are associated positively—as one increases, the other increases, or negatively, as one increases, the other decreases. The study of diabetics mentioned here tested a positive association: the more internally controlled people are, the more knowledge they will have about their conditions. The study of time estimation and fever tested a negative association: the more fever present, the less accurate will be the estimation of time.

"Strength" of a relationship is a statistical measure of how much of the variation in one variable (say diabetic knowledge) is accounted for by the other (locus of control). One hopes to be able to explain all of the variability in the dependent variable by the independent variable, but it never happens. Variables are related in more or less degree, and there are available numerous statistical procedures to test the relationships mathematically and determine what the chances are that the relationship found is a true (reliable, stable) relationship, or is due to chance or random error alone.

In addition to testing the hypotheses themselves, data analysis usually includes other tests of relationship not specifically laid out as hypotheses. For example, certain sample characteristics may be examined to see if the relationship found overall in the sample holds for people of different ages, or lengths of illness (in the case of the study of diabetics, for instance) or other factors of interest.

Statistical tests of relationship (correlations and other measures) are notoriously difficult to interpret, especially when they are only moderately strong or weak. In general, weak correlations may mean that the more important variables were not tapped, and this possibility is a conceptual one that should be seriously evaluated. But correlations and their strength are a function of some technical things like sample size and precision of measurement too, and these limitations have to be part of interpretation of data as well.

Sometimes an artifact of measurement makes interpretation of correlations even more thrilling. The direction in which the measurement scale is defined has to be remembered. (One can be surprised to find how often an investigator loses sight of her/his own data!) Scales can be set up in reverse order, with the conceptually lowest point on it receiving the highest numerical score. A scale of emotional welfare, for example, might rule that the more negative adjectives checked—anxious, afraid, miserable, unhappy, blue—the higher the score. Thus a low score means high emotional welfare, and a high score means low emotional welfare. Correlating this variable, using this scale, with other variables scaled in a positive direction (the higher the score, the more of the variable there is) will result in peculiar statistical findings (negative correlations) which are not negative at all. The researcher is then required to translate the findings into understandable form.

INTERPRETATION

Testing an hypothesis means setting things up so that when the data are in and analyzed, the claim can be made that other things that might have caused the association found are ruled out, such as bias, halo effects or spurious relationships. Ruling out bias and unreliability is a matter of careful operational definition and data collection. Spuriousness, when it happens, is a conceptual problem.

A spurious association is one in which the relationship between two variables is really explained by a third variable. For example, an association between preoperative fear and recovery room behavior may really be a relationship between personality type and fear and between personality type and behavior. That is, personality type really causes both fear level and recovery room behavior. Similarly, there is a high correlation between infant mortality and out-of-wedlock pregnancy. Yet variability in both can be explained by socioeconomic factors. In other words, poverty is strongly associated with both infant mortality and unwed motherhood, so the relationship between the later two is spurious (22). Spurious associations can be ruled out in advance only through analysis of the problem to be sure that the most directly related variables have been picked for the hypothesis, and through replication (see next section).

It is a nasty shock to new nurse-researchers that research never *proves* anything. That is, results can be interpreted to indicate more or less relationship between variables, in one direction or another, but absolute proof, or truth, is quite a distance away from that. It is especially difficult to interpret findings in association-testing studies because the desire is to find causal relationships, yet the data and study design do not lend themselves directly to causal interpretation. Of the three conditions necessary to make causal interpretations (concomitant variation, time order and random assignment), only concomitant variation is automatically part of association-testing studies. Concomitant variation simply means correlation, or association between variables, which is what is being tested in association-testing studies. The social scientist Blalock says it well:

. . . correlation analysis cannot be directly used to establish causality because of the fact that correlations merely measure covariation. . . One of the basic aims of any science, however, is to establish causal relations. Regardless of one's philosophical reservations concerning the notions of cause and effect, it is extremely difficult to think theoretically in any other terms. . . We can ascertain . . . the degree to which [two variables] vary together, and it is also sometimes possible to note the time sequence involved. From these two pieces of information we may make causal inferences if we wish.

If our theory is able to show a logical connection between the two variables . . . we need not be too unhappy about making the intellectual leap to causal interpretation. On the other hand, if we can find no theoretical reason for directly connecting the two events, we are ordinarily more hesitant. (23)

In clinical research, it is often fairly easy to establish the time order of variables. To claim a causal relationship, one variable (the cause) has to occur before the other (the effect). For example, preoperative personality type occurs before postoperative behavior and it would be hard to make a case that postoperative behavior causes personality type (except maybe in the case of brain damage resulting from anesthesia or surgery). To keep the researcher humble about inferring causal relationships from noncausal studies, it is fun to remember the apochryphal story of the storks and chimneys. The legend that storks bring babies grew up because people in Belgium noticed an association between storks nesting on chimney tops and a new baby in the house. It turns out that babies bring storks: when a new baby arrives, more fires are lit to keep the baby warm, and the warmth of the air coming up through the chimney attracts storks to nest there.

If we always scrupulously guarded against ever inferring causation from association-testing studies, a number of important findings would be disregarded. Smoking and cancer, for example. While there are no experiments on human beings where some people are assigned to smoke heavily over years, and some are not, it is almost universally accepted now that smoking causes lung cancer and other nasty conditions. Yet the evidence on which that interpretation is made is a series of association-testing studies. The intellectual leap to causation is not difficult, however, since the time order of the variables is quite clear.

Association-testing studies are sometimes done when it is not possible to introduce a variable and measure its effect, as in the case of smoking. Similarly, it is not possible to randomly assign some people to have mental illness to test the relationship between social class and mental illness. It's not possible to assign some parents to have multiple sclerosis and some not, to see what effect that handicap has on their children's body images. So we either have to live with the possibility of spuriousness in inferring causation or go ahead and make the intellectual leap.

Hypothesis-testing as theory-building is an attempt to be able to say that whatever the relationships found are, they are real relationships, character-istic of the phenomenon in general, not just peculiar to one sample in the one study. The extent to which it is possible to make this claim is conditioned by how the sample was selected, the reliability of measurements and data collection procedures as well as the absolute strength of the statistical relationship at the end. In a technical sense, generalization should be made only when it can be demonstrated that a sample was selected in a way that makes it truly representative of other empirical samples. In real life, the characteristics of other samples are often simply not known, so generalization to a population means to a hypothetical population of people like the ones selected in the present sample. Unlike some studies of very large population groups (such as studies of voting behavior or social attitudes of different kinds), in clinical research we simply do not know the parameters of the theoretical population of which the sample is a part. In voter studies, it is possible to compare the demographic characteristics of a sample (race, age, sex and the like) to known populations because such data are available. In a study of diabetics and their knowledge and control of their diet, we have no idea what the demographic data on the population of diabetics are.

The researcher is always in an anomolous position in generalizing from association-testing studies (or any other kind, for that matter) (24), so some balance is achieved between claiming absolutely that the findings are reliable and true, and humbly weaseling out with some too-harsh criticism of one's own sampling method.

REPLICATION

It is not possible to replicate—repeat—factor-searching or relation-searching studies. Indeed, it doesn't make any sense to think of doing it, since those methods are used when there is no available information on a given topic, and if there is such information from previous factor-searching or relation-searching studies, then there is no reason to repeat them. The methods used for exploratory studies are not repeatable anyway, depending as they do on letting the data collected lead the method.

On the other hand, hypothesis-testing studies are (or should be) repeata-ble. It is only through repeated tests of the same hypotheses, and, it is hoped, repeated confirmation of the original findings that confidence can be placed in the credibility of the hypotheses.

Replication means "repeating the same study under different unique conditions," (25) or carrying out the original study exactly as it was in terms of research approach, method, instrument and data-gathering technique on another sample from the same population (26). Replication helps theory development by giving additional evidence that the findings from the original study will hold up (or won't) under repeated tests.

In clinical research, replication is a powerful tool for theory development not just in the sense of confirming previous findings, but in developing more subtle understanding of the research problem under study (27). Since often in clinical studies the parameters of a population are not known, so it is not known how representative a given sample is, repeating the study is the only way to build up additional information about the extent to which the findings are applicable to groups other than the first sample.

There is often a feeling among new investigators that to replicate a study means the investigator has no original thoughts of her/his own. On the contrary, repeating a study may be as creative an effort as designing a new study in a new situation, and may be even more demanding. Refining conceptualization of a problem, tightening up a study design, perhaps including some additional variables to help make the relationships found more specific, analyzing the data more rigorously or simply bringing new eyes to see a research problem can be enormously engrossing. And being able to conclude something new and perhaps more precise about a relationship once found is very satisfying. Thus, there is a special obligation in association-testing studies (and other hypothesis-testing designs) to make sure that the details of how the study was done are sufficiently spelled out that the study can be repeated by another person, using only the information in the final report. The researcher is also obligated to advance the cause of theory development by pointing out explicitly what should be changed or altered, or tightened in a replication study (28).

NOTES

1. Abdellah, Faye G. and Eugene Levine: *Better Patient Care Through Nursing Research.* New York: Macmillan, 1965; Wandelt, Mabel: *Guide for the Beginning Researcher.* New York: Appleton-Century-Crofts, 1970.

2. Treece, Eleanor and J.W. Treece: *Elements of Research in Nursing* (1st edition). St. Louis: C.V. Mosby, 1973.

   The use of "survey" in this reference is confusing, since it tends to mean the kind of data collection employed in things like the Gallup poll. For this book, such "surveys" are not research at all, but are data collection. Treece and Treece also include case study and other methods in with "survey approach," whereas in this book, case studies are factor-searching studies. Readers should pay particular attention to how terminology is used, here and in any other research methods book, because there is not uniform agreement, or even uniform understanding.

   See also, Fox, David J.: *Fundamentals of Research in Nursing.* New York: Appleton-Century-Crofts, 1966, Chapter 9.

3. The most numerous examples of association-testing studies in the nursing literature are studies of nurses, such as studies attempting to correlate personality patterns to choice of clinical specialty, and studies of the relationship between school performance or other factors and performance on State Board Examinations. Since the present book is focused entirely on studies of patient care, these examples are not included, but the interested reader should take a look at the last five years or so of *Nursing Research* for examples of the method.

4. Lowery, Barbara and Joseph P. DuCette: Disease related learning and disease control in diabetics as a function of locus of control. *Nursing Research,* 25:358–362, September–October 1976.

5. Elms, Roslyn R.: Recovery room behavior and postoperative convalescence. *Nursing Research* 21:390–397, September–October 1972; see also, Elms, Roslyn R.: Prediction of post-surgical nursing needs. USPHS Grant # NU 00199, August 1977. (Harris College of

Nursing, Texas Christian University.) The relationship of personality type to behavior is contained in the latter study.

6. Alderson, Marjorie J.: Effect of increased body temperature on the perception of time. *Nursing Research*, 23:43–49, January–February 1974.

7. Olgas, Marya: Relationship between parent's health status and body image of their children. *Nursing Research*, 23:319–324, July–August, 1974.

8. Hollingshead, August and Fredric Redlich: *Social Class and Mental Illness*. New York: John Wiley & Sons, 1958.

9. Muhlenkamp, Ann F., et al.: Perception of life change events by the elderly. *Nursing Research*, 24:109–113, March–April 1975.

10. Elms, see Note 5.

11. Lowery and DuCette, see Note 4.

12. Muhlenkamp, see Note 9.

13. The logical fallacy of affirming the consequent is seen in the following syllogism:

All dogs have four legs.
This animal has four legs.
Therefore, this animal is a dog.

The fallacy in the argument is, of course, that animals other than dogs have four legs.

14. An elegant prospective study in the sequence of life stress and illness investigations is Rahe, R.H., et al.: Prediction of future health change from subjects' preceding life changes. *Journal of Psychosomatic Research*, 14(4):401–406, December 1970.

15. Nuckolls, Katherine B., et al.: Psychosocial assets, life crisis and the prognosis of pregnancy. *American Journal of Epidemiology*, 95(5):431–441, 1972.

16. Lowery and DuCette, see Note 4.

17. Muhlenkamp, see Note 9.

18. See Treece and Treece (Note 2) for example.

19. Cohort studies are also often "natural experiments" (see next chapter).

20. For an excellent discussion of problems of measurement of life change including this halo effect, see Brown, W., et al.: Life events and psychiatric disorders. Part I: some methodological issues. *Psychological Medicine*, 3(1):74–87, February 1973.

21. Roth, Julius: Hired hand research. *American Sociologist*, 1:190–196, August 1966.

22. Another spurious relationship, isolated by Jones, is between social class and outcome of psychiatric treatment. Lower social class patients have poorer outcomes, but this is due to clinicians not being as skilled with lower-class patients, not to social class itself. See Jones, E.: Social class and psychotherapy: a critical review of research. *Psychiatry*, 37(4):307–320, September 1974.

23. Blalock, Hubert: *Social Statistics*. New York: McGraw-Hill, 1960, p. 337.

24. "Generalization" is sometimes used to mean "application of a general concept or idea to a relatively new object or situation." This definition is confusing and is closer to a nontechnical, lay use of the word than to the technical meaning used in this chapter. See Abdellah and Levine (Note 1), p. 702.

25. Selltiz, Claire, et al.: *Research Methods in Social Relations*. New York: Holt, Rinehart & Winston, 1959, p. 46.

26. Fox, see Note 2, p. 258.

27. Batey, Marjorie V.: Some methodological issues in research. *Nursing Research*, 19:511–516, November–December 1970; Downs, Florence S.: Some critical issues in nursing research. *Nursing Forum*, 8(4):392–404, 1969.

28. This discussion of replication is continued in the next chapter as there are some different issues with experimental studies.

7

Causal Hypothesis-Testing Studies

INTRODUCTION

Like association-testing studies, causal hypothesis-testing studies are at the third level of theory, the situation-relating level. Unlike association-testing studies, they allow statements about the causal relationship between variables. Both associational statements and causal ones can be elements of prescriptive theory, though neither by itself is a prescription.

Causal hypothesis-testing studies are most commonly called "experiments," or explanatory studies (1). The term causal hypothesis-testing study is used here to make clear the distinction in hypothesis-testing studies between the correlational, survey or association-testing ones covered in the last chapter, and tests of cause-and-effect relationships.

The development of nursing research itself is quite recent, and the use of experimental designs in clinical research even more recent. One of the first reports of an experimental study was Dumas and Leonard's test of the effect of nursing on the incidence of postoperative vomiting, published as recently as 1963 (2). In their discussion of the use of experiments in clinical research, Abdellah and Levine remark that until the Dumas and Leonard study, it was assumed that doing a classical experimental study in a clinical situation was practically impossible because the situations themselves were not capable of the kind of "control" that is ultimately desired in experimental design (3). By now there are quite a number of causal hypothesis-testing studies in the nursing literatue, demonstrating that they can be done, and done with elegance, when clinical wisdom can be combined with methodological rigor (4).

Perhaps another reason why the causal hypothesis-testing study was somewhat slower to be seen in clinical research in nursing (and even slower to be seen in any numbers) is that early experiments often tested the effect of one nurse's nursing against "regular hospital nursing." The nurse was often specially trained in nursing process, and while the "experimental nursing" was derived from theories and guided by explicit formulas, it still amounted

162

to that nurse putting her own practice on the line. If the hypothesis was not supported (the experimental nursing wasn't better than the comparison group), the nurse could only believe she/he was a failure (5), though that's not the appropriate interpretation of the findings. In the early days (only ten years ago or so!) of experimentation in nursing practice, it took some courage for nurses to make the kind of commitment to systematic study that experimental testing of one's own practice took (6). Later studies could profit from increasingly well-developed theory and methodological refinement so that the test became less personal.

Clinical tests of nursing practice had to await development of testable nursing theories, and those did not begin to appear with any specificity until Orlando's book in 1960 (7). Now there are available theories not only from nursing, but from social psychology, physiology, child development and many other fields that make possible causal hypotheses for clinical problems.

The method for testing causal hypotheses has been around for some time (8). Early studies developed in agronomy, tested the effect of different combinations of soil, light, fertilizer and seed on plant production. Beautiful designs could be used with nonhuman experimentation, but it was some years before application to human problems was made.

LOGIC OF CAUSAL INFERENCE

The outcome of a causal hypotheses-testing study is a tested statement of cause and effect, including how likely it is that all other things being equal, the results occurred by chance alone, rather than as an effect of the designed manipulation.

To infer a causal relationship, three things are necessary—concomitant variation, time order of variables controlled and *ceteris paribus*—"all other things being equal"—alternative explanations ruled out.

Concomitant variation means that the two factors in the hypothesis are varying together. The reader may wonder how this is different from the varying together in association-testing studies. It isn't. However, concomitant variation is only one of the conditions necessary in causal hypothesis-testing studies.

Time order means that X (the cause) must occur before Y (the effect). This condition is built into the study designs by deliberately introducing X at one point and measuring its effects later. This deliberate manipulation is one thing that distinguishes causal hypothesis-testing studies from association-testing. Only in causal hypothesis-testing studies is it possible to introduce the variable X and measure its effects.

Ceteris paribus means that all other possible causes and sources of *systematic* variation are ruled out (9). Other factors are allowed to vary randomly, and statistical treatment takes them into account. But the only systematic variation desired is that within the X and Y variables. These three conditions are met or approximated through the use of various experimental designs and through data collection and analysis techniques.

The ultimate wish in causal hypothesis-testing studies is to be able to claim that the independent variables—the cause—is a *necessary* and *sufficient* condition.

A necessary condition is one which must be present if the phenomenon of which it is the cause is to be present. If X is a necessary condition for Y, then Y will never occur unless X has happened. For example, exposure to the poliomyelitis virus is a necessary condition for paralytic polio, for without exposure, the disease does not occur. A sufficient condition is one in which Y always follows X, whenever the cause is present, so will be the consequence. For example, destruction of the optic nerve always causes blindness. Something can be either necessary or sufficient, or both. In the examples above, since exposure to the poliomyelitis virus does not always cause paralytic polio, exposure is just a necessary condition. And since blindness may be caused by a number of things besides destruction of the optic nerve, destruction is not a necessary condition. Since it is rarely possible to establish that something is both a necessary and sufficient condition, other kinds of conditions are examined (10).

A contributory condition is one which increases the likelihood of something occurring but does not guarantee it. A contingent condition is one under which a given variable is a contributory cause of a given phenomenon. Alternative conditions are additional contributory conditions. For example, patients who are highly anxious (contributory condition) are more likely to experience relief from pain through nursing care. Unexpected happenings (contingent condition) increase anxiety. And patients who are "internally oriented" (alternative condition) are less likely to experience the effects of nursing. Identifying alternative conditions is a major drive for research. When such conditions are apparent, it is possible to reconceptualize the hypotheses to take account of new information. For example, one could now predict that under conditions of unexpected occurrences, patients who are *either* highly anxious *or* externally oriented will be more likely to experience relief from pain through nursing.

A causal relationship is accepted when the dependent variable varies with the independent variable, when the cause occurs before the effect and when all other things that might have caused the relationship are ruled out. In real life, it is difficult indeed to rule out all other things that might have made the relationship happen, so there are statistical procedures that help decide whether it is probable that the relationship found is a real one, not due to random error or chance alone.

RESEARCH PROBLEMS

Problems for causal hypothesis-testing studies are of the What will happen if . . . ? variety. Instead of concentrating on the natural variation in the situation, a new variable is introduced so that its effect can be measured.

Therefore, causal hypothesis-testing studies come from a sense that some new thing—a procedure, a treatment, a nursing process—might improve patient welfare, and the desire is to see if it will.

Early studies in nursing practice research took particular interpersonal theories to develop special approaches to patients in various kinds of crisis situations. The investigators wondered, "What will happen if patients are given an opportunity to express their feelings of anxiety before surgery. Will they recover better?" (11) Or, "What will happen if parents are given a chance to discuss the hospitalization of their child with a nurse. Will they be less anxious and therefore better able to care for the child in rooming-in?" (12) Later studies refined the independent variable using audiovisual means of preparing patients for surgery (13) or threatening procedures (14), or developing special kinds of preparation given at different points of stress in the patient's preoperative stay (15). In all these studies, the investigators had a notion that something ought to work better than the nursing care usually given, and they designed studies to see if the new approach really did produce decreased patient anxiety and increased patient welfare.

A whole group of causal hypothesis-testing studies have dealt not with an interpersonal nursing approach, but with various kinds of nursing activities to see if they made a difference to patients. For example, a pediatric nurse tested the effect of a planned program of physical exercise of newborns on their growth and development (16). Two obstetrical nurses tested the effect of different kinds of nipple preparation on mothers' success at breast feeding (17). Another team of nurses applied topical insulin to decubitus ulcers to see if they would heal faster (18).

Some lovely causal hypothesis-testing studies have grown out of studies of nursing rituals—things that are done more or less automatically for patients without any real basis in scientific reasoning. One investigator tested the effect of warmed versus nonwarmed tube feedings, wondering whether it was really necessary to warm the foods (19). Others have looked at urinary catheterization and irrigation to see whether the procedures dictated by hospital procedure manuals (as well as nursing education programs) really work (20).

Other experimental studies have tested the effect of aspects of nursing practice so old that they are hardly commented upon, since it is assumed nurses have always done them. Studies have looked at the effects of touch with acutely ill adult patients (21), and tactile stimulation with newborns (22). Here the effort conceptually is to bring to consciousness a nursing "treatment"—touch—that is rarely consciously prescribed.

Still other investigators have tested the effect of new systems of care: primary nursing (23), VNA follow-up of discharged mental patients (24), or group therapy by nurses (25).

There are numerous other examples that could be mentioned, but for now the point is that causal hypothesis-testing studies offer the opportunity to invent a new way of working with patients (or resurrect an old way) and test it to see if it really achieves the predicted consequences in patient behavior or welfare. The new procedure is deliberately introduced into the normal situation, and the effect of it is measured later.

Problems for causal hypothesis-testing studies may come either from clinical experience or from previous work, theory, and the like. What makes a clinical problem a candidate for causal hypothesis-testing is whether the independent variable can be introduced into the situation, with formal predictions about its effects.

BACKGROUND/CONCEPTUAL FRAMEWORK

Whether the clinical problem comes from one's own practice or from previous theory or research, the theory that guides the hypothesis has to be presented. A case has to be made for why the new procedure or treatment or approach ought to work, and why, therefore, a prediction that it will have certain effects is being made.

Often the theory for causal hypothesis-testing is an extension of other kinds of theory, but applied in a new situation, or applied to a real-life clinical problem. For example, social psychology theory predicts that people in stressful situations attend more directly to the way they feel and to the situation around them, and perhaps do not think or reason as clearly as they might in a nonstress situation. This theory could be used to define nursing approaches to prepare patients for stressful events—surgery or procedures (26). Or theory from developmental physiology might suggest that premature infants might develop faster if their environment could be made to approximate some aspects of the fetal environment, especially a gentle rocking motion and the sound of a heartbeat. The nurse-researcher could then create such an environment and see if it has the predicted effects (27). Or, clinical experience in psychiatric nursing might lead some nurses to rethink the treatment possibilities that are available to chronically ill psychiatric outpatients and design new ones that seem better suited to the level of social functioning, living circumstances and even to the nature of chronic psychiatric illness than insight-oriented or supportive psychotherapy (28).

What the problem is an instance of will help decide the kinds of theories that are applicable, or will help the investigator search for potentially useful explanatory concepts. Causal hypothesis problems can be conceived of essentially in two ways: as instances of amelioration of untoward patient states (pain, stress, discomfort and so on), with the effort directed to define from theory ways to relieve pain or whatever; or, they may be conceived of as instances of nursing approaches, with the choice of situation in which to test the effect of the approach being simply a matter of finding a situation that allows the test (has enough variation). In the first conception, the researcher feels the problem as, I want to be able to relieve patients' pain, and goes about inventing ways to do that. In the second, the researcher thinks, I have invented this new nursing approach for people in stressful situations, and she/he finds a stressful situation in which to test it.

However the problem is construed, the theoretical background behind both the approach and the dependent variable is developed in some detail. The relationship between the hypothesis and the theory from which it derives must be made explicit; otherwise, interpretation of the data will suffer. Eventually, when the data are all in, the researcher will want to take the empirical facts found (differences between experimental and control groups) and translate them into theoretical terms, to elaborate or refine the knowledge that got the study started in the first place.

Thorough theoretical work before the study begins is especially important in causal hypothesis-testing studies, given the state of existing predictive knowledge in nursing. We are still at a fairly early stage in developing lines of inquiry with sustained research on a few topics and banks of tested hypotheses. Nursing preparation for surgery or procedures has probably received the most attention (29), with perhaps studies of nursing approaches to patients in pain running second (30). Few other areas or topics can claim more than a very few studies, which means that it is quite possible to invent new approaches to patient problems that simply will not work because the theory is not developed far enough, the measurements aren't sensitive enough or something else is lacking. Therefore, the theoretical background part of a causal hypothesis-testing study should be as full and thought-through as possible in advance so that if the findings do not support the hypothesis (or even if they do), one has a chance of figuring out *why*. At this point in the development of nursing knowledge, negative findings may be as useful as positive ones, at least in refining theory for future use (if not in increasing the researcher's mental health).

In other words, theory development for causal hypothesis-testing studies provides the logic and reasoning that explain how the hypothesis got to be stated as it was, and also gives enough of a framework of ideas that when the findings are in, they can truly be explained. The effort in experimental studies is not only to find out if something works, or doesn't, but to find out why. And why is always a theoretical question.

STUDY DESIGN

Causal hypothesis-testing studies are the third level of inquiry—situation-relating, or predictive (31).

In causal hypothesis-testing studies the *independent* variable is introduced at one point in time and its effects on the *dependent* variable are measured. Independent variable means the experimental event or condition. Dependent variable means the variable measured as effect. Two other terms used in conjunction with experimental design are *antecedent* variable and *intervening* variable. Antecedent variables (background variables) are those things which occur before or are already present before the introduction of the independent variable; intervening conditions are those that take place between the independent variable and the measurement of the dependent variable. The diagram on page 168 illustrates the time sequence.

Variables

| | Introduce | | Measure |
| Antecedent | Independent | Intervening | Dependent |

Time→ |----→ ---→| ---→ ---→- | ---→ ---→ | ---→ ---→-|- →

Antecedent variables might include things present in the situation itself or within the sample. For example, in a study of the effect of nursing on relief from pain, duration of pain before nursing, site of incision, usual level of activity of the patient, unusual upsets on the ward and so on would be antecedent conditions. Intervening variables occur in time between independent and dependent variables and in a study of the effect of preoperative nursing on postoperative distress, surgery itself would be an intervening variable, along with the kind of anesthesia, length of time in the operating room and so on. The importance of collecting data on antecedent and intervening variables will be discussed later.

Experimental designs (causal hypothesis-testing studies) are based logically on the "classical experimental design" devised by Sir Ronald Fisher (32). In this design, there are two groups, an experimental and a control group, to which cases are assigned randomly. Measurements are taken before the introduction of the experimental treatment and again afterwards for both groups, and the difference between the groups in terms of before-after change is analyzed. With this classical design it is possible to determine how alike the two groups were to begin with, and, therefore, how big a difference the experimental treatment makes. The classical experimental design might be diagrammed as follows:

Time----→----------------------------------

Independent Variable Administered

| | *Measure* | | *Measure* |
| | *Before* | ↓ | *After* |

Experimental Group

Control Group

The classical experimental design is also called a before-after design with two groups. It is particularly appropriate when the dependent variable is something that is continuously present but varying. For example, pulse-respiration rates are frequently chosen as dependent variables. The rates can be counted before administration of the treatments, then counted again at some time after the treatment.

Some dependent variables occur only once and cannot be measured before introduction of the treatment. In these cases, a variation on the classical design is used—the "after-only" design with two groups. The after-only design is diagrammed as follows:

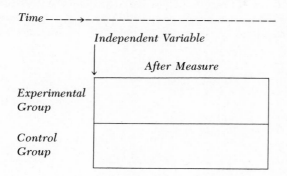

In this design, a group of people are randomly assigned to one of the two conditions, the independent variable is administered and both groups are measured later. For example, since postoperative vomiting by definition occurs only after surgery, it can only be measured then. Therefore, special preoperative nursing care is given to one half the group, the other half receives the usual care and both groups are measured after surgery. The disadvantage of the after-only design is that it is impossible to determine how much "change" is brought about by the independent variable and how much would have been there anyhow. This disadvantage can be overcome by knowledge of how likely the desired outcome is to be expected normally. For example, postoperative records of a large number of patients experiencing different types of surgery could be examined to obtain a baseline measurement of the frequency of vomiting in different surgical categories. Then this frequency could be used to determine how much difference the experimental treatment makes in vomiting rates.

The after-only design is also sometimes used when measurement before the introduction of the independent variable might affect the independent variable itself. This is the so-called pretest effect. For example, suppose an investigator chose anxiety as the dependent variable. She would like to administer a scale to all patients before offering certain patients nursing care, then measure the patients with the same scale after nursing. However, just administering the scale may have an effect like the effect of nursing and the "real" difference between the groups caused by nursing alone could not be determined.

When it is suspected that administering a before measure might have an effect all its own, another variation of the classical design can be used. With this design it is possible to separate the pretest effect from the combined effect of pretest and experimental treatment from the effect of the treatment alone. As shown in the following diagram, there are four groups in this design: the first group is given the before measurement; the second group gets the before measurement plus the experimental condition; the third group gets just the experimental condition; and the fourth groups gets neither the before measurement nor the experimental treatment. All four groups receive the after measurement, and people are randomly assigned to one of the four groups.

Time ----→ --

	Measure Before	*Measure After*
Pretest Only		

Independent Variable ↓

Pretest plus Experimental Condition		
Experimental Only		
Control		

In all these designs, the groups are different people. Another kind of design uses the same group of people, with the experimental and control conditions applied alternately or in random order. This design is especially appropriate when there is reason to believe that there would be such wide differences among people in their response to the treatment (or in antecedent variables that might be related to how the treatment is experienced) that a more rigorous approach using each person as his own control is needed. These designs, therefore, are called "own-control" designs. They are often seen in operant conditioning studies where a baseline of behavior is taken, then a method is used to alter behavior, then measures are taken of its effect. Other examples include some studies of touch during labor (33) when there is reason to think that touch might be experienced differently across people, with so much variation that it would be difficult to tell how much variation is due to the touch itself. An elegant own-control design was used to test the effect of different kinds of nipple preparation (34). Here, breast feeding mothers were given instructions to prepare one nipple (left or right) randomly assigned and not to prepare the other, then comparisons were made. The own-control design is particularly appropriate in this situation where skin condition, complexion, body weight and other variables, if allowed to vary across people, might be so different that it would be hard to tell the effect of the treatment itself.

One group before-after designs are sometimes used when it is not possible to withhold the designed treatment from one group to compare it with another. In this design, the baseline or before measure is taken, and it is assumed (given sampling procedures) that the differences found in the dependent variable can be traced to the introduction of the independent variable. This design is sometimes seen in evaluation studies where a whole new system of care has been introduced (say a community mental health center, or a neighborhood clinic) and where data on the population before are available from statistical banks (mental hospital admission rates or birth statistics).

Probably the weakest possible design is the one group, after-only design, also seen in evaluation studies. Here, data on the population before the new approach was introduced are not available, so the group is measured after only. This design is sometimes called a "natural experiment" when it is used to determine the effect of such things as natural disasters—floods, fires and so on—or other events occurring naturally (or unnaturally, depending on your point of view), such as airplane hijackings or mass kidnappings.

"Natural experiment" is also applied to studies that are more like orthodox experimental designs except for random assignment. These kinds of studies are discussed in the section on sampling, later in this chapter.

Other possible study designs simply expand the classical experimental design by adding more groups or more measures of the dependent variable. For example, instead of giving a new nursing approach to one group and not to another, a study might be designed to compare three different nursing approaches: an experimental approach designed to relieve stress by expression of feeling, and instructive approach and "normal hospital nursing" (35). Or three different nursing approaches to patients in pain might be tested, each one defined by different "orientations" to the patient (36). Or one-shot versus "stress point" preparation of children for surgery might be tested with four groups: one group receives a combination of systematic preparation, rehearsal and supportive care prior to each stressful procedure; a single-session preparation is administered to another group after admission; a third group receives consistent supportive care given by one nurse at the same points as in the first condition, but no systematic preparation or rehearsal, and a control condition including none of the special preparatory or supportive activities (37).

The classical design may also be extended by taking several measures of the dependent variable across time. For example, a study might test the effect of preoperative preparation not only on immediate postoperative behavior, but on long-term behavior, especially in children after they return home (38).

Finally, there is the *factorial* design. This design makes use of information about antecedent conditions which might interact with the independent variable in some systematic manner. The principle of factorial design involves something similar to stratifying. For example, a study of the effect of preoperative teaching on postoperative ventilatory functioning took two antecendent variables—age of the patient and smoking—into account, since it could be guessed that age and smoking might be related to ventilatory function quite apart from the effect of the independent variable (39). The independent variable was individual or group preoperative teaching, and three different measures of ventilatory functioning were taken before and after surgery (40). When it is possible in factorial designs to know the antecedent variables of interest in advance, one can assign patients within the classification groups (age, smoking) to the treatments randomly, producing equal numbers in all the groups. When it is not practical to do this, data may still be analyzed in terms of the predetermined factors.

A factorial design might be diagrammed as below:

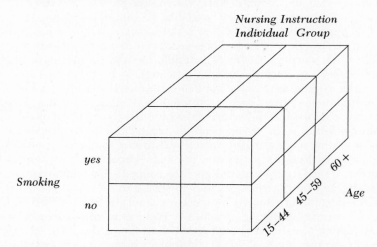

Within each box in the diagram, before and after measures are taken, and it is possible to determine with modern statistical techniques what the different effects of the treatments are in people who do or don't smoke, in people of different ages and so on. It is also possible to tease out the "interaction effects," that is, the effects of two or more variables in combination.

Note that factorial designs are quite complicated and require rather large samples. In the example above, it would take twelve patients just to get one in every group. To have enough patients to use appropriate statistical tests might mean a very long data collection period, or the participation of quite a few nurses doing the preoperative teaching (as was the case in the study cited). When antecedent variables can be identified in advance and "controlled" by factorial designs, this is a very powerful design for testing causal hypotheses.

A "control group" is defined as a group of subjects who do not receive the new independent variable at all, and in whom it is assumed that variation present is simply natural variation. The addition of a control group to various treatment groups is desireable, but not always practical or justifiable. Sometimes withholding a treatment from one group cannot be justified on ethical grounds. Sometimes, particularly when nursing approaches to be tested are rather subtle distinctions among interpersonal behaviors, a control group is not necessary when the theory is confined to the nursing approaches themselves, and the groups are "comparison groups." And sometimes a control group is simply impractical or otherwise questionable (see the section on Setting and Chapter 11).

A "good" causal hypothesis-testing study is one in which the theory is well developed, the hypothesis logically derived and the design is rigorous enough to give a fair test of the effect of the independent variable.

Setting

Most considerations in selecting a setting for causal hypothesis-testing do not differ from any other kind of study. The setting has to contain the thing being measured (patients in pain or whatever) and has to be accessible to the investigator. There are sometimes different problems of access for experimental studies in settings where research is not normally carried out and where those in a position to grant access might be worried about their patients being "experimented on." In addition to assuring that all patients will be informed of the study, its purposes and their responsibilities, and given the opportunity to decline to participate without consequences to their care, researchers have sometimes found that it is necessary to pay some attention to the reactions of those in the setting, either to gain access or to be sure the research moves smoothly and does not disrupt the natural situation.

Faced with the possibility that one group of patients will be offered an experimental procedure and it will be withheld from another group, people who have not had much contact with research before may be disturbed at what seems like unethical conduct. When the to-be-tested independent variable is something conceived of as "better" than whatever is now the case, researchers are sometimes hard put to explain why it is still necessary to test the new treatment to see if it works.

It can be argued that it is ethically more sound to test rigorously new procedures before adopting them than to continue to carry out ritualistic practices without question (41). But experience suggests that this is not a very powerful argument when people may be worried about the image of their institution or about the rights of their patients.

There are two other considerations in setting selection that are particular to experimental studies.

To test a causal hypothesis about the difference between, say, two forms of treatment, one has to be sure that the two forms are indeed different. One group cannot be "contaminated" by the other. Preventing contamination may be a particular problem in inpatient settings, especially where there are multiple-bed rooms. For example, a study of preoperative preparation might have to be designed so that patients who experienced the special preparation would not have contact with those who didn't. Or a study of nurse practitioner care, contrasted to physician care for nonurgent medical problems, might have to be designed so that the patients in the nurse practitioner group were not seen by physicians, and the physician patients never saw the nurse practitioners. If these kinds of precautions are not taken, the independent variable is muddied and chances are that there will be less difference on the dependent variable than there would have been if the groups were "clean."

Another peculiar problem in experimental studies has to do with the nature of control groups. Studies are often designed to test a particular special nursing treatment against "normal nursing care," or "routine care." For example, a study of nursing care to chronic psychiatric outpatients tested the effect of a nurse-run socialization program against the routine care, medication maintenance clinic to which patients came once a month for prescription refills. Part of the nursing program was to offer support by visit or telephone to patients between meetings of patient groups. But it turned out that in the medical maintenance group, patients who experienced difficulties and called the service between appointments were also handled by the same nurses, probably in the same way (42). Thorough knowledge of how a clinical setting normally operates will obviate these kinds of problems.

Sampling

As in other kinds of studies, sampling criteria are specified first. In addition to the usual concerns of setting sampling criteria and representativeness, causal hypothesis-testing studies are particularly concerned with whether the sample will be capable of variation in the dependent variable. If the occurrence or level of the dependent variable is already low, there will be little chance for the independent variable to lower it, no matter how "strong" it is. For example, postoperative vomiting rates differ with different kinds of surgery, the use of antiemetics and the use of nasogastric tubes. In a study testing the effect of preoperative vomiting, patients with nasogastric tubes and antiemetics would be excluded. The sample chosen for this study would have to include a group for which there would be the possibility of lowering the rate of vomiting. If orthopedic patients are known to have a very low rate, say 10 percent, nursing cannot be expected to lower rate much. On the other hand, if gynecological patients have a fairly high incidence of vomiting, say around 60 percent, they would make a good sample for testing this hypothesis.

To repeat, causal hypothesis-testing studies aim to have all things, besides the experience of the independent variable, equal, or at least varying randomly. Applied to sampling, this generally means that samples for experiments are homogeneous—to hold constant some of the important factors. This is in part for economic's sake. To allow everything possible in a sample to vary randomly (unsystematically) would require an enormous sample just so that more than one case of a given kind would appear and be used for comparison purposes. For example, testing the hypothesis that nursing care will relieve pain might suggest allowing any patient with any kind of pain to appear in the sample. The sample then might include children and adults, medical and surgical patients, patients before and after surgery, patients with intractable or manageable pain, different diagnoses and conditions, different races, social classes, ethnic backgrounds, previous hospital experience and so on. Since it is important not only to test the hypothesis, but also to explain the results in terms of a *few* alternative conditions, samples are usually limited to a small number of important characteristics. The few important characteristics are either allowed to vary randomly, or they may be controlled by equalizing the treatment groups (see "matching," later in this section).

Again, in order to generalize the findings from a causal hypothesis-testing study sample to the larger population, the sample has to be randomly selected. Most often in nursing research, accidental or convenience samples are chosen simply because with the variables being tested it is often difficult to be able to identify and draw from a given population. While a randomly selected sample is necessary for generalization, it is not strictly necessary for testing a causal hypothesis. Random assignment is absolutely essential however.

Random assignment means that whether any one patient gets the experimental or control treatment is determined randomly without respect to any of the patient's characteristics. The purpose of random assignment is to allow characteristics that might be systematically related to the independent or dependent variable to vary randomly. If all patients of one kind were assigned to the experimental group and all patients of another kind to the control group, it would be difficult to tell whether the effects of the independent variable were attributable to its variation or whether the groups were just different to begin with. Random assignment does not attempt to equalize the groups, although given enough cases the groups will be relatively equal. Rather, it attempts to assure random rather than systematic variation of important factors. Statistical tests can take into account such random variation, but they cannot account for systematic bias.

Random assignment can be done in a number of ways. Perhaps the simplest is just flipping a coin for every person admitted to the sample—heads means experimental group, tails means control group. Given enough people, the groups will end up with fairly even numbers. If the sample will be small, block randomization, or alternate assignment with a random start, may be used to be sure that the groups will have equal numbers in them. (Equal sized groups are not really necessary, but they seem so much neater, somehow.)

Block randomization means that a randomization scheme is worked out before the data are collected. The first step is to decide how many patients will comprise the total sample. Then, knowing how many treatment groups there will be, a table of random numbers or some other device can be used to determine which patient will go in which group. For example, suppose there is to be a total group of forty-five. Then, one could read down a table of random numbers and put the first fifteen numbers (between 1 and 45) in the first treatment group, the second fifteen numbers (between 1 and 45) in the second treatment group and so forth. There is no reason to assume that the sequence in which the patients' numbers appear has anything to do with any other characteristics that might be related to the independent variable.

A second way of assigning a patient to a group is alternate assignment with a random start. The group that the first patient will be in is determined by a flip of the coin, and thereafter, every other patient goes in the other group. If the flip of the coin says that the first patient will go in the experimental group, the second will then go in the control group, the third in the experimental group, the fourth in the control group and so forth. Again, there is no reason for assuming that the order in which a patient is taken into a sample has anything to do with any systematic relationship to the independent variable. It is the possibility of systematic relationship to the independent variables that is worrisome in causal hypothesis-testing studies, since one wants to conclude that all other things except that variable were not related to whatever variation in the dependent variables is found. Alternate assignment with a random start is not strictly "random" assignment, but it is good enough approximation when the researcher is very sure that the alternate assignment is not varying with some antecedent variable which also happens to vary alternately. For example, if a secretary who makes patient appointments in a primary care clinic automatically alternates assigning patients as they arrive to see a nurse practitioner or a physician, then alternate assignment of patients in that clinic will mean that all patients in one group will be nurse practitioner patients and all patients in another group will be physician patients.

In own-control designs, the order of the treatments is determined randomly (most often alternately). For example, in a study of touch in labor, the nurse might apply maximum touch to one patient in the first contraction, then minimum touch in the next and so on, alternating touch with each contraction. The next patient would receive the reverse order of touch-no touch. In the study of preparing the breast for breast feeding, whether the left or right breast was given the special preparation was determined randomly (43).

To avoid contamination of treatment groups, sometimes patients in particular rooms will be automatically assigned to an experimental group and patients in other rooms to control groups. This is fine as long as there is no pattern in how patients are assigned to rooms by the admitting office. Sometimes patients admitted on certain days of the week are assigned to the experimental group and patients admitted on other days to the control group. This too is fine, as long as there isn't some systematic pattern to when patients are admitted, such as a particular physician's instructions that all his patients are admitted on Mondays and Wednesdays or something.

On occasion, the control treatment is done for the entire group at the same time, then an experimental treatment is introduced and the entire experimental group data collected. This might be done, for example, when a whole staff of nurses will be taught a particular kind of nursing approach, and its effect tested. Here it is assumed that patients who experienced the control treatment in, say, January and February, are no different from the experimental group patients who were in the setting in April or May.

There are other approximations of random assignment that may be used when practical considerations dictate or when truly random assignment is not possible. Any alteration of random assignment weakens the claim that "all other things were equal," so serious thought has to go into both the decision to alter the assignment and the interpretation of the data afterwards.

One study used a clever approach to random assignment to test hypotheses about the effect of nurse practitioner care compared with physician care on patients with certain standard conditions. To keep the two groups—nurse practitioner and physician patients—clean, the sample of physician patients was obtained using the time the nurse practitioner (who happened to be the only one in the clinic) was on vacation (44). It can be assumed that when she chose to take her vacation was not related to any particular patient characteristics.

Another study of nurse practitioner practice compared both with physician-alone practice and with NP-MD team practice took advantage of the known fact that new patients were assigned by a secretary to nurse practitioners and physicians according to who had an available appointment period open, a fairly good approximation of random assignment. In this study, it was not possible to do a strictly random assignment, since all the practitioners already had large case loads who could not be reassigned or turned over to anyone else to open up appointment slots to be handed out randomly (45).

Some natural experiments can take advantage of natural variations in assignment of patients to treatment groups, as long as there is some reason to think the assignment approximates randomness. For example, a study of the architecture of hospital units tested the effect of two different kinds of nursing stations on interruptions during change of shift report (46). Here, the treatment groups were the two nursing stations and staffs in them, and it could be assumed that whatever patterns of interruption there were were not related to the particular configuration of people who worked there or visited that unit.

Other natural experiments are somewhat like retrospective association-testing studies, but with a defined, introduced, independent variable. For example, a study of the effect of nurse pulse-taking on cardiac arrhythmia in coronary care patients examined monitor tapes to define those instances of arrhythmia that occurred when the nurse was physically taking the patient's pulse from those that occurred at other times (47). It could be assumed that when the nurse elects to take the pulse directly is determined randomly.

It is a common misapprehension that the purpose and effect of random assignment is to produce *equal* groups, that is, groups which are equivalent on all important antecedent variables. All random assignment does is provide an equal opportunity for patients to be in one group or another one. This allows antecedent variables to vary unsystematically (randomly), where their variation can be taken into account in statistical procedures. Whether the groups turn out to be equal or not is quite another question (48).

In the long run, random assignment will tend to produce groups which are fairly evenly distributed on the important background variables. But sometimes, as in the case of small samples, there will be no long run, and more specific ways to equalize the groups may be desired. Then it is possible to make use of information about which characteristics of the sample it is important to distribute equally. Pairs of patients who occupy the same position on the important variables are selected and the members of the pairs randomly assigned to the groups. Suppose, for example, that the hypothesis to be tested predicts that a certain nursing approach will lower patients' anxiety on admission to the hospital. The factors in the patients' backgrounds that might be important are previous hospital experience, diagnosis and age. Previous hospitalization might be groups with "no previous experience," and "with previous experience" (exclusive of maternity admissions). Diagnosis might simply be "major" or "minor" surgery, or perhaps "cancer suspected" or "no cancer suspected." Age might be grouped into decades—twenty–twenty-nine, thirty–thirty-nine, forty–forty-nine and so on. Then pairs of patients are picked (preferably at the same time) who are in the same categories of the variables. A patient who is forty–forty-nine years old, has no previous hospital experience and in whom cancer is suspected will be matched with another patient in the same categories and so on. Then, which member of the pair goes in the experimental or control group is determined randomly, by a flip of the coin or some other device. The data from this kind of study are treated in terms of the matched pairs, with the scores of one member of the pair compared with the scores of the other member. Matching produces nonindependent samples and calls for the use of special statistical procedures for matched pairs. This kind of matching is called *precision matching*.

Another form of matching is *frequency matching*. Here, rather than matching people case-for-case, the groups are equalized on the overall frequence of occurrence of the important variables. For example, if one is interested in the effect of nursing support on success in breast feeding, it might be important to be sure that both the experimental and control group had the same proportion of rooming-in and nonrooming-in mothers in them.

To make the groups equal on this variable, one might randomly assign within the two categories. The first rooming-in mother to come along would be assigned by coin flip to one group or another, and afterwards, all rooming-in mothers would alternately go in one group or the other. The first non-rooming-in mother would also be assigned by a coin flip, then as other nonrooming-in mothers appeared, they would alternately be assigned to experimental or control groups. In the end, the groups would be equivalent on this variable. This method is a combination of stratifying with random assignment.

Another way to achieve the same end is sometimes used. Instead of stratifying and randomly assigning within classes of the variables of interest, sometimes the researcher just begins as usual randomly assigning people as they come along. Then at some point, the groups are surveyed to see how they are stacking up in relation to rooming-in; for instance, if one group is short, the next few people who are rooming-in would automatically go in that group. The assumption is that the order in which people appear in the sample is itself random so that constituting groups this way still amounts to random assignment, but this process is clearly not as rigorous as it might be.

The major disadvantage of using precision or frequency matching is loss of cases that cannot be matched. The study design is also more complicated the more variables are included in the matching procedure, and data collection time may lengthened waiting for pairs to appear. The disadvantages are outweighed by the contribution to the rigor of testing hypotheses by having more assurance that the groups are initially as alike as possible on the important variables, especially in small samples.

Sample size is no less an issue in causal hypothesis-testing studies than in any other, and because in these studies the total sample is broken down in the various groups of the independent variable, sample size becomes even more important. It is possible to test adequately causal hypotheses with very small samples, as there are statistical procedures developed especially for small samples and independent groups. But in a small sample, each case carries more weight than in larger samples, so that if even one sample unit acts very different from others in its group (had a very high or very low reading on the dependent variable, for instance), the effect is more than if the sample were larger.

There is often an attempt to create equal sized groups in experimental studies. Equal groups are not really necessary either to test the hypothesis or to use statistical procedures. In small samples, coin tosses to assign each patient to groups will probably not produce equal numbers in each group, which is why alternate assignment or block randomization may be used instead.

Operational definition-independent variable

As in any hypothesis-testing study, all the variables that are going to be treated in the hypothesis or research questions are provided with operational definitions and ways to be measured. In experimental studies, there are particular considerations in the operational definition of the independent variables, the one that is introduced and the one whose effect is measured in the dependent variable.

Studies which test the effect of nursing approaches (as opposed to procedures or techniques) demand that the approach be spelled out in enough detail so that it can be repeated by other investigators from the material contained in the final report alone. This can be difficult, especially when the approach is something like "supportive care," or "nursing support," or "nurse-patient interaction." Theories about such concepts, including their definitions and properties, are not yet well developed in the field, though it is often assumed that nurse readers of research reports will know intuitively what nursing support means.

Two major types of definition of the independent variable can be seen in the literature (49). The first attack on the problem of defining nursing is to define it by reference to either interpersonal theory or nursing theory. Thus, there are references to someone's theory of nursing interaction in fairly general terms: _____'s nursing theory guided the experimental approach. In this theory, the nurse deliberately shares her own perceptions, thoughts and feelings with the patient to validate the patient's experience and help define his need for help. A second method of defining and standardizing nursing approach has been to use a script which the nurse just follows in administering the nursing treatment.

The difficulty with the first method is, of course, that unless the reader thoroughly understands the theory being tested, it is difficult to figure out what exactly was done with patients, much less to repeat the study. The problem with the second method is that it can be difficult clinically to adhere to a script when the patient's situation doesn't fit what was scripted. Further, a script approach represents a somewhat smaller increment of theory construction.

As nursing research has become more sophisticated, we now see clearer statements of nursing approach appearing in the literature, statements that lie somewhere between the theory-only approach to definition and the script. The following is one of the better examples:

. . . the total experimental intervention can be subdivided into two parts: (1) information-rehearsal and (2) the supportive relationship established between the nurse and the child and parents. The information-rehearsal component includes the descriptions and explanations of hospital routines, sequences of events, procedures, sensory experiences, various staff roles, appropriate patient and parent roles, along with the special techniques for communicating this information effectively . . . and play techniques for younger children . . . The desired supportive relationship . . . is one of trust and confidence, which presumably is achieved with a warm personal approach, encouragement, reassurance, reinforcement of appropriate behavior, along with a genuine expression of interest in the individual child and parent as unique persons. This interpersonal mode has been characterized as the "expressive function" of nursing. . . . (50)

Several recent studies have used audio-tape, or tape with slide presentations of information to test the effect of such preparation on postoperative behavior, or other patient behavior during difficult procedures (51). The advantage of this method is that it is standard, and the same information is given in the same way to all patients in the experimental group. The disadvantage is that there is no opportunity for the patient to interact with the voice on the tape if the patient might have information needs or feelings quite apart from the prescribed information or approach.

Devising operational definitions for the independent variable in patient care research is a "damned if you do, damned if you don't" situation. One wishes to respect the clinical situation, including the patients' individual and idiosyncratic behavior, needs, wishes and so on, but at the same time, one wants to keep the experimental approach as standard as possible. Another tactic that has been used (but only in two studies so far) has been to define the independent variable, when it is nursing approach, by categories of an interaction analysis scheme (52). Here, the verbal interaction between nurse and patient can be classified into various categories, and those categories can be used to define different approaches to the patient. For example, the categories of the Nurse Orientation System (NOSY) classify verbal interaction of the nurse as orientation to the patient as a feeling (emotional) person, as a thinking-evaluating person or as a being-doing person. Nursing approaches can be designed (and have been) using various combinations of these categories: in one group, nurses are oriented to the patient in all three dimensions; in a second group, only the thinking and being-doing orientations are used; in a third group, only the being-doing dimension. The categories are defined broadly enough to give standard guidelines to the nursing approaches, but not so broadly that immediate patient responses or an individual nurses' interactional style cannot be accommodated.

Defining the control treatment in causal hypothesis-testing studies is just as important as defining the experimental approach, and receives somewhat less attention than it should in reported studies. The easiest way to define the control approach, when there are only two groups, is to define it as the absence of the experimental treatment. Then additional information should be provided if possible about what the patients who are randomly assigned to the control treatment did get, if they didn't get the experimental approach. The point to be reinforced here is that it must be clear that the experimental approach and the control approach are indeed different; otherwise it is not possible to conclude anything from the results. When normal (or routine) nursing care is the control treatment, there should be some effort to describe that, including, if appropriate, information on who, of the nursing staff, was involved—RNs, aide, LPNs and so on. The study from which the definition of the experimental approach was quoted earlier contains a very good description of the control treatment:

On admission to the ward, the parents and child saw the admission nurse (a part time LPN who did admission procedures for all patients throughout the hospital). The child was weighed and measured and his vital signs recorded . . . During the afternoon, an anesthesiologist reviewed the child's chart and wrote orders for medication. He did not routinely see the parents or child . . . No specific nursing contact, except during change of shift was made with the child or parent unless a problem arose. No preoperative instruction was given. . . . Overall, the nursing contact, except for answering call lights and special requests by parents, was limited for this type of patient. . . . In general, the nurses were friendly, courteous, and concerned in their interactions with parents and children. However, there was no formal preparation nor systematic attempt to determine parents' and children's informational and emotional needs. (53)

More than one comparison treatment may be tested as a control on the investigator's personality. For example, one group of patients might receive a "deliberative" nursing approach, administered by one nurse. The same nurse might work with another group of patients, not using the deliberative approach, but providing information, and generally being her usual self. A third group might receive the "normal nursing care." In cases such as this, all the nursing approaches have to be defined and the difference among them made clear (54).

Hypotheses

As in association-testing studies, causal hypothesis testing-studies contain formal statements of relationships and prediction. In the case of causal hypothesis-testing studies, the prediction is of a particular kind of relationship, not merely correlational, but causal. The particular effects predicted to happen as a result of the independent variable are what are contained in the causal hypothesis.

Causal hypotheses can be either directional or not. That is, the hypothesis may simply state that there will be a difference (in the dependent variable) between the experimental and control group, but not exactly what the difference will be. Or, the hypothesis may predict the direction of the difference: lower anxiety, fewer complications, earlier discharge or whatever. On the whole, stating directional hypotheses is a stronger test, since the direction of the difference is probably implied in the theory anyhow. For example, a study of the effect of nursing on postoperative vomiting really predicts that a certain kind of nursing will lower the vomiting rate, not raise it, so it makes no sense to state a nondirectional hypothesis of difference.

If a study is testing the effect of more than one experimental approach, the direction of difference among the various experimental groups is stated too. Wording such hypotheses can get cumbersome; patients who experience a deliberative approach will have smoother recovery than patients who experience an informational approach, and both groups will have smoother recovery than patients who experience routine nursing care. If a rank order of the difference among treatment groups is implied, it should be made explicit, worded as clearly as humanly possible.

How the hypothesis is worded is a matter of taste and common sense. In the literature, one finds some hypotheses stated in very operational terms: patients in Group A will experience less (or more) _____ than patients in Group B. Other times, the hypotheses are translated into plain English: patients who receive a nursing approach designed to allow them to express anxiety and obtain information will have less postoperative vomiting and smoother recovery from surgery. If the hypothesis is stated as the second example here is, then following it should be a statement of operational definition that makes clear exactly what data will be taken as evidence of the existence of, say, "smoother recovery."

It is important to worry a bit about how best to state an hypothesis not only so that it makes sense to the reader later, but so that the investigator really knows what is being predicted, and what data will be considered as having supported the hypothesis or not. For example, a study might predict that a certain kind of nursing would reduce complications of recovery. But does reduce mean that there will be fewer of them, or that the ones that occur will be more minor? The relationship between the hypothesis and its statement of dependent variation predicted and the operational definitions to be used for the dependent variables has to be very specific.

Again, as in association-testing studies, there is no point in stating the hypotheses in the null form.

Instruments/Measurements

Measurements of the dependent variables are critical in causal hypothesis-testing studies. Evidence of the reliability and validity, as well as the sensitivity and precision of instruments, has to be provided. Standardized forms, procedures, protocols or instruments help guarantee that some sources of systematic error are ruled out, and it is systematic error that one wants to eliminate so that "all other things (besides the systematic variation of the independent variable)" are equal.

There is a relationship in causal hypothesis-testing studies between the degree of difference in the conditions of the independent variable and the precision of measurement of the dependent variable. In general, the bigger the difference in the conditions of the independent variable, the less precise may be the measures of the dependent variable, and the effect will still show up. The smaller the differences in the independent variable, the more precise must be the measure of the dependent variable to pick them up.

For example, a study testing some form of high-powered nursing approach, done by a highly skilled, specially trained nurse compared with "routine nursing care" may be able to depend on rather gross measures of the dependent variable since the difference between the experimental and control conditions is so great. On the other hand, a study testing the effect of rather subtle differences in nursing approach, all administered by the same nurse, may require more sensitive and precise measures. This does not mean that if one is proposing a study where there will be large differences between experimental treatments one can rest easy and use messy measures of the dependent variable. Precision and sensitivity are to be aimed for in any kind of study.

It is a nice touch in causal hypothesis-testing studies to supply measures of the independent variable too, when appropriate. Tape recordings of nurse-patient interaction, or observations by unbiased observers, or some other evidence that the experimental procedures were indeed carried out as specified contributes to the rigor of the study. These measures are particularly important in studies in which someone other than the investigator will carry out the prescribed treatments, like the children's mothers, or perhaps other nurses or even the patients. For example, a study of the effect of teaching antepartum exercises on length of labor has to depend on the patient actually *doing* the exercises, and it is well to build in a way to collect data on that, if possible.

There is a peculiar problem sometimes in causal hypothesis-testing studies analogous to the halo effect discussed in the last chapter. The problem doesn't have a formal name, but might be called "check versus effect." What is meant is that on occasion a variable can be measured as if it were an effect of the independent variable when in fact it is a check on whether the independent variable was carried out as specified. For example, a study tested the effect of a certain nursing intervention on relief from pain (55). The nursing treatment specified that the nurse would explore with the patient alternative ways to relieve pain other than the ordered p.r.n pain medication. Then dosages of pain medication were measured as an indirect measure of "pain," but also as if the medication were an effect of the independent variable, when in fact giving (or not giving in this case) the medication was specified *as part of* the independent variable. In another study of the effect of a nursing approach in reducing disorientation in postcoronary surgery patients, a nursing treatment was designed so that the patient was systematically and regularly given reorientation to time, place and person (56). But the treatment also specified that when the nurses noticed a patient becoming disoriented, the reorientation program would be immediately instituted. Then measures were taken of, among other things, number of instances of disorientation in both the experimental and control group. But because immediate reaction to disorientation was part of the independent variable, numbers of such episodes can't be used as a measure of the dependent variable.

Careful attention to the operational definition of the independent variable and its relationship to the theory being tested can prevent some interesting problems. A study of different kinds of sensory input on time estimation provides an interesting example (57). An elegant piece of theoretical work led the investigator to hypothesize that people who receive a regular, under-standable kind of sensory input (a tape-recorded radio drama) would estimate time intervals more accurately than people who received either meaningless sensory input, or "no input." The last group of people were simply to lie on a bed in a quiet room, with no special sound. The results did not come out the way predicted because, as the investigator found, the "no input" situation wasn't really no input. People in a quiet room will listen for sounds—planes overhead, traffic, noises, footsteps in the hall, in order to keep their time orientation, and short of a sensory deprivation chamber, a "no input" situation is just "different input."

Another study with a nice example of the same problem tested the effect of vitamin C versus a placebo on prevention of colds. The investigators randomly assigned people to receive ascorbic acid pills or a substitute sugar pill, but were out-foxed by the sample who could clearly tell the difference in taste between the slightly bitter vitamin C pill and the definitely sweet sugar pill. Subjects knew, therefore, which group they were in, invalidating the blindness of the study (58).

Data Collection

In this kind of study, data collection aspires to be objective. Since the only thing that is supposed to vary systematically is the independent variable, all other sources of variation are checked on, controlled or allowed to vary randomly. Other sources of variation besides the independent variable include antecedent variables, intervening variables, sources of error in sampling or assignment and within the data collection processes. Antecedent variables are taken account of through sampling and assignment. Sources of error from intervening variables are assumed to vary randomly in the experimental and control groups. However, it is always a good idea to identify as many of these intervening variables as possible and have some data on them so that one can check on what happened between the independent variable and measurement of the dependent variable.

Sources of error in measurement may be within the instrument itself or within the measurer or data collector. If the questions asked the experimental group in an interview are different from those asked the control group, this would be a measurement error. If the data collector collects data differently from the experimental group than from the control group, this would be a measurer error.

Measurement errors are minimized by having standard measurement procedures, instruments or techniques. Measurer errors are minimized through the use of blind observation where the data collector does not know which group the patient is in, and/or does not know the hypothesis. It is assumed that if a data collector knew what group the patient was in, or knew the hypothesis, he might unconsciously treat patients differently depending on their group assignment. Blind observation lends more rigor to causal hypothesis-testing studies by assuring that at least one source of systematic error is controlled. It is possible to set up the data collection procedure in such a way that the person administering the experimental variable does not even know the treatment that is being given, much less the group that the patient is in. This is called a "double blind" study and is most often done in connection with drug research. In this case, the people who are giving the experimental drugs or placebos do not know what drugs they are giving since the drugs are given false labels or names. Similarly, the people who are measuring the effect of the drugs and the subjects themselves do not know which drugs have been given. The random assignment of drugs to subjects is done by someone outside the project. Double blind studies are most often used to guard against the possibility that the investigator's commitment to the efficacy of a particular treatment has more effect than the treatment itself. Double blind studies are rarely used in nursing because the kind of treatments involved require that the investigator know what the treatment is.

It is important that data be collected on the independent as well as the dependent variable. While the latter is used as the primary test of the hypothesis, data on the independent variable can be used not only to help illustrate the operational definitions, but also to help validate that the experimental treatments were in fact different and were carried out according to their definition.

Since the experimental variable in nursing research is so often nursing care itself, causal hypothesis-testing studies can be extremely painful to conduct. It may seem to the investigator that she is putting her own practice on the line—which she is. Some evidence from psychology suggests that is not all "bad," at least from the point of view of results. When an investigator is committed to a certain approach and when she herself is conducting the study, no matter how carefully she defines the independent variable, her commitment to it may carry the most weight. This is the so-called experimenter effect (59) or placebo effect. Such commitment also helps explain why some replications of causal hypothesis studies fail to achieve the same support for the hypothesis. Other investigators may not be as invested as the first one, so replicated studies don't turn out the same way. Although thinking in terms of commitment rather than operational definitions tends to mess up the study, the implications for nursing practice may be just as firm, whether the findings suggest that commitment plus certain treatments or that certain treatments alone achieve the predicted results.

A phenomenon related to the experimenter effect is the Hawthorne effect which means that even the fact of being part of a study can achieve the predicted results with or without special treatments (60). The Hawthorne effect is named after a series of industrial experiments done some years ago. The researchers were varying the working conditions of a group of assembly line workers, changing lighting conditions and so forth and looking at the effects on work output. They discovered that no matter what they did, production increased. Even when the lighting in the room was reduced to barely candle power, work increased. They finally decided that the attention being devoted to the workers was by itself enough to produce the desired results—a finding that has obvious implications. Still it is well to be on the lookout for possible evidence of a Hawthorne effect in nursing research. Just measuring patients on the dependent variable regardless of whether they've been exposed to a special experimental condition may convey something about interest or caring for them.

The more closely a research design approximates practice, the more relevant the findings are likely to be. This goes not only for the selection of measurement variables, settings and so on, but also for the conduct of the independent variable. Early experiments in nursing practice tended to compare the results obtained when one or two expert, specially trained nurses worked intensely with patients with the results obtained by staff nurses carrying out their usual jobs. While this may make an excellent situation for testing a general hypothesis, the findings may be out of reach for the great majority of nursing practitioners. In addition, such comparisons are odious to staff nurses as a group and do nothing for public relations between researchers and practitioners. An independent variable defined so that the nurse has unlimited amounts of time to spend with patients may be method-ologically sound but totally useless to practitioners. Therefore, it is important to chose concepts to test that are applicable to and accessible to practice as it now is as well as to operationalize them so that they can be carried out in natural practice situations. There are now several studies in the nursing literature that make this point exquisitely (61).

As in all studies, informed consent from the subjects under study must be obtained formally. There are special considerations in obtaining informed consent in experimental studies, covered in detail in Chapter 11.

Data Processing/Analysis

It is wise in any study, but especially in causal hypothesis-testing studies to set up in advance, before data are collected, "dummy tables" for how the data will be analyzed. Such tables are conceptual aids to help clarify exactly what numbers will be plugged into the tables later, and what differences will be tested. A dummy table is simply the outline of what will become the real table, without the numbers in it. For example, a study testing the effect of nursing on postoperative vomiting in a two group, after only design, might have the following dummy table:

	Vomiting	
	Yes	No
Experimental		
Control		

(Frequencies)

The numbers of patients in each cell of the table would then be compared.

A before-after, two group design might have a dummy table that looks superficially like the one above, but the numbers to be inserted in it are not frequencies (obviously, there are the same number of people before and after) but are actual readings. For example, a study of topical insulin applied to decubitus ulcers might measure the size of the ulcer in centimeters before applying the insulin, and at a period after, producing the following table:

Decubitus Ulcer Size

	Before	*After*
With Insulin		
Without		

Thinking up dummy tables may seem a kind of infantile tactic to use, but experience suggests that researchers get much more clear about what it is the hypothesis predicts and how the data will be analyzed if forced to use these kinds of visual aids in advance. It is possible to get so involved in one's own research that one forgets some kinds of basic things, like exactly what is going to be counted and compared.

Details of data processing are thought through in advance because how the data will be processed and analyzed has implications for how it will be collected.

To prevent yet another kind of systematic error, data processing might be done by someone who does not know what group the patients are in or who has no connection with the study. If the investigator herself processes the data she may unconsciously slant it. This is probably not a very serious source of error—errors in data collection or measurement are more serious—but if the investigator wants a really rigorous study, blind data processing might be built in. The same issue can be handled by making sure that no identifying data (patient name, characteristics, group assignment) appear on the data collection sheets. Instead, code numbers picked at random can be used and data transferred to machine cards with the group assignment being the last thing entered.

Analysis procedures will depend on the type of study design, the number of variables and measurements and the number of groups. In general, differences between the groups are calculated and appropriate statistical techniques are available to determine how likely it is that the differences have occurred by chance alone.

Both the antecedent and independent variables are examined, the first to determine how alike the groups were to begin with, the second to validate that the condition necessary for testing the hypothesis (variation in independent variable) was achieved. Although in this kind of study the major focus is testing the particular hypothesis, other hypotheses can also be generated for future testing. Such hypotheses may come from an intensive examination of the antecedent variables and the independent variable, if it is possible that the treatment works better for some people than for others.

Analysis of the data that does not specifically pertain to the hypothesis is always a good idea, for it may clarify the findings or point the way for future studies or changes in practice. Such data might consist of an anecdotal record kept by the investigator, including thoughts on the measurements, on the conduct of the research, on a reconceptualization of the problem or anything else. A study is never just the data that were collected, but the data may serve as a jumping-off point for new ideas or new theories about nursing practice.

Data on possible intervening variables should also be examined. Random assignment helps assure the random (versus systematic) variation of antecedent variables. The effect of intervening variables may be minimized by measuring the dependent variable as soon as possible after the independent variable is administered. The longer the time between the introduction of the independent variable and the measurement of the dependent variable, the more possible it is for other things to have happened that might affect the outcome. For example, in the preoperative nursing-postoperative vomiting study mentioned earlier, there were some twelve hours between nursing care and the measurement of the dependent variable in the recovery room. Any number of things could have happened in between that would have had an effect on the findings. When it is known that there will be such a long lapse between measurements, it is wise to collect data on possible intervening variables. For instance, one might ask patients to recall what happened to them or what they did between the time the nurse left and the time they were prepared for surgery the next morning.

The problem of "uncontrolled situational variables" has received some particular attention (62). When intervening variables cannot be controlled by sampling or time of measurement, data may be analyzed later to see what, if any, effect they had on variation in the dependent variable. In the study cited here, the investigators found that type of surgery was related to number of doses of analgesic, occurrence of fever and other signs of infection, length of postoperative hospitalization and anxiety on admission; duration of anesthesia was related to ability to void after surgery, for example. It happened in this study that the effect of these uncontrolled situational variables was greater than the effect of the nursing intervention.

It is a thin study indeed in which only data pertaining to the hypothesis are analyzed. Strictly speaking, only those data are really required to be analyzed, but the movement toward future research and toward prescription may be enhanced much further if alternative, contributory or contingent conditions can be identified.

At the end of a causal hypothesis-testing study, one wants to be able to conclude not only that something worked, if it did, but *why*. When an hypothesis is supported by the data, the explanation will be found in the theory that began the study. When the hypothesis is not supported, explanation has to be found as well.

INTERPRETATION/CAUSAL INFERENCE

Three things are necessary to make causal inferences: concomitant variation, time order and *ceteris paribus*, "all other things being equal." With evidence that these conditions have been met, the investigator can make a claim for causal interpretations, assuming the results came out as predicted. This does not mean the hypothesis has been *proved*. Hypotheses are never proved—they are tested and either supported or not supported by the data. "Support" means that the probability that the findings happened by chance alone—that is, that the independent variable did not have the predicted effect—is less than some preset level, usually 5 or 1 percent. The greater the probability that the predicted effect did occur, the more tenable the hypothesis is. The greater the evidence that all other things were equal, the more confidence one has in the findings.

Hypotheses are usually considered supported or not on the basis of statistical significance. But statistical significance is not the only test that can be applied. Findings can be statistically significant and practically irrelevant, or they can be less than statistically significant but theoretically important. Statistics is not a substitute for thinking. For example, suppose a study tested the effect of various kinds of nursing practice on patients in pain (63). One of the measures used might be amount of pain medication taken (this is a different study from the one cited earlier in check versus effect). There might be a statistically significant difference in the predicted direction in amount of pain medication, measured by equivalent dosages of morphine (a formula available in the literature). The actual mathematical difference might be, say, 2 milligrams, which is less than one-quarter of a normal dose of morphine, and therefore probably clinically irrelevant. Here, because the measurement is so precise, very small mathematical differences can become statistically significant.

On the other hand, suppose that the same study used judgments of verbal and nonverbal behavior to determine whether patients felt worse, the same or better following the nursing intervention. Suppose further that the nursing interventions were rather subtly different interactional approaches to the patient. The data came out this way (with a sample size of 30) (64):

	WORSE	SAME	BETTER	
Experimental Group I	0	1	9	10
Experimental Group II	0	1	9	10
Experimental Group III	0	1	9	10
				30

What this says is that no matter what the approach was, patients tended to feel better. While this is a negative finding in terms of no statistically significant difference, it may be clinically meaningful, since it says that any one of the three approaches produces the same effect, and all the effects are in the direction of betterness for the patient.

When findings come out negative, that is, when the data do not support the hypothesis, the burden is on the investigator to figure out why. In general, the explanation might come from the theory itself, the operational definitions, assignment of patients to groups or sampling, errors in measurement or data collection, imprecision in measurements, or inadequate statistical treatment of the data. All sources of explanation should be consciously surveyed.

Sometimes the theory that one is working with is just plain wrong. For example, a study tested the effect of psychiatric nursing group treatment with chronically ill psychiatric outpatients who were all already stabilized on medication (65). The control group did not have the nursing treatment, but had available a monthly medication clinic. The investigators had developed a theory that said that it would take two years of following these patients to detect the effects of the nursing treatment, because it takes chronically ill psychiatric patients a very long time to identify with the group and establish trust. The results showed no big difference between the experimental and control groups, and what differences did appear showed the control patients, those simply obtaining medication refills once per month with no other treatment, doing better. Reanalysis of the theory indicated that the nature of chronic illness had probably been misinterpreted, and that the nursing groups had the effect of keeping the patients dependent, so that they did not increase their socialization in the community, whereas the patients who received no real treatment were forced to find some socialization elsewhere.

Problems in operational definition have been discussed earlier. Sampling may be an explanation for negative findings, for example, in a case where the sample of people chosen did not have enough of the target condition—stress, anxiety or something—to allow the nursing treatment to lower it much. Or samples might be drawn from certain settings where the nursing care is really superb already, so that a special kind of nursing intervention would not be all that different from "routine nursing care" on this unit.

Review of assignment of people to groups, even when random, may contribute to understanding why an hypothesis was not supported. In the study of chronically ill psychiatric patients mentioned before, it happened that patients in the control group were more often employed as the study began than patients in the nursing group, so they automatically scored higher in socialization and occupation ratings, and it could be suspected that their employment status itself contributed to a higher quality of life. Strictly speaking, random assignment always works when it is truly done randomly, and when the sample is large enough. Analysis of data should take into account how even the groups were to begin with, and systematic variations in group characteristics may be an argument for replication with a larger sample.

Data collection errors were covered in the section on data collection. Imprecision of measurement means that "real" differences between groups are not found because the measures used were not sensitive enough to find them. And errors in data analysis may also contribute to negative findings. This may mean that the wrong statistical procedure was used, or that some mathematical manipulation of the data masked real effects (66).

The investigator's clinical knowledge and sense of the setting in which data were collected may lead to other explanations for negative findings. Most commonly, negative findings can result when there is too little difference between the experimental and control treatment because something in the setting is contaminating the groups. This can be an odd, if welcome, result of previous research. For example, studies have shown that preoperative preparation, especially in gynecological surgery patients, can make quite a difference in their postoperative course. Suppose a head nurse and her staff in a certain surgical service decided simply to implement a standard preoperative preparation routine, without fanfare or publicity, but clearly using the results of the research. The next researcher who tries to do a preoperative preparation study in that setting would find that the control or routine nursing patients were already getting preoperative preparation, which might wipe out the theoretical difference between the experimental and control groups (67).

Very recently, examples of studies in which the desire is to obtain negative findings (or no difference between groups) are beginning to appear. These studies deal with the effect of nurse practitioner practice in realms previously the province of medicine, and the hypothesis is essentially a null hypothesis: patients in primary care situations who receive nurse practitioner care will have no different outcome than patients who receive physicians' care (68). (This is the one excuse for an hypothesis in the null form.) If indeed the findings are that there is no difference, at least in medically related variables, the hypothesis is supported rather than rejected.

These studies are an interesting example not only of a case when negative findings are positive, but of how the choice of variables to measure may illuminate, in an interesting theoretical way, conceptual problems to be sorted out in later studies. The theory behind any causal hypothesis-testing study has to match up the designed experimental procedures with appropriate target variables, appropriately measured. In the case of the cited nurse practitioner studies, the interest was in the effect of nursing on *medical* variables—morbidity and mortality. The theory in these early studies did not encompass the notion that nursing might have a different effect than medical practice, if *nursing* variables, that is, variables on which a case can be made that nursing might have an effect because they are more traditionally in the province of nursing's special skill, had been included. Such nursing variables might include things like compliance, comfort, patient knowledge or satisfaction with care. The lesson to be learned is that in devising theory for a causal hypothesis-testing study, and then deriving operational definitions of variables to be tested, one needs to think about what the independent variable might possibly effect and pick variables where there is a theoretical (as well as empirical) reason to think they might be decent measures of effect.

REPLICATION

To build up confidence in causal hypotheses, studies need to be repeated. Only through replicating studies under different unique conditions can we begin to accept a predicted relationship with any real degree of surety. Replication is especially important in the kind of causal hypothesis testing study found in nursing where one nurse does the experimental treatment and the question is always whether another nurse could achieve the same results.

There are essentially two kinds of replication: *literal replication,* in which the original study is exactly duplicated by the same investigator, and *operational replication,* in which the sampling assignment and experimental procedures are duplicated by another investigator (69). Interpretation of data from replications, especially when the findings do not turn out the same as in the original study, is a facinating experience (70). Smith suggests that several factors must be taken into account in analyzing replication results—the subjects, the apparatus, the material, the procedure, the physical setting, the psychological atmosphere, the experimenter and the subject-experimenter interaction (71). It may be that the samples of people, even when the same sampling criteria are used, just turn out to be different because of geography or other circumstances. The apparatus and material are the experimental treatments, and the procedure, how they were administered, as well as how the data were collected. It is quite difficult to figure out differences among experimenters, especially if such differences are matters of appearance, personal style and the like, and differences among studies in physical setting or psychological atmosphere may be ephemeral at best. One potential difference between repeated studies that would fall under "subject-experimenter interaction" (in studies in which that interaction is not itself the independent variable) is in how the people are informed about the study. For example, a well-known study of the effect of information on perception of stress did not replicate. The second group of investigators discovered that while they had told potential subjects when recruiting them that the study was about pain, the first investigator had not, and it could be suspected that this prior knowledge of subjects made a difference in how they perceived the testing situation.

In a replication study, it is legitimate to try to tighten up on procedures or tools that the original investigator noted needed some work. When this happens, however, results have to be interpreted in light of whatever the changes were that were made.

Causal hypothesis-testing studies are the most powerful ways to establish cause-and-effect relationships, though not necessarily the most powerful studies that can ever be done. As always, the basic value of any study depends on how the design is related to the problem. If a clinical problem is not a causal relationship one, then experimental studies are the wrong approach. As we shall see in the next chapter, it takes all kinds of studies, and all kinds of information, some of it cause-and-effect, some not, to build toward prescriptions for practice.

NOTES

1. Abdellah, Faye G. and Eugene Levine: *Better Patient Care Through Nursing Research.* New York: Macmillan, 1965.

2. Dumas, Rhetaugh G. and Robert C. Leonard: The effect of nursing on the incidence of postoperative vomiting: a clinical experiment *Nursing Research,* 12:12–15, Winter 1963.

3. Abdellah and Levine, see Note 1, pp. 578–579.

4. For comments on development of experimental designs in clinical research, see Leonard, Robert C.: Developing research in a practice oriented discipline. *American Journal of Nursing,* 67:1472–1475, July 1967. Wooldridge, Powhatan, et al.: *Behavioral Science, Social Practice and the Nursing Profession.* Cleveland: The Press of Case Western University, 1968. Also Wooldridge, Powhatan, et al.: *Methods of Clinical Experimentation to Improve Patient Care.* St. Louis: C.V. Mosby, 1978, pp. 151–156; Leonard, Robert C., et al.: The application of behavioral science to patient care as illustrated by the etiology and control of stress in clinical settings. In Verhonick, Phyllis J. (ed.), *Nursing Research* (Vol.1). Boston: Little, Brown, 1975, pp. 93–122.

5. I was party to many discussions of the psychology of clinical experiments of one's own practice, as a graduate student under Prof. Robert C. Leonard. Prof. Leonard's point always was that the personal element should not enter into scientific tests of patient care practices, and certainly a nurse was not a failure, or a success, depending on how the results of an experiment came out. Yet, we were naive in those days and many students worried that if the results did not come out as predicted in their study, they would be graded down, which never happened, of course.

6. Some of the early studies with experimental designs include Mahaffy, Perry R.: The effects of hospitalization on children admitted for tonsillectomy and adenoidectomy. *Nursing Research,* 14:12–19, 1965; Elms, Roslyn A. and Robert C. Leonard: Effects of nursing approaches during admission. *Nursing Research,* 15:39–48, 1966. Moran, Patricia A.: Parents in pediatrics. *Nursing Forum,* 2:25–37, 1963; Tryon, Phyllis A. and Robert C. Leonard: A clinical test of patient centered nursing. *Journal of Health and Human Behavior,* 7:183–192, 1966.

7. Orlando, Ida Jean: *The Dynamic Nurse Patient Relationship.* New York: G.P. Putnam's Sons, 1961.

8. Campbell, Donald T. and Julian C. Stanley: *Experimental and Quasi-experimental Designs for Research.* Chicago: Rand McNally, 1963, especially pp. 1–2.

9. Wooldridge, et al., see Note 4 suggest that *ceteris fortuitus* is the more accurate expression (p. 147). *Ceteris paribus* means "all other things being equal" while *ceteris fortuitus* means "all other things being accidental," more in keeping with the concept of randomness. A very nice distinction which readers are urged to pursue.

10. The discussion of necessary, sufficient, and other conditions is paraphrased from Selltiz, Claire, et al.: *Research Methods in Social Relations.* New York: Holt, Rinehart & Winston, 1960, pp. 81–82.

11. Dumas and Leonard, see Note 2; see also, Dumas, Rhetaugh G. and Barbara Anderson:

Research in nursing practice: a review of five clinical experiments. *International Journal of Nursing Studies*, 9:137–150, August 1972.

12. Mahaffey, Perry R., see Note 6.

13. Lindeman, Carol A. and Betty Van Aernam: Nursing intervention with the presurgical patient. *Nursing Research*, 20:319–332, July–August 1971.

14. Johnson, Jean E.: Psychological preparation for endoscopic examination. *Gastrointestinal Endoscopy*, 19:180–182, May 1973; Johnson, Jean E. and Howard Leventhal: Effects of accurate expectations and behavioral instructions on reactions during a noxious medical examination. *Journal of Personal and Social Psychology*, 29:710–718, May 1974.

15. Wolfer, John A. and Madelon A. Visintainer: Pediatric surgical patients' and parents' stress responses and adjustment as a function of psychological preparation and stress-point nursing care. *Nursing Research*, 24:244–255, July–August 1975.

16. Porter, Luz: The impact of physical-psychological activity on infants' growth and development. *Nursing Research*, 21:210–219, May–June 1972.

17. Brown, Marie Scott and Joan T. Hurlock: Preparing the breast for breastfeeding. *Nursing Research*, 24:448–451, November–December 1975; see also a thoughtful letter to the editor by Ramona Mercer, *Nursing Research*, 25:222, May–June 1976, and a not-so-thoughtful letter on the same study by Betty Countryman, *Nursing Research*, 25:267, July–August 1976.

18. Van Ort, Suzanne and Rose M. Gerber: Topical application of insulin in the treatment of decubitus ulcers. *Nursing Research*, 25:9–12, January–February 1976.

19. Hanson, Robert L.: Effects of administering cold and warmed tube feedings. In Batey, Marjorie V. (ed.): *Communicating Nursing Research: Collaboration and Competition* (Vol. 6), Boulder, Colorado: WICHEN, 1973, pp. 136–140.

20. Cleland, Virginia, et al.: Prevention of bacteriuria in female patients with indwelling catheters. *Nursing Research*, 20:309–318, July–August 1971.

21. McCorkle, Ruth: Effects of touch on seriously ill patients. *Nursing Research*, 23:125–132, March–April 1974.

22. Kramer, Marlene, et al.: Extra tactile stimulation of the premature infant. *Nursing Research*, 24:324–335, September–October 1975.

23. Felton, Geraldene: Increasing the quality of care by introducing the concept of primary nursing: a model project. *Nursing Research*, 24:27–32, January–February 1975.

24. Vincent, Pauline and Janet R. Price: Evaluation of a VNA mental health project. *Nursing Research*, 26:361–367, September–October 1977.

25. Beard, Margaret T. and Patsy Y. Scott: Efficacy of group therapy by nurses for hospitalized patients. *Nursing Research*, 24:121–124, March–April 1975.

26. The social psychology theories referred to in this example are discussed in Johnson, and Johnson and Leventhal (see Note 14), and are greatly oversimplified here.

27. Barnard, Kathryn: Effect of stimulation on the sleep behavior of the premature infant. In Batey, Marjorie V. (ed.): *Communicating Nursing Research*, pp. 12–33, see Note 19.

28. Slavinsky, Ann: Final progress report to the Division of Nursing, USPHS Grant # NU 00370, *Nursing with Chronic Psychiatric Outpatients*, 1977; see also Slavinsky, Ann and Vivian Romoff: Consumer participation. *Journal of Nursing Administration*, 3:14–19, May–June 1972; Romoff, Vivian and Ann Slavinsky: A new approach to an old problem: nurse therapy for lower socio-economic chronic psychiatric outpatients. *Perspectives in Psychiatric Care*, 11 (1):10–15, 1973; Slavinsky, Ann, et al.: Back to the community: a dubious blessing. *Nursing Outlook*, 24:370–374, June 1976.

29. Dumas and Leonard, see Note 2, and Dumas and Leonard, see Note 11; Mahaffy, see

Note 6; Johnson, and Johnson and Leventhal, see Note 14; Johnson, Jean E.: Effects of structuring patients' expectations on their reactions to threatening events. *Nursing Research*, 21:499–504, November–December 1972; Visintainer, Madelon A. and John A. Wolfer: Psychological preparation for surgical pediatric patients: the effect of children's and parents' stress responses and adjustment. *Pediatrics*, 56 (2):187–202, August 1975; Anderson, Barbara, et al.: Two experimental tests of a patient-centered admissions process. *Nursing Research*, 14:151–157, Winter 1965; Schmitt, Florence E. and Powhatan Wooldridge: Psychological preparation of surgical patients. *Nursing Research*, 22:108–116, March–April 1973; Egbert, Lawrence D., et al.: Reduction of postoperative pain by encouragement and instruction of patients. *New England Journal of Medicine*, 270:825–827, April 16, 1964. Johnson, Jean E., et al.: Sensory information, instruction in a coping strategy, and recover from surgery. *Research in Nursing and Health*, 1:4–17, April 1978; Johnson, Joan E. et al.: Altering patients' responses to surgery: an extension and replication. *Research in Nursing and Health*. 1:111–121, October 1978.

30. Meyers, Mary E.: The effect of types of communication on patients' reactions to stress. *Nursing Research*, 13:126–131, Spring 1964; Moss, Fay and Burton Meyer: The effects of nursing interaction upon pain relief in patients. *Nursing Research*, 15:303–306, Fall 1966; McBride, M. Angela: Nursing approach, pain and relief: an exploratory experiment. *Nursing Research*, 16:337–341, Fall 1967; Davitz, Lois J.: Inferences of physical pain and psychological distress. *Nursing Research*, 19:388 401, September–October 1970; Davitz, Lois J. and Sydney Pendleton: Nurses' inferences of suffering. *Nursing Research*, 18:100–107, March–April 1969; Diers, Donna, et al.: Effect of nursing interaction on patients in pain. *Nursing Research*, 21:419–424, September–October 1972.

31. Sometimes a distinction is drawn between "prediction" and "control," the former applied to survey (association-testing) designs, the latter to experimental design. The distinction is made apparently to make clearer the purpose of noncausal hypotheses-testing as prediction, and the purpose of causal hypothesis-testing as controlling variables.

32. Fisher, Sir Ronald: *The Design of Experiments*. London: Oliver and Boyd, (8th edition), 1951. Actually, the "classical experimental design" in Fisher is a two-group, after-only design, but since the before-after, two-group design is the most often referred to as "classical," this mistake is preserved here.

33. Saltenis, Ieva-Jurate: Physical touch and nursing support during labor. Unpublished master's thesis, Yale University School of Nursing, 1962.

34. Brown and Hurlock, see Note 17.

35. See Elms, Roslyn R.: Effects of varied nursing approaches during hospital admission: an exploratory study. *Nursing Research*, 13:266–268, Summer, 1964. Also, Elms and Leonard, Note 6.

36. Diers, et al., see Note 28.

37. Visintainer and Wolfer, see Note 29.

38. *Ibid,* and Wolfer and Visintainer, see Note 15.

39. Lindeman, Carol A.: Nursing intervention with the presurgical patients: effectiveness and efficiency of group and individual preoperative teaching—phase two. *Nursing Research*, 21:196–209, May–June 1972.

40. In the study cited, "site of surgery" was also used as a classification variable, *ex post facto*, making a 2x2x3x3 factorial design, which is too complicated to try to diagram!

41. Wooldridge et al., see Note 4, p. 188.

42. Slavinsky, see Note 28.

43. Brown and Hurlock, see Note 17.

44. Komaroff, Anthony: Nurse practitioner management of common respiratory and genitourinary infections, using protocols. *Nursing Research*, 25:84–89, March–April 1976.

45. Molde, Susan: Nurse practitioners and physicians in primary care: evaluation in an urban university hospital medical clinic. Unpublished master's thesis, Yale University School of Nursing, 1976.

46. Gagneaux, Vickie and David V. Shaver, Jr.: Distractions at nurses' stations during intershift report. *Nursing Research*, 26:42–46, January–February 1977.

47. Mills, Mary E., et al.: Effect of pulse palpation on cardiac arrhythmia in coronary care patients. *Nursing Research*, 25:378–382, September–October 1976.

48. It can be argued that surveying the antecedent variables of treatment groups after data are collected to see if the random assignment "worked" is not legitimate. The appropriate test of whether random assignment works is to look at the assignment procedure itself. If it was done correctly, and truly randomly (or if it can be determined that even with alternative assignment after a random start, that there are no alternatively varying phenomena in the setting), then how the groups actually turn out is irrelevant, and is taken into account in statistical procedures as random variation. (Robert C. Leonard, personal communication.) If precision matching has not been used, nor random assignment with stratification, I believe it is valid to look at the antecedent variables, not to see whether random assignment worked so much as to tease out of the findings some possible hints for future research. We know far too little about what, in patients, might be related to either independent or dependent variables, so *ex post facto* analysis of all data, including antecedent variation, may give some valuable clues for replication.

49. This discussion is paraphrased from Diers, et al., see Note 30.

50. Visintainer and Wolfer, see Note 29, pp. 189–190.

51. Lindeman and Van Aernam, see Note 13; Johnson, see Notes 14 and 29.

52. See Diers, et al., Note 30 and Conant, Lucy: An exploratory study of nurse-patient give and take. Final progress report to USPHS, Division of Nursing, Grant NU 00181, 1967.

53. Visintainer and Wolfer, see Note 29, p. 191.

54. How the groups are named can be important. In McBride's first study, see Note 30, the groups were named "deliberative" nursing, "friendly" nursing, and "automatic" nursing. The first two were done by the investigator herself; the last was "routine nursing care." McBride had the experience of reporting back her study to the nursing staff, with negative reactions, since it appeared that their nursing care was not only "automatic," it was unfriendly.

55. Tarusuk, Mary Ann B., et al.: An experimental test of the importance of communications skills for effective nursing. In Skipper, James K., Jr. and Robert C. Leonard (eds.): *Social Interaction and Patient Care*. Philadelphia: J.B. Lippincott Company, 1965, pp. 110–120.

56. Budd, Suzanne and Willa Brown: Effect of a reorientation technique on postcardiotomy delirium. *Nursing Research*, 23:341–348, July–August 1974.

57. Smith, Mary Jane: Changes in judgment of duration with different patterns of auditory information for individuals confined to bed. *Nursing Research*, 24:93–98, March–April 1975.

58. Karlowski, Thomas T., et al.: Ascorbic acid for the common cold: a prophylactic and therapeutic trial. *Journal of the American Medical Association*, 231:1538–1542, March 10, 1975.

59. Rosenthal, Robert: *The Experimenter Effect in Behavioral Reseach*. New York: Appleton-Century-Crofts, 1967.

60. See Chapter 3 of this book. Also, Wooldridge, et al. see Note 4, p. 32.

61. Healy, Katherine: Does preoperative instruction make a difference? *American Journal of Nursing*, 68:62–67, January 1968; see also almost anything written by Carol A. Lindeman (Note 12, for example). See also Elliott, Jo Eleanor: Research programs and projects of

WICHEN. *Nursing Research*, 26:277–280, July–August 1977. WICHEN has piled up an enviable record of research stimulation and production in studies of nursing practice under the direction of Carol A. Lindeman and Janelle Kreuger.

62. Johnson, Barbara, et al.: Research in nursing practice: the problem of uncontrolled situational variables. *Nursing Research*, 19:337–342, July–August 1970. See also Wolfer, John A.: Definition and assessment of surgical patients' welfare and recovery. *Nursing Research*, 22:394–401, September–October 1973, for discussion of the Johnson paper and other related problems.

63. This example is a real one, but not of a dependent variable. See Diers, et al., Note 30.

64. This is a real example. McBride, see Note 29.

65. Slavinsky, Ann, see Note 28.

66. One of the mathematical manipulations used in before-after experimental designs is "change scores"—subtract the "after" score from the "before," then compare the two groups, experimental and control, on how much change there was. There is some argument in statistical camps about whether change scores are the right way to analyze data, or whether repeated measures analysis of variance is. The latter technique makes use of more information, the former is easier to calculate by hand, if that's a consideration.

67. This is a real story. Two nurses on the gynecological unit at Yale New Haven Hospital started quite on their own a program of preoperative preparation for surgical patients, using a group technique. Also at the same hospital, research on preparing children for surgery, using tours and rehearsals, led to instituting hospital and operating room tours for children and their parents as a matter of course.

68. See Spitzer, Walter O., et al.: The Burlington randomized trial of the nurse practitioner. *New England Journal of Medicine*, 290:137–142, February 1974; Wolfer, see Note 61; also comments on the distinction between "medical" and nursing variables, not in the context of the expanded role, but in discussing nursing practice in terms of its major focus on supportive care.

69. Lykken, D.T.: Statistical significance in psychological research, *Psychological Bulletin*, 70(3):151–159, 1968. In Lykken's article he notes a third kind of replication: "constructive replication"—formulating new methods, sampling procedures, measurement and data analysis. I have left out this third kind of replication which seems only to confuse things, since it seems clearly a different order of "replication."

70. Diers, et al., see Note 30, for example.

71. Smith, N.C.: Replication studies: a neglected aspect of psychological research. *American Psychologist*, 25:970–975, October 1970.

8

Toward Prescription-Testing Studies

Creating prescriptions for testing in practice and developing tested prescriptive theory is the logical extension of the other kinds of theory development and testing covered in the last four chapters. However, the discussion of prescription-testing here will necessarily be more tentative than previous discussions of kinds of studies, since there are not available in the literature tested examples, or even expositions of the method. Therefore, this chapter presents an overview and restatement of the idea of prescriptive or situation-producing theory (1), then a consideration of what a prescription might look like, then some deductions about the kinds of study design that might test prescriptions for practice.

There has been some debate in the nursing literature about whether there can be such a thing as "situation-producing theory," and whether it is testable or not (2). The notion of prescribing nursing in such a way as to bring about new and desired states of affairs makes conscious the sometimes half-conscious professional commitment and obligation of the practice professions. To take the kind of knowledge produced in testing other kinds of theory, including predictive theory, and use that information in the service of improving practice is a leap of faith. To make the inferential leap from a tested, accepted prediction into a real change in the way patient care is delivered means literally leaping over a rather large intellectual chasm, yet nurses and nurse-researchers are often unconsciously or intuitively aware of what in a real situation might have to be studied or changed to implement a tested predictive theory. What prescriptive theory does is offer a way to put that intuition to work consciously, with purpose, systematically to devise a kind of theoretical entity that goes beyond prediction.

But to think in terms of prescriptive theory is dangerous, in some sense, since as will be seen later, it demands the deep involvement in practice of the researcher, or the deep involvement in research of the practitioner. The separation between research and practice becomes explicitly counterproductive when the researcher thinks about devising and testing prescriptions,

199

and she/he may feel a loss of highly valued distance, thought of as objectivity. The clinician, on the other hand, may feel the loss of art and intuition as the bases for changes in practice, when forced to think through, in abstraction, the elements of practice that have to be articulated in prescribing to meet goals.

Prescriptive theory, as presented here, has two major elements: statement of goals, and a "survey list" of elements or aspects of prescription to achieve the goals (3). The goals are states of affairs considered desirable to be achieved, and the prescription is a way of writing out the aspects of activity for the goals to be achieved. This way of thinking about knowledge or theory is quite different from the kinds of theory dealt with in previous chapters, and the ways of thinking about research in prescriptive theory are, therefore, different also.

Prescriptive theory is normative theory; that is, it contains *within the theory* conceptions of desirable states to be manufactured, or norms or goals. And prescriptive theory sets out ways to meet those stated goals which take into account many kinds of relationships among aspects of the survey list in a highly complex way.

The elements of the survey list are agency—who or what performs the activity; patiency—upon whom the activity is performed; framework—in what contexts the activity takes place; procedure—process, or how the activity is done; dynamics—why, or with what motivations or energy sources the activity is done; and terminus—the end points of the activity.

This way of thinking about nursing theory and practice makes the most sense when the nursing activity is thought of as a *system of care* (4). Indeed, using the prescriptive theory terminology and point of view almost forces one to consider even a relatively simple nursing activity in its larger context, as a system of care. Nursing, then, in the sense of nursing practice, would be a very large number of interlocking systems of care, with perhaps similar goals, but different ways of defining operationally the aspects of the survey list. Thinking of nursing practice as systems of care brings into conscious awareness the context within which nursing is done, and makes available for change, as well as for intellectual consideration, things that ordinarily are not thought of as relating directly to achievement of nursing goals, such as motivation of its practitioners, the quality of leadership of an institution, or economics, geography, legislation or reimbursement practice.

The point can be made more clear by a detailed discussion of one system of care already available in nursing—primary care nursing.

SYSTEM OF CARE: PRIMARY CARE NURSING

For purposes of this illustration, primary care nursing is considered to be the work of the nurse practitioner in ambulatory care, rather than inpatient practice. The nurse practitioner's work includes traditional aspects of nursing practice, as well as the expanded role of nursing in aspects of patient care more traditionally the exclusive province of medicine, such as health history taking, physical examination, ordering and interpreting laboratory tests, managing chronic illness and minor acute problems, recommending prescription of medications and evaluating the treatments prescribed.

Originally, the goal of inventing this new role for nurses was to increase access to primary care (first contact and continuing care), improve the quality of outpatient care, and implicitly, decrease the costs. It was also expected that if nurses could take on some of the functions previously assigned to physicians, while continuing their nursing work, there would also be more efficient use of scarce health manpower resources (5).

The words usually used to conceptualize this kind of work indicate that the focus was initially on the *activities* and the *role* of the nurse practitioner. That is, the nurse practitioner would learn to perform some new activities, such as physical examination, and would take on a new role and with it new responsibilities for relatively independent judgment in areas of patient care not usually in the province of nursing. A good deal of research has now been done on the nurse practitioner's activities and their effect, and on the new role, and considerable literature has piled up documenting the effectiveness of this kind of practice, as well as the raging controversy it has stimulated in nursing circles (6).

To date, nearly all the research on nurse practitioner practice has been confined to the study of the nurse practitioners' medical or technical care—the new aspects of her role. To the extent that the research aim was to document that nurses could safely and effectively carry out the practice of clinical medicine, the research accomplished its purpose, and stimulated federal legislation to support nurse practitioner training and perhaps soon, third party reimbursement for these kinds of nursing services. Yet the limited conceptualization of primary care nursing has automatically limited it as prescription, an instance of how theoretical issues affect real problems.

It is now possible, after some ten years of experience with this new role for nurses, to think of nurse practitioner practice, or primary care nursing not simply as a new set of activities done by new people, or simply as a new psychological and sociological role, but truly, as a new *system of care* which deserves and dictates study as a system, as well as studies of how various parts of the system fit together.

Using the prescriptive theory terminology, primary nursing care includes considerations of agency: Who are nurse practitioners? What is their training? Does it matter whether the postbasic additional role expansion learning is based on a diploma, a bachelor's degree or a higher degree? The scope of knowledge in both nursing and clinical medicine of the nurse practitioner becomes an issue. Just how much does the nurse practitioner need to know about, say, biochemistry? Human development? Neurology? Pharmacology? How does the nurse practitioner understand her/his role and responsibilities, and, therefore, how much responsibility and authority will she/he take on?

The patiency aspect of nurse practitioner practice as a system of care includes considerations about the kinds of patients (by disease, condition, age, economic circumstance, cultural background, gender, health history, vulnerability, compliance pattern and so on) who are served by the nurse practitioner. Patient acceptance of the nurse practitioner is another variable.

The framework aspect of primary care nursing has received very little attention as a subject of research, though numerous articles have dealt with legal restrictions on nonphysician practice and on some variables in clinical settings which enhance or detract from the nurse's ability to practice to the limits of her knowledge, such as physician acceptance, local protocols or policies, hospital privileges, interprofessional relationships, and economics. Framework includes all of these things and more.

In a system of care, all of the possible variables that might affect progress toward the goal of improved access and quality and decreased costs of primary care would be subject for consideration. Such variables might include geography—rural areas or underserved inner cities have been more willing to experiment with the use of nonphysicians than tertiary care-oriented medical centers. The policies of health insurers become an obvious factor in the extent to which nurse practitioners are put in place if the practitioner or the institution cannot bill and recover money for the services rendered. More subtle social factors, such as an increasing consciousness of women as patients and as health care givers, may have an impact. Nurse midwifery as a form of primary care practice has received considerable publicity recently, for example, as women as patients have begun to demand women as clinicians as an alternative to male dominated, highly technical obstetrical practice. Similarly, women as nurses have sought opportunities to have more independent responsibility in their work, and have broadened the original scope of nurse practitioner practice beyond well-child and chronic illness care to include acute care and care of patients with multiple problems.

In a given setting, other aspects of the framework might come to light, such as the support systems within the setting—nursing administration or clinic administration; allocation of office space and equipment; access to additional learning; involvement of nurse practitioners in all of the activities of the service, including grand rounds, patient conferences and other public presentations. The nature of physician attitude, as well as consultation, may effect the extent or scope of primary nursing care practice. Policies of the institution, hospital by-laws, care protocols, utilization review procedures are all part of the framework. The extent to which nurse practitioners participate in both clinical and administrative decision-making may also have an impact on their practice.

The procedure aspect of nurse practitioner practice has received considerable attention in the research literature, but primarily the technical aspects of care, rather than the totality of care. Here, "procedure" means how the nurse practitioner does her work and includes not only activities of technical care, such as taking a health history, doing a physical examination, differentiating between normal and abnormal findings and so on, but also the "art of care." (7) The latter would include interpersonal process—for example, the way in which the nurse practitioner involves the patient in decision-making, in patient teaching or self-care. It would also involve how the nurse practitioner assesses the ability of the patient to carry out the treatment plan, his compliance, his motivation, the extent to which he is financially and psychologically able to understand and follow a prescribed regimen. Procedure would also include the ways in which the nurse practitioner assesses and deals with the nonmedical aspects of care, such as counseling, teaching, patient advocacy and the other parts of care more traditionally thought of as nursing. Clinical decision-making would be a part of procedure, and would include considerations about how the nurse practitioner decides when the limits of her/his knowledge have been reached and when a consultation with a physician or a referral is indicated. The extent to which nurse practitioners collaborate with other professionals, including physicians, social workers, psychiatrists, community agencies, administrators, lay and professional groups (AA, or other such self-help groups) would also fall into procedure.

Dynamics means the energy source for the system of care and includes not only the motivation behind the nurse practitioner's work, but the energy behind the entire conception of nurse practitioner work as a system of care. Included in dynamics would be money—federal or institutional support as "input"; altruistic impulses on the part of administrators; community pressures for improved quality of care; the impact of regional health-planning agencies, such as Health Systems Agencies, with their annual health systems plans and implementation plans. Professional and interprofessional politics which serve as energy sources would be included as well.

Finally, terminus as an aspect of prescriptive theory of primary care nursing means units of the system of care, those times which might be measured as the end points of the activity. Here, progress toward the goal is assayed (and perhaps the goal itself is reassessed). Account would be taken of the extent to which the prescribed system of care "works," in improving access to care and quality and decreasing costs. Terminus as an aspect of theory breaks the activity into manageable units.

A "system of care" then, is a set of agents, doing work with patients, in a given sociopolitical context, using certain processes or procedures, with certain sources of motivation or energy, toward measurable end points, all in the service of achieving some desired goal. It is a "system" of care because it is not simply procedures, process or specific agents. Each aspect of the system has an impact on every other aspect, often in highly complex ways, and one element does not exist without the others.

To think of nursing practice in this instance as a system of care makes more understandable the use of prescriptive theory in practice.

A prescriptive theory of primary care nursing would include *all* of the considerations mentioned in all of the elements of the theory, and more besides. Such a theory would have in it not only descriptive information classifiable under one of the elements of the theory, but also predictions and theories and descriptions of how various elements of the theory are linked together. The theory would include tested predictions about the effect of certain activities on patients (agency-patiency); about the effect of institutional attitudes on practitioner effectiveness (framework-agency); about styles of practice (dynamics-procedure) and so on.

One way to visualize prescriptive theory is as a giant spider web. The radii of the web are the elements of the theory—agency, patiency and so on. The threads connecting the radii are the theories or hypotheses or speculations about the relationship among aspects of the theory. The whole spider web is the theory, and when one thread on one side of it is twitched, the whole thing vibrates since the elements are so interconnected and interdependent.

Prescriptive theory only makes sense as a theory about practice—a theory that prescribes so as to bring into reality desired states of affairs. It is, therefore, not testable except in practice, when the prescription, as it were, can be put into action, and progress toward the goal specified in the theory can be measured. Therefore, to test prescriptive theory, an entire *system of care* would be created, its aspects theoretically and operationally defined and its effect measured by how well the system of care is indeed able to bring the goal into being.

Returning to the primary care nursing example, it would appear that the agency and terminus aspects of the theory have received the most empirical attention. The "nurse practitioner" has been defined, her/his training more or less standardized (more in the case of nurse midwives) and there is now quite a body of literature dealing with some termini of nurse practitioner practice—effects on patient care. The framework aspects of nurse practitioner care as a system of care has received attention, but not as articulately as would be desired. For example, physician acceptance has been studied, but not certain other kinds of institutional support systems that seem necessary to make the system of care work, such as ancillary personnel, hospital privileges or access to third party reimbursement. Dynamics has received hardly any attention as an area of systematic study, though it is empirically clear that federal funding priorities have provided considerable energy to nurse practitioner work, as has consumerism. Procedure as an aspect of primary care nursing has been studied, but primarily in the technical care given, not in the art of care. And while terminus has been studied, it too has been primarily in terms of medical outcomes, as opposed to a larger vision of quality of care.

Very little research has been done on how various aspects of the system of care are linked together, and while there have been more than a few evaluations of nurse practitioner practice, to date none has dealt with it as a *system* or even as a *theory*. Rather, evaluations have concentrated on how well putting nurse practitioners into certain settings has met the goal for which they were hired—increased access to care, increased quality and decreased cost. The focus, therefore, has been on the nurse practitioner, not on the practice.

A review of the research to date on nurse practitioners, and some knowledge of how they practice, reveals that the elements of theory as described here are intuitively reasonable; it's just that they have not been considered *theoretical* entities, subject to intellectual work just as any other theoretical concepts are. A good deal is already known, inarticulately, about the aspects of prescriptive theory of primary care nursing. Putting that knowledge into the form of prescriptive theory is a way of opening it up for inquiry, as well as a way of forcing the intellectual work on it that would be necessary for a fully developed prescriptive theory.

If nursing practice can be thought of as systems of care, then how can a whole *system* be studied? Intuitively, it seems as if evaluation research approaches might become useful, since it is that field that has developed most thoughtfully the notion of evaluating entire programs (8).

PRESCRIPTIVE-THEORY-TESTING AND EVALUATION RESEARCH

The first step in testing prescriptive theory, as in any other kind of research, would be to formulate the prescription and the goal. Immediately, this is different from the way in which evaluation research is generally conceived. In evaluation research, the "program"—a new approach to community mental health, a program to reduce highway accidents and so on—is invented, usually by policy makers such as state or federal government officials (Congress) or federal agencies (such as the National Cancer Institute, the National Institute of Mental Health, the U.S. Public Health Service). The program is based on whatever the available data are about need for a program, and the goal is set by the legislation that creates the funding to implement the new programs. This is a political process, however, not a conceptual one. There is little notion of a theory which prescribes the activities to be undertaken to achieve the goal. Rather the decisions on particular agents, are decided by political means (lobbying and so on), and the decision that a program for certain targets (patiency) is needed comes also from a political base, such as the liberal belief in using federal resources to cure social ills or bring needed services to underserved peoples. While it is easier, for purposes of explanation here, to use as examples of program evaluation federally mandated programs, the same considerations would apply to rather smaller examples, including the introduction of nurse practitioners into a given setting. In the latter case, a policy decision is made to employ nurse practitioners, perhaps in an effort to expand services and use physicians more efficiently, perhaps because of a documented shortage of physician manpower, perhaps in an effort to demonstrate the new role that nurses have taken on. The targets of the program might be the general clinic population, the people who use the emergency room for nonurgent conditions, well children or normal obstetrical patients. In any case, the program, here nurse practitioners, is introduced from outside, and introduced essentially in operational, rather than theoretical terms: we need somebody to take care of the normal pregnancies so the doctors can concentrate on the patients at risk.

In prescriptive-theory-testing, the *theory* of the system of care to be tested is the prescription itself, a whole package to be introduced, measured, tested. In program evaluation, the fact that there should be evaluation is sometimes prescribed, but the evaluation is rarely done by the same people who invented the program, and the purpose of evaluation is not to develop theory, it's an empirical purpose—to see if the program "works," so that a decision can be made about whether to put more of that kind of program into place. The purpose of prescriptive-theory-testing, as in any other kind of practice research, is to build knowledge, understanding, upon which changes in patient care for the better may be made. Those changes might indeed mean the spread of prescriptions for practice of systems of care.

In evaluation research, or program evaluation, rarely are all of the elements of the prescription (program) considered in detail as they would be in prescriptive-theory-testing. Indeed, some of the elements may not even be testable, since they, too, are set by whatever the program formulation is. For example, certain mental health programs may stipulate that the target population must be made up of persons with incomes under the official poverty level; or federally supported continuing education efforts in nursing may state that all enrolled students must be registered nurses, or that the programs must be open to LPNs or whatever.

Programs which are to be evaluated through evaluation research rarely contain any specific attention to framework, except as stipulated in the legislation or program guidelines themselves, to dynamics and often not to procedure either. Indeed, Bloch has discussed various models of evaluation and points out the necessity for explicit definition and study of the "process" (procedure) used in the program, and its relationship to the outcome (terminus) (9). When attention is given to these aspects, it is again either stipulated through the political process or otherwise defined in advance in operational terms. For example, programs in community mental health may require that they be operated out of a community mental health center, and not another entity. Dynamics is addressed only in the most tangential way, and it may be safely assumed that the major dynamic, or energy source behind the program, is the federal money which created it.

Suchman, an expert in evaluation research, highlights the differences between evaluation research and nonevaluative research (here, prescriptive-theory-testing) (10). In nonevaluative research, the concept is primary. Observable data are based on some operational definition of the concept, but there are always alternate possibilities for this operational definition, and it is the concept, not the specific operational definition, that is of theoretical interest. In evaluation research, the reverse is true. The specific operations in the program are the main focus of interest and the concept, the underlying theory on which the program is based, may receive little attention. "To a large extent, the specific program activities are the independent variables, not simply indices of these variables, while the dependent variable is directly represented by the specific, observable criteria of change." (11)

In prescription-testing, the motivation is to be able to generalize from the specific situation to the class of situation of which it is one. In the case of primary care nursing, the force is to be able to understand the nature and effect of primary care nursing by studying it as a system of care in one or a few instances, then generalizing to the class of situations of primary nursing care anywhere, anytime.

In program evaluation, the hypotheses (prescriptions) are derived directly and mechanically from the program content and goals, rather than creatively from theories or previous studies. In program evaluation, when the data are in, they are specific to the program evaluated, and not generalizable to other similar programs because there is no theory behind the program to rest such generalizations on. Several evaluations of similar programs may be compared or combined, but each one is an $N = 1$ idiosyncratic situation, not really comparable to the others.

There are also differences in the logic of evaluation and prescriptive-theory-testing. In evaluation, since the goal is preset in advance, the question to be answered is how well the program meets the goal. In prescriptive-theory-testing, the setting of the goal is itself part of the theory, and subject to more than just political discussion about its rightness, efficacy, justification and so on. Further, the prescription to meet the goal derives not from preset means, but from the question, How can I make _____ (the goal) happen? allowing free consideration of numerous alternative agents, frameworks and so on. In prescriptive-theory-testing, the actual agents are the operational definition of the notion of agency, rather than the independent variable as Suchman discussed it above.

Some of the terminology used in quality assurance as evaluation research hints at the possibility that evaluation researchers are searching as are nurses for a theoretical perspective that will match the level of complexity of the empirical reality to be evaluated. Donabedian's division of three modes of evaluation is very frequently cited (12). He distinguishes three types of evaluation—evaluation of process, structure and outcome, and advocates combinations of these three approaches as optimal for complete understanding of a program and its effects. "Process" would be more or less equivalent to procedure in prescriptive theory terms, with perhaps a little of dynamics thrown in. "Structure" is not unlike framework, and "outcome," is patiency and terminus.

Thus, prescriptive-theory-testing and evaluation research bear some resemblance in 1. the notion of testing the effect of an entire program (system) of care and 2. the explicit consideration of the goals to be achieved by the programs. Therefore, some of the very thoughtful work of those involved in evaluation research becomes available for tests of prescriptive theories.

AN EXAMPLE

With this background, let's return to the primary care nursing example and discuss it again, as an instance of how prescriptive theory might be developed and tested.

Goal Setting

Suppose an institution recognized that the way its ambulatory clinic situation was working was not working. A very high percentage of people were using the emergency room for nonurgent reasons; there was demonstrable lack of follow-up of patients when referred to specialty clinics; the physicians who delivered the care were overworked and there was reason to think the ambulatory care was not good. Further, the institution looked around its city and realized that it was unlikely that other sources of ambulatory care were going to develop in the near future, and that the population in its immediate geographic area was rapidly shifting toward newly emigrated relatively poor people, often black or Puerto Rican, and often with multiple social and environmental problems as well as health problems. There were long waits for people to see the few physicians in the primary care setting, and community pressure was building on the institution to deliver better service. At the same time, the institution was taking a look at all its manpower resources and feeling the vibrations from other parts of the country coming from nursing, advocating better use of nurses in nontraditional care patterns.

Note that even how this background information is presented implies some analysis of the problem beyond simply the vague feeling on the part of an institution that something is wrong with its primary care. The first step in developing prescriptive theory research is the same as the first step in any research—defining and analyzing the problem. But what makes the problem different is that it is of a different order than problems which end up at other levels of inquiry. Here the problem is how to *change* an entire system for the better.

Suppose that in this institution, it was decided that a priority for the next few years would be to improve the access to and quality of primary care programs, with decreased costs, to the extent possible. The content of that goal would be elaborated considerably, and the meaning of the element in it teased out: what is "increased access?" What is "primary care?" What is "quality?" To what extent is quality simply quality of medical care, and to what extent does it encompass "softer" quality considerations, such as humanistic care, psychosocial care and so on. In setting goal content, a normative approach would be taken. Who says this is a good goal? What should be the role of, say, a community hospital in meeting the entire primary care needs of its service area? How can a balance be struck between the multiple missions of a medical center for service, teaching and research in this situation? How does the institution fit into a regional framework of service delivery, and, therefore, how much responsibility for primary care should belong to it, and how much to other agencies? With what other important, significant community resources is the institution connected, to provide the threads for either a referral network out, or a referral network in?

Perhaps the reader can already anticipate that, in part, what thinking of systems of care in this way does, is force upon institutions (or anybody in a decision-making capacity) some considerations that are not normally brought to consciousness in deciding about institutional change, or change in service programs (13).

Once the content of the goal is laid out, consideration then turns to the various aspects of prescriptive theory to decide how to design a system of care to bring about the goal specified. The research problem is, How can I make _____ happen? Probably, the first step in considering elements of the theory would be to consider patiency, since the problem springs from a discrepancy between what the need is, for services, and what is currently the state.

Patiency

The problem, How can I make _____ happen? is now pinned down to, How can I make primary care more accessible and of higher quality and lower cost? But accessible to whom, of higher quality in what ways, and less costly to whom?

To arrive at a theoretical formulation of patiency, from which operational definitions would derive, would be to consider the nature of patiency in the setting already. In theoretical terms, who are the people to be served, and what variables characterize them? Are they old, young, minority, nonminority, poor, not poor, with other sources of care or not, chronically or acutely ill, having available supportive services or social supports or not. Perhaps available data would be used to help define the theoretical patiency, and perhaps those data would be combined with more general theory about such things as population migration and its effect on utilization of services; social attitudes of low-income people toward hospitals; the effect of geography on use of health services as related to ability to delay gratification; attitudes of patients toward various categories of health care workers, men, women, doctors, nurses. What is being aimed for is a theory of patiency, not a definition of exactly the kinds of people who will end up being served by the new program. The operational definition will come later.

Suppose that this theoretical analysis ended with the notion that patiency in this problem probably means, in general, lack of other sources of care, multiple health and social problems, general dependent orientation toward health services, lack of knowledge of alternative ways to obtain needed services, general lack of social and economic resources, orientation toward physician care as "first class" care, either recent emigration to the area, implying lack of knowledge of the social/cultural ambience as well as just plain ignorance of other sources of care, or other explanations (social/cultural barriers) for care-seeking in the public, rather than the private sector.

If this is the theoretical notion of patiency, the next question probably becomes, with this notion, what kind of agency can we prescribe that will be best suited to the care of people described theoretically above?

Agency

Remembering that one of the aspects of goal content is the need to decrease costs, consideration might first be given to simply increasing the kinds of primary care givers already in place in the setting—physicians. Costs would be high, but that might be all right if otherwise physicians are theoretically suited to the theory of patiency developed. But note that emphasis in patiency is not on complicated medical problems for which theory substantiates physicians are best suited. Rather, emphasis in patiency is upon chronic illness and multiple social problems, probably difficulties in compliance with care, and inappropriate use of facilities. What kinds of theories of agency does that imply? Social workers might theoretically be considered appropriate to deal with the social problems, but it is not generally a complaint of social problems that brings people to health institutions.

Theory about what nursing in primary care is suggests that nurse practitioners are trained to deal with chronic illness, but more important (for the theory, not for the politics), the tradition of nursing in dealing with the whole patient, not just his disease, suggests that they might be an appropriate resource. Further, social distance theory might suggest that the patiency defined by the theory might be best combined with theories of agency that minimize social distance (so as to maximize compliance, for example). Further, psychological theories and organizational theories might suggest that when people (nurses) are able to practice relatively independently in their areas of competence, with defined accountability and responsibility, they are likely to have more job satisfaction and to continually improve their practice so as to feel better about it. In contrast, theories relative to physician practice, especially in medical centers, might suggest that physicians are bored with chronic illness and minor complaints, are impatient with social problems and generally not sensitive to environmental or psychosocial stressors in patients. Data would suggest that nurse practitioners are easier to find and recruit than physicians, and that nurse practitioners may be employees and satisfied with that state, whereas the value system in medicine is to move from the employee status to the fee-for-service status, which would mean relatively large turnovers among personnel, perhaps defeating the purpose of the prescription.

Suppose these theoretical considerations then led to a theory of agency which prescribed use of nurse practitioners as primary care givers in this situation, recognizing that in some sense, there is still not a perfect match between agency and patiency, particularly in the unknown area of patient acceptance.

Framework

Thinking through agency automatically brings up necessary theories and realities about framework. For example, if nonphysicians are to be prescribed, what will be the role of physicians? What will be the necessary legal and administrative coverage of the nurse practitioner?

Since at this point, theories that might be useful in developing prescriptions for primary care are few and far between, we can only guess at what other theories might be incorporated into specification of framework. In general, what kinds of personal support systems are necessary to make nontraditional, highly independent work happen? What kinds of organizational considerations would need to be taken into account to both support and monitor the prescribed practices. For example, can it be predicted that affiliating the nurse practitioner with the division of nursing will be more effective (in terms of how the NP works) than making the NP administratively responsible to, say, the department of internal medicine? What theories about reference groups might be brought to bear to predict the need for and use of support systems for agency?

Framework would also include, to the extent possible, theories regarding utilization of health services that might predict success (or not) for the system of care; theories about economic supply and demand in health services; legal theories about personal responsibility and accountability and so on.

Procedure

How will the agents actually do their work? Here, theories about the nature of the practice of clinical medicine—clinical judgment, diagnosis and so on would be included. To the extent possible, theories about interpersonal process, particularly with respect to how patiency is defined, would be stated also. Theories about how to increase patient knowledge, or compliance, would be built in to the prescription. Theories about procedure would also include theories about interprofessional relationships when such theories might predict how role relationships effect service delivery, job satisfaction and the like. Both the scope and limits of practice would be addressed, again in theoretical terms, to be defined operationally later. What is wanted is as much knowledge as possible about what in "procedure" works or doesn't work to increase quality of care, so that those theories can then guide the prescription itself.

Dynamics

What kinds of energy sources will have to be built into a system of care to make it function? Energy sources might include money, reward systems, working conditions (fringe benefits, vacation time, office accommodations), job satisfaction, feedback, power, control, and there are already available some theories that would be useful in specifying dynamics. Theories about institutional change might predict that there are more or less effective ways to introduce new systems of care into existing settings (14). Organizational theories might predict the necessity of involving certain kinds of people both in the decision to institute a new system of care and in monitoring and controlling it. Marketing theories might be useful in predicting how to "sell" the new system of care.

Terminus

Finally, theories about what the end points of the activity in primary care nursing are would be selected and defined. Such theories would take into account the nature of agency, patiency and procedure especially, along with the other aspects of theory. For example, if primary care nursing is considered to include both "care" and "cure," both clinical medicine and nursing, then both must be measurable. Measurement of the effect of the system of care is incomplete if it includes attention only to the clinical medicine parts of patient service. Further, since the activity is conceived of as a system of care, there will be termini which are specific not only to patiency, but to framework or other aspects of the theory. For example, how will the units of activity that relate to the effect on medical education in the setting be defined? Cost? Administrative structure? Again, to the extent they are available, theories that might help define particular end points would be explicated.

The aspects of the survey list have been addressed here as if they were clean and separable. In reality, theories that touch on more than one aspect at a time would automatically be included as relevant.

What we're after in this exercise is devising the elements of a theory which, when defined operationally, will bring desired situations into being. The kind of theory is situation-producing theory, whose aim is to bring about desired states of affairs. Situation-producing theory includes within it many other kinds of theories, from descriptive (for instance, a descriptive theory about nursing process), to predictive (as in a theory of institutional change). But, at the risk of being redundant, the second step in testing prescriptive theory (after defining the problem) is to invent the theory.

The process of inventing situation-producing theory is not unlike the process of selecting or inventing theory for any other kind of study. It's just that the theory itself is so much more complex, and the relationships among aspects of theories so intricate. Therefore, attention is drawn in this chapter to this kind of synthesis of theory as a separate activity, even though the mental processes are essentially the same as in any other kind of study. Note also that to this point we have been talking exclusively about abstract notions. Once the theories to be included in a situation-producing theory are as articulate as they can be at this point, the time comes to define operationally, from the theories, the actual *prescription*.

A prescription is to prescriptive theory as an hypothesis is to predictive theory. It is the empirical statement of the situation to be produced, and the way the terms (survey list) are to be defined for the particular prescription.

Just as in hypothesis-testing studies at lower levels of inquiry, each term in the prescription will have an operational definition, an empirical referent.

In the example we've been using, all of the aspects of the theory will be given real meaning in observable terms, adding up to the prescription.

PRESCRIPTIONS

First, the goal will be translated into empirical terms. "Access to care," "improved quality," "decreased cost" will be given operational definitions. Most likely the process of operationally defining the goal will lead readily to an operational definition of terminus as well. In the example here, the thing to be measured as the end point of the activity might include cost (per patient, per visit, per hour, per minute, per practitioner, whatever makes sense from the theory); quality of care as patient outcome—morbidity, mortality, ability to follow prescribed regimens, comfort, compliance, satisfaction; access to care—not only numbers of new patients seen, but how patients feel about their access to the system. Do they feel the system is responsive, accessible; as patient process—comprehensiveness, completeness, accuracy, sensitivity of care, the extent to which care is tailored to the individual patient's ability/circumstances/condition; impact of the system of care upon other systems (defined operationally perhaps as the residency training program, the administrative system, the nursing system, how are NPs received by other nurses)?

All of the other parts of the prescription would receive similar operational definition. Agency would be defined as nurse practitioner care (with certain kinds of nurses, with certain kinds of preparation, functioning with or without protocols, with certain availability of physician supervision and so on); patiency would be defined from statistical projections of the kinds of patient to be seen, with what conditions, support systems, economic circumstances, cultural background; framework would be a statement of the way in which the system of care is organized within the existing framework, or the existing one is changed to accommodate it; procedure would be defined operationally into perhaps the activities performed (both medical activities and nursing ones), and dynamics would be defined operationally as clearly as possible from whatever theories are available to determine the energy sources.

Note that throughout this discussion, the future subjunctive tense has been used—"would be." What is being proposed here is the way to approach the testing of prescriptive theory, but since there are as yet no studies that have followed this model, it is necessarily tentative. Even evaluation research studies do not entirely fit, given the general lack of theoretical development in them.

A prescription, then, is like an hypothesis in a predictive study in the sense that it is a statement of the relationship among variables of interest. Unlike an hypothesis, it contains the explicit statement that the goal to be achieved is a desirable one, and the statement of the prescription is the way to achieve the goal. While hypotheses in predictive theory may indeed include as dependent variables things that are desirable (decreased pain or discomfort, for instance), the normative statement is outside the theory, not part of it. Further, hypotheses state, If this, then that. . . . Prescriptions take the form, to bring about that, do this. . . . In both cases, the prescription or the hypothesis is a kind of shorthand for the theory of which the hypothesis or prescription is an instance.

PRESCRIPTION-TESTING

Before continuing with the primary nursing care example, it might be well to clarify possible developing misconceptions.

Unlike predictive hypothesis-testing of the effect of nursing, in prescription-testing "nursing" (agency) is not the independent variable, with "patiency" as the dependent variable. Rather the entire *system of care* is analogous to the independent variable, recognizing the reality that the direction of effect is not just nurse to patient, but also patient to nurse, nurse to framework, framework to dynamics and so on and on. Also, "setting," as normally conceived in hypothesis-testing is part, but not all of "framework," and as such is part of the independent variable, not simply a described situation in which a predictive hypothesis is tested.

The concept of "sampling" has no analog in prescription-testing studies. Patiency is not sampling, since patiency is part of the prescription itself. In a conceptual sense, sampling in a prescription-testing study would be picking out the reality situation(s) which implement the prescription, so sample would not mean people, as it usually does, but "situations."

"Intervening" and "antecedent" variables are also part and parcel of the independent variable in the sense that usually such variables are considered part of "patiency" or "framework." In testing prescriptions, antecedent variables would become situations which existed before the prescription was implemented, and might be considered part of the history of the institution, or perhaps even the philosophical background behind the prescription. Intervening variables in predictive hypotheses are those things which occur between the administration of the independent variable and the measurement of the dependent variable. In prescription-testing, variables would not intervene, they would simply be part of the description of the implementation of the prescription. Another meaning of intervening variable sometimes used in predictive studies is "alternative explanations"—other things that explain the findings. Such other things are most often variables outside the hypothesis itself. In prescription-testing, such variables are included in the system of care from the beginning, and are not, therefore, intervening. For example, it may be that something in the framework interferes with the implementation of primary care nursing. But since the framework itself is part of the independent variable, whatever happens within it is grist for the theoretical mill, to be monitored with formal data collected, to be massaged theoretically, to be changed if it isn't following logically from the theory, but not to be considered as outside the hypothesized relationship.

Once a prescription is devised, it can be tested. The test of a prescription would be how well it does indeed bring about the desired state of affairs stated in the goal content. In hypothesis-testing, the effort is not only to see if the hypothesis does predict what it's supposed to, there is also an effort to explain *why* the hypothesis does or does not predict. In prescription-testing, there is the similar assignment not only to see if the prescription results in the desired ends, but why it works (or doesn't). Therefore, tests of prescriptions would be designed so that theoretical explanation can be done.

There is no reason to think that some of the steps in the research process would be different in testing prescriptions for practice (15). Analysis of the problem, as the first step, would begin with a perceived discrepancy between a perhaps unstated desired state of affairs and what things are really like. Analysis of this discrepancy would resolve to a statement of the problem in the form of How can I make _____ happen? Probably along the way to this conclusion it would begin to be suspected that the answer to how to make achievement of a goal happen is to implement a new system of care; that is, the problem would lend itself to potential solution through this kind of change. Once the problem was stated in this form, recognizing that a prescription-testing study would be called for, the next step in the research process—developing the conceptual framework follows easily.

How the conceptual framework would be developed has been covered earlier in this chapter, though not under that heading. For a prescription-testing study, theories of the various aspects of the survey list would be drawn upon to bring to conceptual awareness those aspects. Many kinds of theories would be used, ranging from descriptive theories through tested causal theories, with the purpose of making clear in theoretical terms the "system of care" to be implemented as prescription. The attempt would be to put forward as thorough an understanding, again in abstract terms, of the system as system (as well as each aspect of the survey list independently) as possible, since eventually this theoretical background will be used to help explain why the system of care does or doesn't work.

Then, each element in the theory considered important to testing the prescription would have to have its operational definition. Here, just as in studies at other levels of inquiry, there would be some selection of theories to use, some picking out of the ones thought to be most useful, more appropriate, or best suited for describing the system of care. It would be impossible to provide operational (or even conceptual) meaning to every single way of thinking about, for example, framework, so there would have to be some editing of available material to a manageable handful. Unlike studies of predictive hypotheses, operational definitions would be provided for *all* aspects of the system, not just an independent and dependent variable.

An important part of the conceptual work at this point would be consideration of what evidence will be taken to indicate how well the goal was achieved. Even knowing in advance that achievement of a goal is, in part, a matter of judgment (just as is deciding on support or nonsupport of a predictive hypothesis), it would be critical to spell out in advance general notions about goal achievement. Further, it would be crucial to lay out in some detail why the goal set is a good goal, and what the theoretical consequences are of adhering to that goal. Consideration of alternate goals, discarding some, adopting others, would lead to a fuller understanding of just what it is that is desired, including some limitations on the tendency to grandiose goal setting.

All of the theoretical material would be distilled to a statement of the prescription. Such a statement could probably not be as simple as stating a causal hypothesis, given the more complex nature of a prescription. But the conceptual material would have to be reduced to a one-paragraph exposition of goal and prescription which would encapsulate all the reasoning behind it.

Once the prescription was stated, the study design would be outlined. The level of inquiry would be situation-producing, the fourth level of inquiry.

Testing a prescriptive theory would mean putting the prescription into operation and measuring progress toward goal achievement. Dickoff and James cite three purposes of prescriptive theory:

> (1) that the activity called for by the theory, if done by the specified agents, will achieve the theory's goal; (2) that guiding activity by this theory will produce desirable results; and (3) that guiding action by the theory is feasible when considered in relation to the worth of the goal achieved and the costs of achieving that goal. (16)

The three purposes lead to three kinds of tests of the theory: testing for "coherency," testing for "palatability" and testing for "feasibility." Coherency, palatability and feasibility are all empirical questions. Testing the coherency claim would mean, among other things, having a way for finding out whether theory-specified agents are acting as specified; and validating that the activity called for is actually being carried out. Testing the palatability of a prescriptive theory would involve collection of data at the end points of activity and analysis of such data in terms of how close it comes to achieving the preset goal. Feasibility would mean applying human and material cost analysis considerations to the data which show the activity and its outcome, along with assessment of whether the cost of inducing the agents to produce the desired activity is worthwhile in view of what is sacrificed, including other goals left unachieved.

Operational definitions of all the aspects of the prescription would be supplied and data gathered on them. Probably the aspects would all have several or even many measurements and the parameters of the goal itself would require considerable clarity.

The validity of the prescription-testing (or credibility) would not rely on the conditions for causal inference as experimental studies do. Rather, the validity would be in the correspondence between the theories of aspects of the survey list, their operational definitions and the specification of goal. Unlike other kinds of studies in which it is assumed that operational definitions are "accurate," "complete" or "valid," in prescription-testing, especially in the early days of it, the force of the analysis of data would be on the relationship between theory and data as operation. And much effort would go into relating various aspects of the prescription to each other, as well as to terminus and goal, so as to build increasingly precise and logical connections. Perhaps some kind of conceptual weighting procedure would be used, to help figure out which aspects of the survey list in a prescription are most crucial for progress toward the goal, which ones should be developed further or altered, and which can be left less well developed for the particular goal.

It could be assumed that the general rules that guide data collection and measurement in any study would also operate in prescription testing— objectivity, reliability and so on. But because prescriptions would always be tested in practice with clinical considerations of highest priority, perhaps new measurement or data collection criteria would emerge—like "relevance" (of a measure), or "clinical usefulness," even "clinical bias."

Prescription-testing studies could only be done in practice settings, when they deal with prescriptions for practice. They could not be done in a laboratory, though someday when computer science is sufficiently advanced and when the theories that might go into a prescription are, it is possible to imagine simulation studies. Since prescriptions are intended to achieve real-life goals, in real situations, it makes no conceptual sense to try to test the theories in laboratory situations, especially when the aspects of prescriptive theory that might turn out to be the most important, such as framework, differ so much from laboratory to real situation.

It would probably be the case that many different kinds of data would be collected on various aspects of the prescription. It may even be that a team of researchers would be needed, or that there would be considerable use of information not usually considered research data, such as procedure books, minutes of meetings, discussions of patients in grand rounds or public information releases, as well as interviews, attitude measures and any of the standard forms of data. Especially in the early days of prescription-testing studies (from tomorrow on), it could be suspected that a good deal of nonquantitative data would be collected, and plans for analyzing it made. At this point it is not even possible to guess at what exact kinds of data processing or analysis techniques would be used, though it might be suspected that something like the "field research conference" of factor-searching studies might be a major analytic tool. That is, the researchers (who would also include the clinicians) would meet formally for discussion of information as it developed, or at other points, with specific attention being paid to the aspects of the prescription in some defined order. These discussions would then become data as well.

It might also be suspected that the proper vehicle for reporting a prescription-testing study would be a book rather than a shorter form. The report would of necessity be lengthy, given the amount of theory to be addressed and explained, the method and the "results."

The roles of researcher, in the usual sense, and clinician, in the usual sense, might require some particular attention. The role of the practitioner as theoretician would be critical, which might make the role of the researcher less methodological than consultative to the clinical theoretical process. The researcher would have to be engaged enough in the practice situation to understand it, and to understand especially the goals, and the practitioners would have to be articulate enough to be able to communicate the essence of the prescription's implementation, even when that essense is more descriptive than conceptual. And both would have to realize that some of the conventional notions of research method do not apply in prescription-testing studies, and free enough to explore different ways of thinking about "science" and scientific method. Asking a lot, perhaps!

Using the situation-producing theory model and the prescriptive ideas both offers the opportunity to look in a new way at practice changes and forces attention systematically to theoretical and methodological issues that might otherwise not surface. Yet further development of the method must await some trials and errors in application, as well as further discussion of the method of prescription-testing *as method*.

OTHER EXAMPLES

The primary care nursing example was chosen deliberately as some kind of middle-ground concept between a notion which is more intuitively a "system of care," and rather smaller "systems" of care more like those which are tested in experimental studies of the effect of nursing. It can be seen from the lengthy discussion here that it is possible to conceive of simply a change in agent (nurse practitioner) as in reality a much more complicated change in the system of care. In this section, some other examples will be presented, though not discussed in detail.

There are some changes in the health care delivery system that are intuitively "systems" from the beginning. The hospice concept makes a nice example (17). The hospice notion in the United States is derived from the work of Dr. (and nurse and social worker) Cecily Saunders at St. Christopher's in England. Here, the "problem" was felt as a discrepancy between the care that terminally ill people received, and that which they seemed to need more. This problem then was translated into the goal of improving the care to terminally ill patients through explicitly changing the system of care from acute-illness, technological, cure-oriented health delivery system, to a system based more on an understanding of patiency and recognition of the facts that terminal illness is not curable, that high technological intervention simply prolongs discomfort, that patients should participate in decisions about their life and their death. A whole new system of care developed, over some years, called "hospice"—literally a way-station on a journey. The new system of care was different from the existing ones in agency (more use of nonphysicians), patiency (patient participation), framework (low technology, settings designed to be peaceful but growth producing, slow paced, tuned to patient needs), procedure (pain control as opposed to medical intervention, among other things), dynamics (recognition that helping a person die with dignity is as important as cure, and as reimbursable), and terminus—effect on patients, families, and other systems. Separate buildings or programs, called hospices began to spring up, and as the concept of hospice developed, additional theoretical notions began to undergird it—notions about the kinds of agents to plug in, the kinds of patients, involvement of families, relationships with existing systems, marketing, architectural design, measurements of effect and so on.

What has now become known as the "hospice movement" is a nice example of prescription, and of a system of care. But there are other, less dramatic examples within nursing itself. Primary nursing is a good instance. Primary nursing has been defined as ". . . the delivery of comprehensive, continuous, coordinated and individualized patient care through the primary nurse who has autonomy, accountability and authority to act as the chief nurse for her patients." (18)

Buried in this definition are a number of aspects of prescriptive theory as a system of care, though clearly not all aspects are explicit. The agency— primary nurse is identified. Patiency is obviously patients, though further writing about primary nursing suggests that patients may be chosen or otherwise assigned by the primary nurse on the basis of their needs, matched with the primary nurse's skills, making a somewhat more subtle definition of patiency. Framework is not addressed in the definition, though considerations of framework (numbers of staff, for example), are explicit in some studies of primary nursing (19). Procedure is explicit (in theoretical terms) in the definition: comprehensive, continuous, coordinated, individualized patient care. Dynamics are hinted at by reference to autonomy, accountability, authority. Terminus is not addressed at all but would presumably be the end points of the activity, measured in job satisfaction, efficiency, effectiveness, cost and patient outcome. The goal of primary nursing is improved patient care. The labeled goal: "the patient, not the tasks, is the central focus of the nurse, and accountability of nurses for their patients is paramount" (20) is really *procedure*.

Most studies of primary nursing have dwelt upon patient outcomes, measures of nurse performance and job satisfaction and cost. Research on primary nursing as a system of care might also include its effects on other systems of care (the medical care system, for example, or the administration).

Another intuitively comprehensible example of a system of care that could be translated into prescriptive theory is milieu treatment (the "therapeutic community") in psychiatric practice (21). Milieu therapy makes a nice example because "agency" in this system of care is very complicated because it is closer to being agen*cy* than agent, as is more often the case. Agency includes agents—doctors, nurses, social workers—but the agency is in reality the "milieu," a highly complicated and structured social system.

Finally, it is also possible to conceptualize rather smaller parts of nursing practice (smaller than primary nursing, or primary care nursing) as systems of care. Even something so relatively "small" as preoperative preparation, discharge planning or transfer from intensive or coronary care to floor care can be conceptualized as systems of care. Trying to do so reveals how very complicated nursing practice is, and how important it may be to take deliberately into consideration all the aspects of the survey list.

For example, preoperative preparation has been studied rather more than most nursing activities, but generally only as a set of procedures—anxiety reduction, patient teaching and so on. Yet conceiving of this activity as a system of care makes hitherto inarticulate ideas conscious. For example, if preoperative teaching is a system of care, what is its framework? To what extent do things such as surgeon's wishes, or competition from anesthesiologists make or break preoperative preparation? To what extent do certain patient variables—type of surgery, previous experience with hospitalization or surgery, sex, age, suspicion of malignancy—predict that preoperative preparation will "work" or not? How about agency? Conceptually, who does, or should do preoperative preparation? An RN? With a BSN? An aide? A team leader? A primary nurse? Why?

Despite the focus of present research on preoperative preparation as procedure, there is still more to be thought through theoretically about the nature of procedure. What, exactly, is "preoperative preparation," and how exactly is it done, so as to achieve the goals set by the theory? Similarly, dynamics could be stipulated as well as terminus.

The same kind of reasoning could apply to other nursing activities, perhaps even all of nursing activities, which would then make nursing *per se* a set of systems of care, not a bad way to think about it.

What is intriguing about using the prescriptive theory approach to reconceptualize the nature of nursing is that it takes appropriate account of how inordinately complicated the practice of nursing is, in its social context and contract, in its purpose and in the measurement of its effect. If we are serious about using nursing research to develop the knowledge base on which changes in practice can depend, then eventually we will need to consider in theoretical terms the nature of practice and its context, and use those theories to build prescriptions for change which can then be measured. Any prescriptive theory will include many predictive theories, descriptive information and untested speculations. But to the extent that among the missions of nursing in these times is to change the nature of the health delivery system, we may turn to prescriptive theory for explicit notions of how to do that from data, rather than from opinion.

AFTERWORD

It must be emphasized that the material in this chapter is a tentative formulation of prescriptive-theory-testing, to be reconceptualized as the formulation is used to guide research in patient care. There is a great deal more conceptual and methodological work to be done before methods for testing prescriptions for practice achieve the level of sophistication now apparent in methods for testing predictive hypotheses.

The models of levels of inquiry, matched to study designs used in this book, offer the opportunity to put into perspective the many kinds of clinical and research problems and studies that may be done to eventually arrive at situation-producing theories to bring into existence new and desired states of affairs in patient care. To reiterate the major idea here, research in nursing practice is ultimately for the purpose of changing the practice of health care for the better. On the way to prescribing those changes, there well may be thousands of studies and years of thinking on a given topic, to build up the body of theoretical knowledge from which prescriptions may be derived. On the other hand, there is already a great deal of information available that could be used in arriving at prescriptions—knowledge not necessarily about the topic at hand, but information about conceptually related matters. Further, there is the experience of nurses which, when brought to a level of conceptualization, can help define the various aspects of a prescription, and more important, can help assure that the prescription is realistic, or that the realities may be shaped in certain ways not yet done to make the implementation of the prescription possible and researchable.

NOTES

1. Dickoff, James and Patricia James: A theory of theories: a position paper. *Nursing Research,* 17:197–203, May–June, 1968. A complete list of the citations relative to prescriptive theory is contained in Note 2 at the end of Chapter 2 and will not be repeated here.

   However, in one article, Dickoff and James explicitly warn against too-easy use of the term "prescriptive theory" for situation-producing theory. For the purposes of this chapter, I have ignored that warning, but suggest that readers pursue the argument for themselves. See Dickoff, James and Patricia James: Theory development in nursing. In Verhonick, Phyllis J.: *Nursing Research,* (Vol. I). Boston: Little, Brown, 1975, pp. 45–92.

2. The debates about the nature of theory in nursing are cited in the notes at the end of Chapter 2, especially Notes 10, 11, 48 and 49.

3. See Note 1.

4. The phrase "system of care" is not used here in the technical systems theory sense, but rather in the sense of an organized collection of agents and activities, joined together for common purpose to achieve similar goals.

5. The literature on nurse practitioners is now extensive. Some useful collections are Bliss, Ann and Eva Cohen: *The New Health Professionals.* Germantown, Md.: Aspen Publications, 1977, and Yale University School of Medicine, Office of Regional Activities and Continuing Education. *An Evaluation of Policy Related Research on New and Expanded Roles of Health Workers.* (An annotated bibliography.) New Haven: Yale University School of Medicine, 1974; Edmunds, Marilyn: Evaluation of nurse practitioner effectiveness: an overview of the literature. *Evaluation and the Health Professions,* 1:69–82, Spring, 1978; Diers, Donna and Susan Molde: Some conceptual and methodological issues in nurse practitioner research. Unpublished paper.

6. Though research on nurse practitioners is very recent, already there are some "classic" studies:

   Bates, Barbara: Doctor and nurse: changing roles and relations. *New England Journal of Medicine*, 283:129–134, July 19, 1970.

   Duncan, B., A. Smith and Henry Silver: Comparison of the physical assessment of children by pediatric nurse practitioners and pediatricians. *American Journal of Public Health*, 61:1170–1178, June 1971.

   Farrisey, Ruth: Clinic nursing in transition. *American Journal of Nursing*, 67:305–309, February 1967. This article reports, belatedly, the first known experiment in the expanding nursing role.

   Lewis, Charles and Barbara Resnick: Nurse clinics and progressive ambulatory patient care. *New England Journal of Medicine*, 277:1236–1241, December 7, 1967.

   Sackett, David, et al.: The Burlington randomized trial of the nurse practitioner: health outcomes of patients. *Annals of Internal Medicine*, 80:137–142, February 1974.

   Spitzer, Walter, et al.: The Burlington randomized trial of the nurse practitioner. *New England Journal of Medicine*, 290:251–256, January 31, 1974.

   Slome, Charles, et al.: Effectiveness of certified nurse midwives: a prospective evaluation study. *American Journal of Obstetrics and Gynecology*, 124:177–182, January 15, 1976.

   Levy, B., et al.: Reducing neonatal mortality with nurse midwives. *American Journal of Obstetrics and Gynecology*, 109:51–58, January 1971.

   Runnerstrom, Lillian: The effectiveness of nurse midwifery in a supervised hospital environment. *Journal of the American College of Nurse Midwives*, 14:40–50, May 1969.

   Perrin, Ellen and Helen Goodman: Telephone management of acute pediatric illness. *New England Journal of Medicine*, 298:130–135, January 19, 1978.

   The development of training programs for nurse practitioners is addressed particularly in:

   Silver, Henry, et al.: Program to increase health care for children: pediatric nurse practitioner program. *Pediatrics*, 39:756–760, May 1967.

   Januska, Charlotte, et al.: Development of a family nurse practitioner curriculum. *Nursing Outlook*, 22:103–108, February 1974.

   Storms, Doris: *Training of the Nurse Practitioner: A Clinical and Statistical Analysis.* North Haven, Conn.: Health Services Research Series, 1973.

   Two of the most articulate critics of the nurse practitioner movement have written about their thoughts:

   Rogers, Martha: Euphemisms in nursing's future. *Image*, 7(2):3–9, 1975.

   Schlotfeldt, Rozella: Planning for progress. *Nursing Outlook*, 21:766–769, December 1973; also, On the professional status of nursing. *Nursing Forum*, 13(1):15–31, 1974.

   And of course the basic document on expanding roles in nursing is the Report of the Secretary's Committee to Study Extended Roles for Nurses, *Extending the Scope of Nursing Practice*, DHEW (HSM) 73–2037, November 1971.

7. On the "art of care," see Brook, R., et al.: Quality assurance today and tomorrow: forecast for the future. *Annals of Internal Medicine*, 85:809–817, December 1976.

8. There are massive amounts of literature on evaluation and evaluation research, and on quality assurance, which is one of its branches. Perhaps, the most often cited reference is Donabedian, A.: Promoting quality through evaluating the process of patient care. *Medical Care*, 6:181–202, May–June 1968.

   More comprehensive material on evaluation research is contained in the two-volume *Handbook of Evaluation Research*, edited by Elmer L. Struening and Marcia Guttentag,

Beverly Hills: Sage Publications, 1975. In Volume I, particularly useful articles for this chapter are Weiss, Carol H.: Evaluation research in the political context (Chapter 2), and Campbell, Donald T.: Reforms as experiments (Chapter 5).

9. Bloch, Doris: Evaluation of nursing care in terms of process and outcome: issues in research and quality assurance. *Nursing Research*, 24:256–263, July–August 1975.

10. Suchman, Edward A.: Principles and practice of evaluation research. In Doby, J.T. (ed.): *An Introduction to Social Research*. New York: Appleton-Century-Crofts, 1967.

11. *Ibid.*, p. 330.

12. See Note 8.

13. It is interesting to fantasize about how much easier it might be to make the kinds of changes in the health care system that seem necessary, if a prescriptive theory approach were taken. Among other advantages of this way of thinking about some things is that it makes the most troublesome aspects of institutional change—aspects of the framework—matters of rational inquiry rather than matters completely of political power relationships. Further development of the notion of dynamics could also lead to new ways to think about changes in the system. Instead of deciding on a new service, for example, on the basis of who has the power or control, consideration of dynamics might rest on who wants to do the activity, and why they want to. Experience with nurse practitioner practice in a medical center setting, for example, makes one aware that the nurse practitioners actually like to care for chronically ill people, with continuity of care, where those patients are seen as uninteresting by the physician staff, surely a difference in dynamics.

14. In fact, one such theory deals with how to introduce nurse practitioners into a new setting. See Lewis, Charles E. and Teresa Cheynovich: The clinical trial as a means for organizational change: report of a case study. *Medical Care*, 14:137–145, February 1975.

15. Dickoff and James (and Joyce Semradek) have written extensively on research methods for nursing, but their articles do not address directly research in prescriptive theory. See Dickoff, James, Patricia James, and Joyce Semradek: 8-4 research: A stance for nursing research—tenacity or inquiry. (Part I) Designing nursing research, eight points of encounter. (Part II) *Nursing Research*, 24:84–92 and 24:165–176, March–April and May–June, 1975.

16. See Dickoff, James, Patricia James and Ernestine Wiedenbach: Theory in a practice discipline. *Nursing Research*, 17:415–435 and 545–554, September–October and November–December 1968, p. 549. See also Diers, Donna and Mimi Dye: Situation producing theory. University of Kansas Medical Center (Kansas City): *Proceedings Second Nursing Theory Conference* (C. Norris, ed.), 1969, especially pp. 38–39.

17. For a discussion of the hospice concept, see Chapter 50 in Henderson, Virginia and Gladys Nite: *Principles and Practice of Nursing*. New York: Macmillan, 1977, pp. 1929–2007. The Chapter is written in collaboration with Florence S. Wald. See also in the same book, pp. 1951–1954 on hospices.

18. This definition is taken from Marram, Gwen, et al.: *Cost Effectiveness of Primary and Team Nursing*. Wakefield, Mass.: Contemporary Publishing, Inc., 1976, p. 2.

19. *Ibid.* See also Daeffler, R.J.: Patients' perceptions of care under team and primary nursing. *Journal of Nursing Administration*, 5(3):20–26, 1975; Felton, Geraldene: Increasing the quality of nursing care by introducing the concept of primary nursing: a model project. *Nursing Research*, 24:27–32, January–February 1975.

20. See Note 15, p. 2.

21. The literature on the therapeutic community is voluminous. The basic reference is Jones, Maxwell: *Therapeutic Community: New Treatment Method in Psychiatry*. New York: Basic Books, 1953. See also, Fleck, Stephen: Residential treatment for young schizophrenics. *Connecticut Medicine*, 26:369–376, 1962; also, Rubenstein, Robert and Harold Laswell: *The Sharing of Power in a Psychiatric Hospital*. New Haven: Yale University Press, 1966.

9

Measurement and
Measurement-Testing Studies

INTRODUCTION

A distinction can be made between studies aimed at producing "content," or substantive information, and studies aimed at inventing or testing measurements or methods. Though the design of the studies may be the same, the purpose and outcome are different. In general, content studies assume (or provide information about) the reliability and validity of measures used in order to test hypotheses. Measurement studies assume the truth of the hypothesis (or the reality of comparison groups) to test the validity of instruments. The study designs may be identical in form, but the purpose of the study and the inferences drawn from it are quite different.

A distinction can also be made between measurement and data collection (though the dividing line is not so clear). Data collection assumes that a measurement, or tool, has already been developed, tested, validated, and the concern is then with how it is applied in collecting information. Measurement implies here the construction of tools to provide quantitative evidence of the existence or degree of concepts operationally defined. And in general, there are two sources of error in measurement: one, in the measurement itself (unreliability, invalidity), and the other in the way the measurement is applied, or measurer error (1). The first will be covered in this chapter, the second in the next chapter.

LEVELS OF MEASUREMENT

Measurement implies quantitative information. Qualitative data—narrative description for example, is not "measurement" as the term is used here.

Four levels of measurement can be distinguished, and in each one different kinds of numbers emerge, and, therefore, data analysis depends on level of measurement. Statistical procedures appropriate for one level of

224

measurement aren't for another. The four levels of measurements are nominal, ordinal, interval and ratio (2).

In the *nominal* level of measurement, categories are named and the numbers used are simply the frequency of appearance of units in the categories. For example, the dimension "religion," can be divided into categories—Protestant, Roman Catholic, Jewish, Greek Orthodox, Russian Orthodox, Buddhist and so forth. The categories are simply named in no particular order, and there is usually no implied quantitative dimension underlying the categories. Catholics are no higher, or lower, than Protestants, for example. It is also assumed that everyone in one category is the same, with respect to that dimension: all Jews are equally Jewish.

Diagnoses are another example of nominal categories. Appendicitis, duodenal ulcer, arthritis, hyperthyroidism, hypertension, diabetes and so on are simply named categories, with no order implied. Categories for the analysis of nurse-patient interaction are also nominal categories (3).

When there is an order to the categories, the level of measurement is called *ordinal*. Here the categories are named and ordered, but the difference between one category and another is not known mathematically. For example, patients might be asked to grade themselves as very nervous, moderately nervous, a little nervous or not at all nervous. A person who grades himself as a very nervous is more nervous than a person who grades himself as moderately nervous, but we don't know just how much more nervous he is. Again, it is assumed that everyone who falls into a particular category is like everyone else in that category with respect to that dimension. Every "moderately nervous" person is as nervous as every other "moderately nervous" person.

Social class, as defined by Hollingshead is an ordinal scale (4). Classes range from I (the highest) to V (the lowest) based on a combination of points assigned for education and occupation. Thus, someone who is in social class II has higher social position than someone in social class III, but the exact distance between the two is not known.

In the *interval* level of measurement, categories are named and ordered, and the distance between them is known and equal, but there is an artifical, or arbitrary, zero point. A clinical thermometer is a good example of an interval scale. The "categories" are the degrees and the difference between 98.6° and 99.6° is the same as the difference between 100° and 101° on a Fahrenheit scale. The interval scales have an artificial zero point. On a Fahrenheit scale, there is still some degree of temperature at zero degrees, which is what the scale is supposed to measure, and the zero point—the freezing temperature of water at certain atmospheric pressures—is arbitrary. Even on a Centigrade scale, zero is artifical. The Kelvin scale is the only available temperature scale with a "true" zero point.

In a *ratio* scale, the categories are named and ordered, the distance between them is known and equal, and there is a true zero point indicating absence of the thing being measured. The Kelvin temperature scale is one example. Many physical measures are examples of ratio scales: heart rate, blood pressure, weight, age, pounds, grams, dosages, inches, centimeters.

The presence or absence of a true zero point is important for mathematical reasons. Without a true zero, it is not possible to multiply or divide scale readings, though one can add or subtract them. For example, a temperature of 100° F is not twice as "hot" as a temperature of 50°, it's just fifty points higher. To say something is twice as much (or half as much) is to multiply or divide. To say a reading is five points higher or lower is simply to add or subtract.

The point can be made clearer by imagining a clinical thermometer which includes not only the Fahrenheit scale, but also the Kelvin scale. "Zero" is −273° F, so a temperature of 50° F is really 323°, and a temperature of 100° F is really 373°. Clearly 373 is not twice 323. If a picture were drawn of such a scale, both 50° and 100° would be in the top piece of the picture, very far aware from "zero."

The "names" or "categories" of interval and ratio scales are the numbers in the scale. 98.6° F is the name of a particular category, and it is assumed that everyone whose temperature registers 98.6° (given that all thermometers read equally) is like everyone else with respect to the temperature dimension.

It should be easy to see that as the level of measurement is increased from nominal to ordinal to interval to ratio, the sensitivity and precision of the measure is increased. For if it is possible to say that one quantity is different in degree and/or direction from another, more information is being conveyed than simply saying two things are in different categories. It should also be noted that a ratio scale has all the qualities of nominal, ordinal and interval scales, that an interval scale has the qualities of nominal and ordinal scales and so forth. This suggests that it is possible to change ratio or interval scales into nominal or ordinal. For example, heart rates are ratio scales. But a group of people could be ranked according to the heart rate and the data analyzed at the ordinal level. The data could even be divided at the median into high and low rates, giving an even lower level ordinal scale. Collapsing data in this way means losing rather a lot of information. If data are available about someone's absolute position on a scale, rank ordering that person obscures the "score."

Sometimes data are collapsed from one level of measurement to the next lower one because even though actual numbers are available, they may not be clinically meaningful. For example, imagine a scale to measure patient anxiety that uses a point scoring system for, say, ten items. Each item is scored 1–5 depending on the patient's answer. Scores can then be summed, to make a range of 10–50 points. But it is probably not the case that a person with a score of 45 is five points more anxious than a person with a score of 40, or a person with a score of 30 one half as anxious as a person with a score of 50. In such a scale, data would probably be collapsed into intervals of five points or so, converting the scale into an ordinal level of measurement.

It is rarely possible to upgrade a lower level of measurement into a higher one. However, change scores are an example of such a maneuver. Even though temperature, for example, is an interval scale, when repeated measures are taken, the change from one time to another can be calculated, and by definition, change scores are ratio scales—there is a true zero point of "no change."

There are two other levels of measurement that do not quite fit in the four mentioned. They are *ordered-metric* and *nominal dichotomous.* Ordered metric scales fall somewhere between ordinal and interval scales and are found in various kinds of measurement of attitude and behavior. Such scales depend on the visual appearance of the scale itself, with "equal-appearing intervals" made equal by how they are typed on a page (5). For example, a scale might be constructed like this:

> *Rate below your satisfaction with the care you have received in this hospital. Circle the number that corresponds to your rating.*

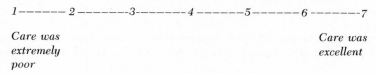

Care was
extremely
poor

Care was
excellent

Here, the numbers are treated as if they were real scores, rather than rank orders which is what they really are, and data are analyzed as if the scale was an interval scale (6). Such scales are a little more than ordinal, by virture of having equal appearing intervals, but a little less than interval, since the intervals only appear to be equal and actually are not.

Nominal dichotomies are measures in which there are only two categories. Gender, for example, can be classified as male or female. When there are only two categories, special statistical procedures that resemble those used for interval scales can be used so nominal dichotomies are treated as if they were interval scales.

There is another quality of interval and ratio scales that has certain technical as well as conceptual ramifications. Scales can be either *discrete* or *continuous.* A discrete scale has no halfway points (or any other gradations) between one category or reading and the next. Continuous scales have actual or theoretical graduations between points on the scale. Number of children in a family is a nice example of a discrete scale (a ratio scale). In theory, there can be 1 or 2, or 4 or 5 children, but not 4.5, or 1.73 or .9. Interestingly, heart rate is another example of a discrete scale. One can have 80 beats per minute, or 81, but not 80.5. Technically, data analysis for discrete scales is supposed to differ from that for continuous scales, but rarely is this condition observed, so we have paradoxical findings that the median family size in the United States is 2.3 children. Examples of continuous scales are everywhere: inches, points, age, centimeters and so on.

The distinctions among levels of measurement and between discrete and continuous scales are important not only for technical reasons in data analysis, but for conceptual reasons as well.

CONCEPTUAL AND OPERATIONAL DEFINITIONS AND MEASUREMENT

Every concept or factor in an hypothesis or research question is provided with an operational definition and a way to measure it. (Except in factor-searching studies, where the attempt is to find the concepts and define them theoretically. Therefore, "measurement," in the sense used in this chapter of quantification, may not apply to some factor-searching studies.) The measurement must derive logically from the conceptual definition, but certain things about the conceptual definition may dictate how an operational definition is devised.

For example, "anxiety" might be an appropriate concept to use according to the analysis of the problem. That concept could have any number of different conceptual definitions, depending on the investigation. And different definitions will imply different measurement or data collection procedures. If anxiety is defined as both a biochemical and psychological phenomenon, different measures will be required than if it is defined strictly as an intrapsychic variable.

Part of deciding on a theoretical definition is determining the scope of the concept. For example, is anxiety something that is either present or absent? Or does it have degrees? Is there an opposite to anxiety—that is, does anxiety just go up from zero to whatever the upper limit is, or is there a "positive" and "negative" anxiety?

The closer an operational definition and measurement are to the concept itself, the better, because the bigger the distance, the more difficult it is to make the inferential leap from data to theory and back. For example, suppose postoperative "stress" is defined conceptually as a psychological state, but the measurement selected is postoperative vomiting. Can one then conclude that those people who did not vomit were not in stress? Or suppose blood pressure increase had been used as a measure of stress. Can it truly be concluded that everyone with increased blood pressure is in stress, as opposed to, say, angry?

Wolfer discusses a number of these kinds of problems with operational and conceptual definitions (7). Among them are the problem of using physiological measures for what are actually psychological concepts; the problem of using indirect measures of patient state, such as observer ratings, chart data or other reports, rather than patient reports; the problem of using measures of staff behavior as if they were measures of patient behavior, as in using a measure of nurse performance as if it were a measure of patient care.

In general, the more directly the concept and the measure are linked, the better. Indirect measures are particularly appropriate when there is no direct way to obtain data on something, as in the case of intrapsychic states where projective tests of various kinds may be used. Otherwise, direct measures will prevent problems of interpretation of data later. For instance, amount of pain medication taken, number of days in the hospital, even number of certain kinds of tests or procedures done on patients may measure staff behavior rather than patient behavior. Number of patient complaints may or may not be an index of "satisfaction" with care, depending on whether the complaints are about the care, the food, the temperature of the room, noise in the hall or whatever. There is even some suspicion that in some circumstances, number of complaints may be a measure of how satisfied, rather than how dissatisfied a patient is, as in a situation in which primary nursing is aimed at patient participation, which is then seen as patients being more assertive to have their needs met. Here, number of complaints might better be a measure of "participation" rather than satisfaction (8).

There are other measurement problems that start as conceptual problems. For example, a study used a list of adjectives on which patients checked the degree to which each adjective applied to their emotional state at several points in time (9). Each adjective had three degrees—a little, some and "a lot." The instrument generally worked well, except that on one adjective, responses were always in the a lot category, meaning there was too little variation. The adjective was miserable, and a little *post facto* common sense revealed that it is not possible to be a little bit miserable. One either is, or isn't. Miserable is one of those states that implicitly always means a lot.

A similar problem can happen with equal-appearing interval scales, if the anchor points (the scale numbers) are defined in certain ways. It is possible to define the bottom and top anchor points of the scale so extremely that they will never be checked. For instance, a seven-point satisfaction with care scale might have the bottom of the scale defined, "the worst possible in the world," and the top of the scale, "the best I could ever imagine." It is very unlikely that people will ever use either of these two scale points, which will sharply decrease what is already a short range of responses from 1–7 to 2–6.

Sometimes an attempt is made to make ordinal scales out of things that really aren't ordered, things that it would be better to leave as nominal categories. For example, a scale of social competence defining living situation with categories such as "lives alone," "lives with parents," "lives with nonrelative roomate," "halfway house or sheltered living" or "total care situation" looks on the surface like a scale, but really isn't. There is no theory that says it is "better" to live alone or with family, and while a total care situation probably does indicate less social competence, living alone doesn't necessarily indicate less than living with others.

One conceptual confusion leading to measurement problems was once fairly common in the nursing literature—the confusion of attitude with behavior (10). One still finds studies in which hypothetical situations are presented to nurse respondents, then the data are taken as measures of actual practice, which they are not. There is nothing wrong with hypothetical situations as measures of what a nurse said she *would* do, but the connection between reported hypothetical behavior and real behavior is tenuous at best.

Other conceptual problems were discussed in Chapter 3. In general, one always has to be wary in using measures developed for one purpose in a study that might have another purpose, since the conceptual derivation of the measure may not fit the present situation. The more the researcher understands about the theory that is behind any measure, the better, and the more appropriate the use of the measure.

MEASUREMENT CRITERIA

Measures may be "good" or "bad," or useful or not along several dimensions. These dimensions are called here "measurement criteria," meaning they are the standards against which any measure is tested. Further, at least for some measurement criteria, there are formal study designs that can be used to provide empirical evidence that a measure is reliable or valid.

The measurement criteria are validity, reliability, meaningfulness, sensitivity, precision and appropriateness. They are defined as follows:

Validity: the extent to which the measurement measures what it's supposed to measure; the extent to which the results found by using the measurement are compatible with other relevant evidence.

Reliability: the extent to which repeated uses of the same measurement on the same sample will give equivalent results; the extent to which two measurers can agree on the reading. First definition = consistency, second = equivalence.

Meaningfulness: the extent to which 1. the phenomena being measured are important (i.e., accessible, controllable) to nursing, 2. the measurement can be used or abstracted from in practice.

Sensitivity: the extent to which the measurement captures the "true" range of the possible variation in the phenomenon being measured.

Precision: the extent to which the measurement can discriminate between individuals; also the extent to which an individual's placement on the measure characterizes him as different from everyone else.

Appropriateness: the extent to which the measurement "fits" the sample.

Validity

Validity has to do with the relationship between the concept being measured and the measurement itself. Validity is defined as the extent to which a measure measures what it is supposed to measure, or the extent to which its use provides data compatible with other relevent evidence. The first definition has been called "internal validity"; the second, "external validity." (11)

There are five types of validity, and a measure may be "valid" according to any of the five, or several in combination. The five types are face validity, content validity, construct validity, concurrent validity and predictive validity. A measure may be tested for any of these types of validity, and the kind of validity reported for a measure is an important index.

Face validity simply means that just on inspection, the measure looks like it is a good indicator of the concept. A measure of relative social position based on education and occupation can be said to have face validity when education and occupation data are indeed collected and somehow summed to produce social class rankings. The only "test" for face validity is expert opinion. One can put together a panel of experts who look over a measure and decide whether it looks as if it measures what it is supposed to, admittedly not a very strong test. Face validity is usually a concern during the phase of constructing an instrument, and measures used in hypothesis-testing studies usually have stronger evidence of validity to have confidence in the findings produced by using them.

Content validity means that the content of the measure can be justified from other evidence, or the extent to which the measure represents in its items the entire range of the concept being measured (12). For example, in order to claim content validity, a tool to measure quality of nursing care has to include items that tap physical care as well as psychosocial, environmental and other kinds of care. The "other evidence" used to justify the content validity of a measure comes from the theory behind the concept being measured, in this case, what conceptual framework is taken on the notion "quality of nursing care."

Construct, concurrent and predictive validity are all much stiffer validity tests. At the present stage in the development of nursing research, they are often beyond the scope of a study that doesn't concentrate specifically on developing and testing a measure.

Construct validity means applying the measure to groups or situations that are known to differ on the construct involved and seeing if the measure picks up the difference. For example, a new measure of blood pressure might be applied to known groups of normotensives and hypertensives to see if it would detect the difference. Or a quality of care measure might be used in two different settings, one known for its excellence of care, one known to be poor. Depending on how big a difference there is between the groups to begin with, a measure may be quite insensitive and still pick up enough difference to claim construct validity. The other problem with this kind of validity test is finding groups that are truly *known* to be different on the dimension of interest.

Concurrent validity is the correspondence of one measure with another of the same phenomenon (13). For example, a new measure of attitude toward pregnancy might be administered to a sample of people, along with an already standardized measure of the same concept, and the results compared. Concurrent validity has a built-in paradox. If one assumes that one measure is already a valid measure, it had to be tested for validity itself at some point, and one would want to look hard at the evidence of the measure's validity before comparing a new measure with it. Further, if there already exists one measure of a given thing and it has tested validity, why invent another one? If the new measure is more economical, practical, simple, precise or noninvasive, the effort put into its construction may be justified.

There are recent reports of concurrent validity testing of patient self-reports versus nursing interviews or other measures done by clinicians, with encouraging evidence that self-reports are as valid (complete, accurate) as other ways of obtaining the same information (14). One study tested the validity of an observational tool for assessing body position and motor activity against a known-to-be-valid machine recording motor activity (15). Here, inventing a way to observe and record body position and activity without using expensive and perhaps inappropriate equipment has clear clinical implications.

Predictive validity refers to the ability of a measure to predict something else. For example, it was once thought that IQ scores could be used to predict performance in college. Children of a certain age group were tested and then followed through college to see if the test really did predict their performance. Volicer has been working with the prediction of stress in hospitalized patients aiming to establish the predictive validity of a tool used by nurses to assess patients before hospitalization (16). Studies have also been done to develop tools to predict recovery from surgery (17). To test predictive validity, it is assumed that the hypothesis (IQ is related to college performance) is true, and the effort is to test the predictive validity of the measure of IQ. Since in clinical research in nursing there are few hypotheses that can be accepted as true, so measures can be tested, examples of predictive validity are so far few in nursing literature.

The stronger the evidence of validity that can be presented for any measure, the more likely are we to believe the results obtained through its use. No matter what the level of inquiry or the precision of a measure, its validity should always be assessed and reported.

Reliability

Reliability refers to the stability and consistency of a measure. It is the extent to which repeated administrations of the instrument will provide the same data, or the extent to which a measure administered once, but by different people, produces equivalent results. (There is a third kind of reliability: the extent to which various parts of a measure measure the same thing, used most often in paper-and-pencil scales or tests.)

Consistency can only be tested in situations where the thing being measured is in itself stable, unchanging over time. For example, judgments of chart data can be tested for consistency because the data themselves do not change from one time to another. Coding of tape recordings or transcripts can also be tested for consistency.

Testing equivalence means having more than one data collector use the measure on the same data, to see how much agreement there is between them. Here, the phenomenon being measured may not be stable, but the data collectors do their measuring all at the same time on the same data. Generally, equivalence is a stiffer test than consistency because it is usually harder to get two people to agree on the same thing than to get one person to agree with himself at two different times (18).

Reliability can be increased by carefully constructing the instrument in the first place to make the amount of inference needed low, to make the categories or classifications mutually exclusive, jointly exhaustive and unidimensional, and to train observers or data collectors in the use of the measure. Using the measure the same way on every case increases its reliability, and keeping observers or data collectors blind to the hypothesis or the treatment groups in an experimental study increases the claim to reliability.

The more information one has to take into account in making judgments with a measure, the lower the reliability. If one has to judge the verbal behavior, nonverbal behavior, posture, tone of voice, speech patterns all at once to come up with a measure of "discomfort," the possibilities for disagreement between observers are considerable. The more an observer or coder has to infer from the empirical data to a classification or category, the larger the chances for disagreement. For example, categories might be developed for body position, with the observer being expected to watch people interact, then classify their position as indicating "hostility," "friendliness," "distress" or something else. The closer the categories are to the real observations, the less possible errors in judgment or assignment of data to categories are.

Equivalence testing can be complicated by some interesting factors. For example, a researcher might choose an individual with whom to check reliability of an instrument, who might have such a different conception of the data that reliability can never be obtained. A study of nurse-patient interaction used a non-nurse coder at one point, with the result that reliability between the nurse and non-nurse was never as high as it was between two nurses, since coding the data depended on one's clinical sense (19).

Interesting problems of equivalence can be found in testing observational measures. The observers not only have to share an understanding of the observational task and the instruments, they may have to be alike in other ways. For instance, if a measure that depends on acuity of hearing is used, the observers have to be able to hear the material in the same way. An odd example of inequivalence occurred in a study using observation of facial expression of laboring women. The observer was to stand at or near the foot of the bed on which the patient was semireclining. A system had been devised to classify particular positions of parts of the face—brows, eyelids, eyes, forehead and so on. It happened that one observer was 6 inches taller than the other, producing a significant lack of agreement on positions of the eyelids especially, since the shorter observer could often see that the eyelids were not quite closed when the taller observer thought they were closed (20).

Training observers can also contribute to inflated estimates of agreement so that reliability checks really test the efficiency of the training rather than the "real" extent of agreement. Similarly, researchers often depend on colleagues or students for reliability testing, and exaggerated agreement can result if the raters already share some common frames of references. Both of these problems are less serious when the instrument is itself well constructed and the amount of inference demanded is low (since training or likeness among observers is most likely to be an issue when inference is called for).

Measures can be reliable without being valid, but cannot be valid without reliability. For example, suppose a blood pressure cuff has a pinhole in it that consistently leaks the same amount of air. Readings obtained from its use will be reliable—that is, will be stable over time and repeatable, but will not be valid. If the pinhole does not leak air consistently, the measure would be unreliable as well.

Reliability can be increased by increasing the sensitivity and precision of the instruments as well (see below).

Meaningfulness

Meaningfulness is defined as the extent to which the phenomenon being measured is important (accessible, controllable) to nursing and the extent to which the measurement can be used or abstracted from in practice. In other words, does the use of the measure tell us anything about nursing practice and could it be used in practice? It may be more important for nursing research to have a rough tool that tells something more important about nursing than to have a very precise tool that says nothing. The scientific conventions that require validity, reliability, precision and so on are not to be neglected, but meaningfulness is also important.

Meaningfulness is attained first through the clear analysis of the problem, where knowledge of nursing as it is, could, or should be will allow statements about how a particular measure could be used in nursing practice; then, by using the measure as "naturally" as possible. This is partly a consideration of study design. If the study is designed to take full account of the normal setting of nursing practice, the possibility that the measure will be meaningful is increased. Taking into account from the beginning the typical skills with which nurses are endowed and tailoring the measure to fit those skills increases the meaningfulness of the measure too.

Evaluating a measure for meaningfulness involves the pragmatic questions of how useful or potentially useful the indicators could be in practice and whether they really tell anything important about practice. Obviously, the standard against which such questions are gauged is nursing practice, and answering them requires an intimate connection with practice.

Meaningfulness is well illustrated in recent reconsiderations of measurements of the effect of nursing (as opposed to the effect of medical care). Studies of nurse practitioners, for example, have often used what are essentially measures of medical practice (morbidity, mortality) rather than measures that might be more sensitive to the effect of nursing, such as compliance, knowledge, return for reappointments, follow-through on referrals or even management of a chronic illness. Measures that tap the differential effect of the nursing care in nurse practitioner work, in contrast to that part of the work that is an expansion of the nursing role into traditional medical practice, are more meaningful to the study of the effect of the whole of nurse practitioner practice (21).

Sensitivity

Sensitivity is defined as the extent to which the measurements capture the true range of possible variation in the phenomenon being observed (22). Imagine a one foot long ruler. Sensitivity deals with the extent to which the ruler is able to pick up "twelve inchness" that is, the extremes of the phenomenon. The sensitivity of a measure depends on the theoretical definition for which it is intended, too. If one chooses a one-directional definition of "stress," for example, assuming it starts with zero and goes up, then the measure has to reflect this. If incidence of vomiting is chosen as the measure of stress, one can justify saying that the more times one vomits, the more stress is present. But if someone does not vomit, can it be said that he is not in stress?

Precision

Sensitivity is related to another measurement criterion—*precision*. Precision is defined as the extent to which an individual's placement on the measure characterizes him as different from everyone else. That is, can the measurement pick up the small differences? If sensitivity is the length of the ruler, precision is the quarter inch marks.

Both sensitivity and precision have to be tempered with meaningfulness. For example, although it is possible to measure blood pressure in halves or quarters of mm. Hg, such precision is clinically irrelevant. A premature drive for sensitivity and precision often characterizes research in disciplines to which systematic study is fairly new. Somehow precision, relevant or not, seems more "scientific." But, at the risk of redundancy, it is better to have a rough tool that tells something important than a precise one that says nothing (23). Once the categories or dimensions of the rough tool are defined, it may be possible to make finer distinctions.

Sensitivity and precision in nominal categories can be increased by attention to making them mutually exclusive, jointly exhaustive and a significant division of the whole. Sensitivity and precision can also be increased by choosing the smallest unit of analysis that makes sense. For instance, categories for classifying verbal interaction can be made more sensitive by making the complete sentence, or even individual words, the unit, rather than a complete paragraph of speech. (Probably individual words as unit is too precise to be meaningful in this example.)

Moving from lower (nominal, ordinal) levels of measurement to higher ones (interval, ratio) also makes measures more sensitive and precise. Similarly, a measure that is really precise but too precise to be meaningful can be made more meaningful during data analysis by collapsing data into larger divisions. If precise mm. Hg are not clinically meaningful, data may be analyzed by grouping readings into intervals of 5 mm. Hg, for example.

Appropriateness

Appropriateness is defined as the extent to which the measure fits the sample. This criterion has to do with the relationship between the operational definition and the sample characteristics. The question asked of measurement appropriateness is, does the sample have the thing being measured? For example, a questionnaire could not be used with people who could not read. Vomiting would be a useless measure with people who have nasogastric tubes.

Considerable methodological concern has recently been raised about the extent to which various measures are "culture bound," that is, have an inherent cultural bias that effectively makes the measure invalid and inappropriate with other sample groups. The recent furor over the use of IQ testing with black children is probably the most obvious example of this kind of question. There are other kinds of culture boundness. Some measures of social competence have been criticized as sexist, or at least as measuring a peculiar conception of social competence in women. For instance, there are some social competence measures on which women score better if they wear skirts and lipstick then if they wear no cosmetics and pant-suits (24). The most used life change instrument has been criticized, oddly enough, for a bias toward normal people. That is, it appears not to be sensitive to the kind of life change that exacerbates illness in chronically ill psychiatric patients, where a bus strike, or the refrigerator breaking down, or a big snow storm may be "life change." (25) Another measure, of problem-solving ability, turns out not to work with chronically ill psychiatric patients either because those who have real difficulty with problem-solving refused even to try to participate in the testing situation (26).

Appropriateness can be increased by careful attention to the sample criteria and selection, by examining any potential measures for cultural bias and by a commonsense evaluation of any instrument for how well it fits the sample.

The relationship between reliability and validity has already been mentioned. Some of the other criteria are also related. Validity does not guarantee meaningfulness, but meaningfulness may increase validity. Generally, sensitivity and precision increase reliability, as long as they go along with careful definitions and an appropriate number of categories.

There are special considerations in nominal categories besides the measurement criteria listed here.

Nominal categories should be mutually exclusive, jointly exhaustive, unidimensional and a significant division of the whole. Categories are mutually exclusive when there is no overlap between them, when every unit to be categorized will fit in only one category. Categories are jointly exhaustive when every unit will fit somewhere, that is, when the categories exhaust the possibilities. Unidimensional means that the categories are all related to one underlying dimension. And categories are a significant division of the whole when they carve up the dimension into pieces that are not so big as to obscure differences, and not so small as to be meaningless for the purpose for which they are intended. If categories are not mutually exclusive, reliability will be compromised. If they are not exhaustive and unidimensional, validity will be in trouble. And if they are not a significant division of the whole, it will not be possible to conclude what one wants from the study.

Overlapping categories can happen when the definitions for the categories are vague or when a good deal of inference is called for in classifying things. For example, "anxiety" and "fear" judged, say, from verbal interaction, would probably not be mutually exclusive categories. Categories can be less than exhaustive if some potential classification is left out, cured easily by adding the category "other" to a list of nominal categories. Making categories unidimensional and a significant division of the whole is largely conceptual work, relating the categories to the problem and the variables under study.

MEASUREMENT STUDIES

In addition to the kinds of studies discussed in earlier chapters, it is possible to conduct studies specifically to develop and test measurements. In contrast to content studies, measurement studies aim not at developing substantive knowledge in the form of "findings," or "results," but at devising and testing ways to measure variables with the hope that the measure may then be used in content studies. Measurement studies are not particularly aligned with any one level of inquiry, so they are treated separately here.

The Delphi Survey of Priorities in Clinical Nursing Research determined that in the opinion of the nurses in research and in administration sampled, the highest priority for nursing research should be developing ways to measure the effect of nursing (27). Abdellah and Levine make a strong plea for more measurement studies or what they call "methodological studies" in nursing research (28). Developing tools for measuring the results of nursing is frequently just part of a larger study, and the tools developed may have little generality outside that study, but may be useful in other studies in the future. Without good—meaningful, valid, reliable—tools, hypothesis-testing is more difficult and less rigorous and the possibility of developing well-tested predictions is undermined. Some people have suggested reasons for the lack of concentration in nursing research on developing tools. Abdellah and Levine say:

The absence of research methodology especially developed for research in nursing can be explained by the highly technical nature of this work. In the physical sciences, instrumentation is often the full-time activity of specialist. . . . as more and more of such specially trained personnel become interested in research in nursing, the output of special methodologies for studies in nursing should increase . . . secondly, . . . to engage successfully in methodological research requires a more creative and ingenious approach than do other forms of research. . . . There is no question that a considerable amount of the effort expended by the researcher in methodological research is intellectual—thinking through the problem and developing ideas—whereas in descriptive and explanatory research much of the effort centers around actual collection and analysis of the data, activities which may not be of a comparable intellectual level. (29)

Methodological research may or may not require any more creativity or intellectual potential than any other kind of study, but the larger point is well taken. Until very recently, there simply were few nurses either trained or interested in developing measures for nursing research. Yet nurses are the most appropriate group to engage in such activity if the measures developed are going to have relevance for nursing practice, for they alone know what will work in the real nursing situation.

The need for tools for nursing research becomes readily apparent during the analysis of problems for research. Nearly always one reaches a point where one has to decide to stop and develop a measure, or trust to fairly superficial, gross measures that are easy to think up or borrow some tool from another science. If the decision is to develop a tool, there are special methodological considerations to be met, just as there are for any other kind of study.

Factor-searching studies are sometimes designed deliberately as the first step in measurement-testing studies. The categories, once developed, can then be subjected to further tests for reliability and validity.

There is no real methodology for testing meaningfulness or appropriateness. To the extent that the measure is related to important, accessible, controllable variables in nursing, it is meaningful. And to the extent that the use of the measure allows specific statements about the nature of the phenomenon, it is meaningful. Judgments about meaningfulness have to be made within the framework of nursing practice and the "test" of meaningfulness is pragmatic.

However, nursing practice is not always going to be the way it is today. In fact, the whole aim of nursing research is to improve practice. Therefore, in judging meaningfulness, one has to take into account not only practice as it is now, but also practice as it could and/or should be. For example, measures that several years ago would have been totally inappropriate for nursing, such as cardiac monitors, are now appropriate, since nursing has increased its responsibility for reading and interpreting data from such equipment. The continuing expansion of nursing functions may lead into whole new areas of measurement that weren't considered before.

The "test" of appropriateness, like that of meaningfulness, is pragmatic: how much, and how good is information gathered through the use of the measure. If there are cases during a validity check that do not fit the measure at all, some redefinition of the sample may be in order. To the extent that the measure can be used on a group of people without excessive difficulty, it is appropriate. If, despite theory that says a given measure would be good, data gathered by using the measure do not show predicted differences, one explanation may be that the measure was not appropriate to the sample. Appropriateness, then, is something that is not often directly tested in a study having just that purpose, but is something that may be discovered in the course of analyzing why a prediction didn't come out the way one thought it would.

Testing Validity

Procedures for testing construct, concurrent and predictive validity are rather more specific and involve the same aspects of the research process as any other study—study design, sampling, data collection, analysis and so on.

Construct validity is tested with a relation-searching design. A sample of people who have different places on the continuum to be measured is selected purposively, or by some other means. The sample may consist of two groups at extreme ends of the dimension, or a number of groups at several places. (This design is the same as the "known groups" design discussed in Chapter 5.) It is known that people are different on the dimension, so the measure is administered to the sample in exactly the same way to every case, just as equivalent data are collected in a more usual relation-searching study. Data from the groups are compared to see if the measure did indeed pick up the differences known to be there. Interpretation of data is based on how much difference is expected and how much was achieved by the measure.

This kind of study was done to test the validity of a tool to measure nurse-patient interaction (30). It was suspected that if the tool was any good, it should be sensitive to differences among patients, so groups of interactions of nurses with different kinds of patients (old versus young, mentally ill versus not, aphasic versus not) were put together. The interactions were coded and the differences indicated that the tool was indeed sensitive to the expected differences.

Concurrent validity is tested through a cross-sectional association-testing design. Instead of having two (or more) different variables as in a usual association-testing study, there are two different measures of the same variable. The sample is chosen randomly so that it will be representative of the distribution of the variable involved, both measures are applied at the same or nearly the same time and the results are correlations. Actually, it is not absolutely necessary that the sample be chosen randomly since the purpose is not generalization. Purposive or accidental sampling can be used instead, as long as there is variation in the phenomenon and a large enough number of cases can be collected.

Predictive validity is tested through either a prospective association-testing or a causal hypothesis-testing study design. The measure to be tested is applied to a group of people, then data about the dependent variable are collected and correlated. Samples may be selected randomly, and if the causal hypothesis-testing design is used, random assignment to groups is done. Data are analyzed for how well the measure predicts other results, assuming the hypothesis is true. The difference between testing predictive validity and testing an hypothesis is in where the assumptions are. Testing an hypothesis assumes the validity of the measure; testing validity assumes the truth of the hypothesis.

For example, a study might test the hypothesis that prenatal factors should predict Apgar scores of newborns. This would be a prospective association-testing study (31). It is assumed that the measurement of "prenatal factors" is valid, and so is the measurement of Apgar scores. However, if one were doing a measurement study to develop a prenatal assessment tool, for example, one would use exactly the same design but assume that the Apgar measure is valid, *and* that the relationship between prenatal factors and Apgar score is in fact true. The research question then becomes, will the new measure of prenatal factors pick up this "truth?"

It is poor form indeed to simultaneously test the validity of a measure and an hypothesis with the same measure. It is impossible to conclude anything from such a study, though it has been tried. If an hypothesis-testing study is being done, one simply has to assume (or it is hoped have some evidence) that the measures used are valid and reliable. One can't test both a measure and an hypothesis at the same time.

Testing Reliability

Reliability can be tested formally with particular kinds of study designs. Consistency is tested by applying the measure to the same set of data twice, with a time lapse in between, and comparing the results for agreement. For example, a method for coding the content of nurse-patient interaction could be applied to some data once, then after a time applied again by the same person to the same data.

Equivalence is tested by having two (or more) people use the same measure on the same people or data at the same time and correlating their results. For example, with a double stethoscope, two people can listen to the same heart rate or blood pressure and compare their readings. Or two people can code the same data simultaneously but without consultation between them and the agreement on the data can be calculated. Or two people can observe the same situation or behavior and compare the ways they coded or scored it. Testing reliability simply means repeating these double observations enough times so that agreement figures can be obtained.

The sample of people or data for reliability checking should include as much of the variation in the phenomenon as possible. It is much easier to obtain agreement on the more normal or usual cases than on the extremes. For example, there is likely to be more agreement on blood pressure readings in the 100–130 range than in the below 90 or above 200 ranges. Samples can be chosen randomly or purposively, since, again, generalization is not the desired end.

Reliability of paper and pencil tests can be tested also. Here, the interest is in determining whether the whole instrument measures the same thing.

The items on the instrument can be divided randomly in half, and each half administered to the same group of people alternately. Then the two halves can be correlated (called the "split-half" method). Consistency can also be tested by administering the measure to a group of people, then readministering the same measure after a time lapse and correlating them (the "test-retest" method). Alternatively, each item may be correlated to the total score, to ferret out items that don't fit the measure.

Various correlational techniques are used to compute reliability estimates. Often simple percentages of agreement are used, and if the data have been examined unit by unit, they probably tell as much as the more complicated techniques. Acceptable levels of reliability depend on the phenomenon being investigated, the precision of the measure and the investigator's own judgment. Usually agreement of 80–90 percent is considered satisfactory (or correlations of .60–.70 and above), but what is acceptable depends on the purpose for which the measure was intended.

Testing Sensitivity and Precision

Tests of sensitivity and precision can be built into designs for testing validity. Sensitivity is assessed by seeing if, when the measure is applied, there are people in categories at both ends of the scale. Assuming that the sample is selected in such a way that potential variation is maximum, there should be cases that would fall into all the categories of the measure. If all the cases are lumped toward the middle, the measure is not very precise. If there are cases that do not fit on the measure at all, it is not very sensitive. Some additional assessment of sensitivity and precision can be made during reliability checking too. Paying attention to patterns of disagreement between coders may illuminate categories that could be more precise. Paying attention to instances of very high agreement may indicate a need for more sentitive distinctions.

In recent years, a good deal of attention has been paid to inventing measures of "quality assurance" in institutional care. As the quality of care has become more and more the focus for hospital accreditation, which itself determines importantly an institution's reimbursement rate for charges for patient care, institutions have been motivated to develop methods by which the quality of care can be measured, and the effect of changes in care demonstrated. The literature in quality assurance is now considerable, and several measures of quality have been tested for validity and reliability, with some success (32).

Inventing measures for nursing research is one of the thorniest problems facing the researcher. One is often tempted to make do with measures invented for other disciplines, particularly attitude indices and physiological measures. While using such instruments is probably time-saving, in the long run the effort spent in developing and testing a measure constructed with nursing in mind will probably lead to bigger payoffs.

The necessity for original, valid and reliable nursing research measures is considered one of the foremost problems for nursing research. Very often in analyzing a problem for research one comes to the point at which one realizes that even though the problem is important, it cannot be studied until a measurement is invented. Though the time and energy necessary to invent measures is considerable, it is probably better to spend the time developing a measure rather than to leap too soon into hypothesis-testing studies with untested measures. Nevertheless, the basket into which any individual investigator wishes to put all the eggs is still a matter of individual choice and analysis of the problem.

A brief summary of the considerations in constructing, using and evaluating measures is presented in Figure 9-1.

Figure 9-1

CRITERION	CONSTRUCTING MEASURE	HOW SEEN IN: USING MEASURE	EVALUATING MEASURE
VALIDITY	Analysis of problem will help show relationship between measure and theory. Literature may help make the connections too.	Use measure in same standardized way on all cases.	Face or content validity should be explicit. In measurement study, construct, concurrent or predictive validity is usually tested.
RELIABILITY	Limit the number of categories or dimensions. Categories should be mutually exclusive and exhaustive. Amount of inference needed for judgments should be kept low.	Standard procedure for all cases. Keep observers "blind" to the hypothesis and treatment group the patient is in.	Usually an attempt is made to see how much inter- intra-observer argument there is. In measurement studies, reliability (agreement) is rigorously tested.
MEANINGFUL-NESS	Analysis of problem, with explicit indications of how theory and knowledge of practice lead one to use certain measures. Explicit indication of where the measure fits with practice as it is and as it should be.	Select a "natural" setting. If study approximates real practice, chances are the meaningfulness of measure will be increased.	Interpret results with reference to practice, further research, theory. How easy or hard is it to use measure, and how much does it tell you?
SENSITIVITY	Analysis of problem to determine the concepts and what they include. Distinguish between what is included in the concept and measure and what isn't. Categories exhaustive.	Standard procedure. Also, systematically record instances where the measure doesn't seem to "fit."	Can test sensitivity in measurement study. Report deviant cases where measure doesn't fit.
PRECISION	As above. Categories should be unidimensional, mutually exclusive. Increase level of measurement.	As above.	As above.
APPROPRIATE-NESS	Specify reasons for selecting the sample criteria—analysis of problem will include relationship of problem to larger problem.	Use (select and treat) as specified. Keep data systematically on cases where the measure doesn't seem to fit or tell enough about what we want to know.	Evaluate findings with respect to hypothesis or question, and measure. Analyze deviant cases with respect to theory and measure including practicality.

NOTES

1. Actually, there is another source of error too—sampling error—discussed here as an aspect of "appropriateness." See Webb, Eugene, et al.: *Unobtrusive Measures: Nonreactive Research in the Social Sciences.* Chicago: Rand McNally, 1966, pp. 23–27.

2. Experience with early drafts of this book indicated that students sometimes (somehow!) think that the levels of measurement match up with the levels of inquiry. That is, students have thought that the nominal level measures belong in factor-searching studies, ordinal level ones in relation-searching and so on. I suppose because there happen to be four levels of inquiry and four levels of measurement, and that in both cases, they are cumulative, supports the confusion. Nevertheless, it should be said out loud: levels of measurement and levels of inquiry are independent.

3. See Chapter 4, p. 117, for example.

4. Hollingshead, August and Fredric Redlich: *Social Class and Mental Illness.* New York: John Wiley & Sons, 1958.

5. L.L. Thurstone is credited with developing the methods of equal-appearing intervals. See Goode, William and Paul K. Hatt: *Methods in Social Research.* New York: McGraw-Hill, 1952, pp. 262–270.

6. A nice, brief treatment of the issue of treating ordinal data as interval data is Jaspen, Nathan: Research q and a. *Nursing Research,* 26:470, November–December 1977.

7. Wolfer, John A.: Definition and assessment of surgical patients' recovery and welfare. *Nursing Research* 22:394–401, September–October 1973.

8. My favorite example of choosing the wrong thing to measure a concept with comes from a study I can no longer find. The investigators were studying postpartum depression, and used "crying in the early postpartum period" as their operational definition. It turned out that crying wasn't associated with anything, including depression, and the authors rather contritely reported that they hadn't thought in advance that women cry for lots of reasons, including depression, but not exclusive to that.

9. Eisler, Jeanne, et al.: Relationship between need for social approval and postoperative recovery and welfare. *Nursing Research,* 21:520–525, November–December 1972. The discovery of the problem with the word "miserable" is in Ms. Eisler's thesis (unpublished Master's thesis, Yale University School of Nursing, 1971).

10. Confusing attitude with behavior has been a particular problem in studies of nurse patient interaction. See Diers, Donna and Robert C. Leonard: Interaction analysis in nursing research. *Nursing Research,* 15:225–228, Summer 1966.

11. Webb, et al., see Note 1, pp. 10–12.

12. For a brief treatment of reliability and validity, see Lindeman, Carol A.: Measuring quality of nursing care: Part Two. *Journal of Nursing Administration,* 6:16–19, September 1976; see also, Batey, Marjorie V.: Some methodological issues in research. *Nursing Research,* 19:511–516, November–December 1970.

13. In the Lindeman article cited above, concurrent validity is treated as an aspect of construct validity.

14. Aspinall, Mary J.: Development of a patient completed admission questionnaire and its comparison with the nursing interview. *Nursing Research,* 24:377–381, September–October 1975.

15. Downs, Florence and Joyce Fitzpatrick: Preliminary investigation of the reliability and validity of a tool for the assessment of body position and motor activity. *Nursing Research,* 25:404–408, November–December 1976.

16. Volicer, Beverly J. and Mary W. Burns: Pre-existing correlates of hospital stress. *Nursing Research,* 26:408–415, November–December 1977.

17. Wolfer, John A. and Carol E. Davis: Assessment of surgical patients' preoperative emotional condition and postoperative welfare. *Nursing Research*, 19:402–414, September–October, 1970.

18. For a long treatment of reliability in interaction analysis, see Diers, Donna and Ruth L. Schmidt: Interaction analysis in nursing research. In Verhonick, Phyllis J. (ed.): *Nursing Research* (Vol. II). Boston: Little, Brown, 1977, especially pp. 94–108.

19. *Ibid.*

20. I was the taller of the two observers. The study was Sharp, Elizabeth S.: Development of a tool to measure patient behavior, USPHS Grant NU 8883, 1963.

21. See Bloch, Doris: Evaluation of nursing care in terms of process and outcome: issues in research and quality assurance. *Nursing Research*, 24:256–263, July–August 1975; see also the section, Quality assurance, by several authors in *Nursing Clinics of North America*, 9:303–380, June 1974; see also Wolfer, Note 7.

22. Precision has also been called "specificity." See, for example, Rodgers, Beckett, et al.: A screening tool to detect psychosocial adjustment of children with cystic fibrosis. *Nursing Research*, 23:420–426, September–October, 1974.

23. Wald, Florence S. and Robert C. Leonard: Toward development of nursing practice theory. *Nursing Research*, 13:309–313, Fall 1964.

24. The concept of social competence is discussed in Slavinsky, Ann, et al.: Back to the community: a dubious blessing. *Nursing Outlook*, 24:370–374, June, 1976; Smith, M.B.: Competence and socialization. In Clausen, J.A. (ed.): *Socialization and Society*. Boston: Little, Brown, 1968; White, R.W.: Motivation reconsidered: the concept of competence. *Psychological Review*, 66:297–333, September 1959; Inkeles, A.: Social structure and socialization of competence. *Harvard Education Review* 36:265–283, Summer 1966.

25. See Slavinsky, Ann: Nursing with chronically ill psychiatric out-patients. USPHS grant # NU 00370, June 1970–December 1974.

26. *Ibid.*

27. WICHEN, *Delphi Survey of Priorities in Clinical Nursing Research*. Boulder, Colorado: WICHE, 1976. See also, Lindeman, Carol A.: Delphi survey of priorities in clinical nursing research. *Nursing Research*, 24:424–441, November–December 1975.

28. Abdellah, Faye G. and Eugene Levine: *Better Patient Care Through Nursing Research*. New York: Macmillan, 1965, pp. 422–423.

29. *Ibid.*, pp. 423–425.

30. Diers and Schmidt, see Note 18.

31. Krigis, Carol A.: Predicting infant Apgar scores. *Nursing Research*, 26:439–442, November–December 1977.

32. One of the best measures, and reports, in quality assurance measurement is Jelinek, R.C., et al.: *A Methodology for Monitoring Quality of Nursing Care*. Report of Phase I of USPHS Contract NIH 72–4299, July 1972. USDHEW Publication No. (HRA) 74–25. See also Hegyvary, Sue and R.K. Dieter Haussmann: Monitoring nursing care quality; nursing professional review; the relationship of nursing process and patient outcomes; correlates of the quality of nursing care (four articles). *Journal of Nursing Adminisration*, 6:3–27, November 1976.

10

Data Collection

INTRODUCTION

Data collection is the phase in the research process in which research comes alive. Up to this point, it has all been planning not doing. Data collection begins the aspects of a project where the real world is encountered and where all the small, practical problems just waiting out there surface to make the researcher's life more interesting.

There's not a whole lot that can be done about some of the practical problems one runs into during data collection. If there is anything to be learned from experience, it's that data collection will always take longer than one thinks it's going to, and that it will always be more difficult than it seems as if it's going to be. Twenty-twenty hindsight says that it is wise to allow more time than one thinks will be needed, and develop in advance some support systems to get one over the inevitable hitches and hassles.

It is rarely as easy to get a sample as one thinks it should be. In spite of broad sampling criteria, it always seems that the first ten people to be entered into the sample don't fit the criteria and have to be dropped. People refuse to participate, fill out questionnaires incorrectly, forget to return for a reinterview, have their surgery cancelled, are discharged early or disappear. Even when the sample is to be obtained all at once, say a whole group of patients scheduled for prenatal appointments the same day, the biggest snowstorm in recorded history will happen and clinic will be cancelled.

Even when the sample can be found and things are progressing nicely on that end, there will be other hitches. A mimeograph machine will break down on the day before 400 questionnaires are due to be run off. Copies of a psychological measurement ordered through the mail are lost somewhere on the New Jersey Turnpike and you can't start without them. A machine that's essential to data collection develops terminal rust. A cassette jams the one and only available tape recorder. The record room can't find the charts you need because the resident has them signed out for *his* research project.

There's nothing to be done about these kinds of practical problems except

246

develop patience and grin and bear it. There are other considerations in **data** collection that do require some advance thinking and planning to assure that the data collected are as accurate a representation of reality as possible.

OBSERVATION AND QUESTIONING

In general, there are two types of data collection—observation and questioning. Under observation is included not only those kinds of data collection that are actually observing, looking, seeing and writing down, but also collecting physiological data and collecting information from existing records, such as charts or log books. Questioning includes interviewing, questionnaire construction and administration, as well as some kinds of self-reports of patients on paper-and-pencil instruments. While the distinction isn't perfect, observation implies a one-way communication—from the subject or patient to the researcher. Questioning implies a two-way communication—questions asked, answered, heard and recorded.

Also in general, observation is used to collect data on behavior, broadly construed, including physiological behavior (heart rate, galvanic skin response, blood pressure, clinical indices of various kinds). Questioning is used to collect data on things that are not observable, such as opinions, attitudes, perceptions, past experiences, feelings and so on.

Planning for data collection begins with decisions about what variables are relevant, how operational definitions for each one are to be provided, and ends with the actual plan for obtaining the information needed. Decisions about what kinds of data to collect follow from analysis of the problem, and are based on a certain nursing sense of the appropriateness to a clinical setting of whatever methods will be used.

The distinction between behavior, measured through observation, and other things, measured through questioning, deserves a few more words. There is some confusion in the literature when responses to hypothetical situations are taken as if they were real behavior, which they are not. Such methods of collecting data are probably better thought of not as behavior at all, but as something closer to "attitude."

On the other hand, data on behavior cannot automatically be taken as reflecting particular attitudes. It is well known that people do not always mean what they say and that their words may not adequately convey the sense of what the feelings are. Actions may not always speak louder than words—they may just speak differently. Observations of what a nurse does with a patient may say nothing about what her feelings were at the time. An increase in systolic blood pressure may or may not reflect a psychological state. The point here is merely to reemphasize the necessity for being clear about what data are going to be taken as evidence of what concept or what factor.

Both observation and questioning as methods of data collection are subject to errors or bias from the subject or respondent and from the investigator or data collector, so there is a special kind of observation or questioning called "nonreactive measures", or "unobtrusive measures" that may also be used in clinical research (1).

OBSERVATION

Observation means gathering data by means of the senses. Although visual and aural observation are most commonly used, it is also possible to observe through tasting, touching and smelling.

Observer Roles

There are two general observer roles that can be distinguished: nonparticipant observer, and participant observer (2). The nonparticipant observer simply observes, but does not contribute to (or detract from) the natural situation. Sometimes the nonparticipant observer is not even in the same room, as when an observation room with two-way mirrors is used.

Participant observation means that the observer is part of the natural situation, taking part in its activities, or otherwise immersing her/himself in what is happening. Anthropological field observation is the model for this kind of observation, though participant observation has now become a major tool for nursing research, especially when the research nurse her/himself is performing as nurse in a situation, testing the effect of nursing on some aspect of patient experience.

There are advantages and disadvantages to either role. Nonparticipant observation may provide more reliable data since the observer is not distracted by being part of the situation and responsible within it. Yet, simply observing and not taking part may not provide data as rich as might be obtained by participant observation. Nonparticipant observation can be agonizing when the situation is clinical and the observer a nurse observing patient care. It is very difficult to "stay in role" and not interfere with or otherwise get into the action, and it is difficult as well not to bring to bear unstated biases that come from one's own sense of nursing care (3). On the other hand, participant observation can be difficult when the observer gets so caught up in the activity that she/he forgets to record observations or unintentionally biases the observations to meet some unstated, implicit internal criteria. Yet participant observation means the observer has access to her/his own thoughts and feelings as data, which may be very useful in interpreting behavior.

Situations may dictate the use of a particular kind of observation. Nonparticipant observation may be more appropriate in a crisis situation in which a great deal is going on and the participants are so involved that they may not be able to maintain distance from the tasks. For example, the emergency room, the delivery room, the operating room are examples of intense, demanding situations. On the other hand, participant observation may be the only type of observation that is appropriate in some situations in which the introduction of another person will distort the situation too much. Therapy sessions and some kinds of physical examinations might be situations in which it is not appropriate to include a third person as an observer.

Time Sampling

A particular problem in observation is that often the behavior of interest is continuous over a very long period. For example, observation is used in some methods of evaluating quality of patient care, where patient care is continuous for any given person from admission through discharge (4). It is obviously impossible to have the same observer present through a continuous hospital stay, and it would be prohibitively expensive to have enough observers to cover enough patients for a meaningful sample (5). So some method of dipping in to the continuous stream of behavior is needed so that observers do not become exhausted (and less reliable), and so that enough data can be obtained. Time sampling is the answer.

Time sampling is like any other kind of sampling, meaning, picking from the entire universe or population of times some segments in which to observe. Depending on the situation, the times might be parts of an hour or a shift, selected randomly, or with some other probability sampling method. If a situation is self-contained, such as labor, or a psychotherapy hour, sections of time may be chosen in such a way that the whole time is well represented. In the case of labor, it might be every fifteen minutes or so, or perhaps every third contraction. In the case of a therapy hours, it might be the first ten minutes, a middle ten and the last ten.

Methods of Recording Observational Data

Observation is nothing by itself—it has to be written down or otherwise recorded and preserved. The simplest method probably is a *checklist* on which the items of interest to be observed are listed, and a check is made if the item occurred during the observation period. There is no great difficulty in setting up checklists. The major point to be remembered is that the items must be clear enough (reliable) so that observers can agree that the thing either happened or didn't. For example, an item "crying" might be too loosely stated, if "tears in eyes" is what is wanted. In general, items should be worded so that as little inference on the part of the observer as possible is required. What this most often means is that items on a checklist are fairly exact translations of visual descriptions—body position, names or numbers of people in the room and their positions, who talked and when, body movements or activities (walking, sitting, standing, lying) and so on. When appropriate, line drawings or diagrams of a setting may be used as aides to the observer, who then fills in on the diagram the positions of people, the actual facial expression or whatever is needed.

Checklists most often just note whether an activity or an item occurred or not during the period of observation. Sometimes the number of times something happened is noted as well, but rarely are there qualitative judgments called for such as how much (or how little or how great or small) a given item was. Qualitative judgments are very difficult to record reliably. What is "a great deal" of something to one observer may be only "a moderate amount" to another.

Checklists are also rarely completely exhaustive of the phenomena observed. Rather, particular aspects of behavior may be chosen on the basis of the theoretical and operational definition of the variables.

On the other hand, *coding* behavior directly from observation does attempt to encompass all of the behavior, by assigning bits of it to the categories of the coding scheme. For example, verbal behavior (conversation) of nurses and patients may be coded directly from observation and the utterances of each assigned to predefined categories on the spot (6). Or the body positions and movements of a client may be coded right in the situation, using a form of stick figure drawings with symbols to indicate direction and force of movement (7).

As with checklists, coding systems must have categories quite explicitly and clearly defined in advance, otherwise observers cannot agree on what they saw or heard. Attempts are also made to limit the amount of inference the observer has to make, but this is difficult at best when working with verbal behavior which must be immediately classified.

Modern technology has produced machines to help record observations. *Video tape* and *audio tape* are becoming used more often in clinical research, and they are an enormous help to the researcher in observation. Problems of reliability of recording observation are diminished considerably with continuous-running tape recording, assuming high quality and high fidelity equipment are used. The same problems of categorizing or classifying the material from tapes exist, but at least the data themselves—the observations—are preserved (8).

A method halfway between tape recording and simply observing is the "behavioral diary." (9) Here, the observer dictates a stream of continuous observations into a small tape recorder, minute by minute, to record continuously the behavioral data. The tape recordings can then be transcribed and categories applied to them, or other analyses done.

Video tape and audio tape may also be used to produce simulated behavior for research purposes. Here, the intent is not so much to classify the behavior of the person being taped, but of the respondent to the simulated behavior (10). Simulations are particularly useful in training observers in a situation in which it is not feasible or practical, or perhaps ethical, to add cameras, microphones and other equipment to the patient care situation.

Mechanical recording is not influenced by feelings, so observations collected through mechanical equipment do tend to be less biased than participant or nonparticipant observation. However, the video tapes must still be interpreted and the biases of the people interpreting the tapes can still reduce the reliability of the data. (Once the equipment is activated, it probably isn't affected by feelings. However, investigators have sometimes been chagrined at the number of times they've "forgotten" to turn on the tape recorder, or turned it to "play" instead of "record," or used the wrong tapes. Such "accidents" may be indications that the method of data collection is wrong for the particular study and the investigator might do well to reconsider. Of course, unfamiliarity with the equipment can also influence the comfort with which it is used. Training in the use of equipment will eliminate some of the "errors.")

When the observer takes the role of participant, it may not be possible to record directly behavior or activity. Process recordings or reconstructions of patient care situations may be used instead. Such methods were once very common in nursing research, but have been used increasingly less as audio tape equipment became available and as people realized the inherent weakness of memory reconstruction.

When memory reconstruction is used, it is possible to increase the observer's retention of data. A format or outline of topics helps. One can tape record a situation, then reconstruct it from memory and compare the reconstruction with the tape. Such comparisons, repeated several times, will point out where the observer is missing data and may suggest special points for the observer to work on. "Ghost recording"—recording as said something the observer only wishes had been said, can be ironed out by such a method. Truman Capote is said to have increased his ability to retain conversation (while preparing *In Cold Blood*) by a similar method.

In any kind of observation, observer training is necessary to increase the reliability of observed behavior. Reliability checks may be done as part of the training period. Training usually starts outside of the real situation with the explanation of the recording procedure, including definitions of categories or descriptors. Observers practice recording behavior together until they may move into the clinical situation and, with the patients' permission, observe a few nonstudy situations until they feel adequately prepared to observe and record data consistently.

The decision on which method to use to record observations depends on the type of study, the problem and the type of analysis that is to be done. Even though transcriptions of tape recordings can miss a great deal of data, depending on the fidelity of the recording, the transcribing equipment and the secretary's ear, transcripts may still be more useful sources of data for certain kinds of studies. Generally speaking, the further one gets from the original source of data (as transcripts are further removed than audio tape recordings, which are further removed from the "real" situation), the less accurate the data are likely to be but the more reliable coding is likely to be. Therefore, if the primary concern is with reliability of coding, one should choose a method of recording data that is inherently more reliable than some other method. The fewer stimuli recorded, the more agreement between judges or coders will result because they do not have so many things to cope with. Studies at low levels of inquiry do not put so much emphasis on reliability, but more on completeness of data. For these studies, any method that is likely to yield complete data is justified.

UNOBTRUSIVE MEASURES

There is a whole set of problems of validity of measurement that is called "reactive" measurement effect; that is, the person observed, or the subject, reacts to the process of measurement in such a way as to make the data produced invalid (11). Webb indentified several such effects: the "guinea pig effect," "role selection," response set, interviewer effects and change in the research instrument (12).

The guinea pig effect is self-explanatory: people being observed change their natural way of behaving because they are being observed. Role selection encompasses a number of things, including what is known in test construction as "social desirability response set," in which people respond to items according to the way they think they are supposed to respond. This kind of role selection may also occur in observation situations in which the subjects being observed take on particular behaviors they think will make them appear "better." Response sets are particular to paper-and-pencil instruments and include the tendency to say "yes" or "no" consistently, no matter what the item is; the tendency to use the middle of the scale rather than the extremes and other kinds of patterned responses that do not reflect true attitudes or opinions of the respondents. Interviewer effects come from reaction to the interviewer her/himself, rather than reaction to the content of the interview; for example, race or sex of an interviewer may make a difference in how people respond. And changes in research instruments over time may invalidate findings; for example, when interviewers become very experienced, they may conduct later interviews differently than earlier ones.

There are various technical ways to reduce reactivity in paper-and-pencil tests. Unobtrusive measures are used to reduce reactivity in observational situations.

Webb's book on unobtrusive measures is full of fun examples of data collected for marketing and sociological research (such as the number of nose prints on the window as a measure of the popularity of museum displays). In these cases, observation is made of things that occur normally and naturally, but may be indications of variables of interest. In most of the examples given, the data are not direct observations of behavior at all, but rather trails left by behavioral patterns. In this sense, unobtrusive measures are something different from simply not telling people being observed what the observer is looking at or for.

In the clinical situation, the chart or medical record is a prime example of unobtrusive measurement, especially when groups of charts are pulled to be examined retrospectively. The chart is nonreactive, and since the data are collected after discharge, or at least when the patient is not in active treatment at the time, charting practice cannot be affected by the data collection procedure. The validity of chart data may be questionable on other grounds, but not on observer effect.

Observations of who sits next to whom in group meetings is another example of unobtrusive measure. The distance of the bedside stand or overbed table from the bedridden patient may be a measure of the patient's social desirability. The number of times a call light is turned on during a given period is an obtrusive measure as well. The reader may think up any number of such ways to collect data without chancing observer effects.

QUESTIONING

Data on attitudes, opinions, beliefs and feelings are obtained through various kinds of questioning, primarily questionnaires, interviews and self-reports.

A questionnaire is a self-administered, paper-and-pencil instrument, designed to be completed by the individual subject. An interview schedule is a set of questions to be asked by the interviewer, who then records the patient's responses. Self-reports are variations of questionnaires. Though the purpose of a questionnaire and an interview is the same—to gather information about specific topics—one method may be better than the other for particular studies.

A questionnaire is usually easier to administer and cheaper because it does not require additional help. Questionnaires are usually sent out through the mail or are handed out and require no other intervention of the investigator. Questionnaires do require a large sample initially because the return rate is considerably lower than the rate for interviews. For a standard mail-out questionnaire, about a 20 to 30 percent return rate can usually be expected, but less than about a 40 to 50 percent return rate is considered unacceptable. There is always a question about whether information from people who return questionnaires is really generalizable to people who don't.

Questionnaire data can usually be expected to be easier to analyze because in order to have ensured that each respondent has the same stimulus to respond to, a great deal of thought must have gone into the construction of the questions and the construction of the categories which respondents check for their answers. Since the categories are already precoded and standardized, it is much easier to count up the number of people that replied to a certain category than it is to analyze open-ended questions. A questionnaire is generally more impersonal, and, therefore, a patient will have more confidence in his anonymity. Usually there is less time pressure on the respondent in a questionnaire.

Questionnaires are usually harder to construct because a great deal of thought must go into the wording of the questions and there is no opportunity to clarify the meaning of a question if the respondent does not understand it. Questionnaires generally miss qualitative anecdotal data because it has been found that people will not respond very fully to open-ended questions on a questionnaire. Nearly all the questions on the questionnaire must be precoded so that the respondent need only check the box with the answer that fits him. Therefore, less formal data that might be interesting are missed.

On the other hand, interviews are generally more expensive because it takes time to train the interviewers and administer the interviews. Interviews are generally harder to analyze because they may have less precoding of the categories and many more open-ended questions. Interviews are generally more personal; therefore, respondents may have lower confidence in the anonymity. On the other hand, interviews may get more relevant responses because the situation is more conversational and more informal. Interviews are more flexible. The interviewer can interpret the question if it appears that the respondent does not understand it. There is usually a higher return rate, with a low rate of people who refuse to be interviewed. Therefore, a smaller sample may be selected to begin with. An interview also does not depend on the literacy of the respondent. In an interview there is more opportunity to assess the validity of the answers by nondirective probes and asking the respondent to say more about a particular answer. Since the interviewer and respondent are face-to-face, it may be easier to detect inaccurate or untrue answers through facial expressions. An interview also gets qualitative data that a questionnaire misses.

There are some general points that apply to either interviews or questionnaires. The information that is desired dictates the questions to be asked. The questions will be determined by the analysis of the problem. The list of research questions that results from analysis of the problem can be broken down into interview or questionnaire items. Another decision to be made is how the data are to be best obtained—in an interview or in a questionnaire. Questions of economy must be considered in deciding whether a questionnaire or an interview is better for a particular study. Availability of a large sample and the time, energy and expenditure necessary to train and pay interviewers are all important factors.

In practice, nurses use interview techniques all the time, whether they realize it or not, because a large part of nursing depends on getting certain information from the patient on which to base decisions for intervention. The techniques for obtaining useful data in research and nursing practice are essentially the same.

Both questionnaires and interviews begin with an introduction in which the purpose of the instrument is explained. Who the interviewer or author of the questionnaire is, what the study is about, what the expectations are for the respondent and the fact that the data will be kept confidential are all explained. Some cases may require being fairly vague about who the interviewer is and why the study is being done in order not to prejudice the answers. If, for example, one is studying nursing care and using interviewers who are nurses, they may not introduce themselves as nurses but might wear lab coats and emphasize their interest in studying patient care practices. It should be clear that the introduction to an interview or a questionnaire does not differ markedly from the usual rapport-establishing aspects of nursing practice. When nurses want to establish rapport with patients, they define the situation for the patient. This is often done by introducing oneself to the patient, explaining what will be done, what he is expected to do and why.

One way to increase the usefulness of the data is to make maximum use of the respondent's frame of reference. For example, avoiding medical jargon respects the respondent's lack of understanding of some very technical terms. Using lay terminology whenever possible helps reduce the intimidating effect interviewers can have over respondents: womb instead of uterus, operation instead of surgery, bandage instead of dressing—as many adequate translations of specialized terminology as possible without being condescending. More generally, the more an interview can be aimed at things that are accessible to the respondent and that he is likely to have experienced or thought of, the better.

One also wants to minimize the defenses of the respondent. This can be done by using questions in a variety of ways. The "some people" technique—Some people feel very anxious about having an operation. How do you feel?—is most common. Hypothetical situations in which the respondent is asked to name his closest friend, then asked how the friend would answer the questions are based on the theory that people choose friends who share their feelings. Similarly, one can ask the projective question—If you had a friend who was going to have the same operation you've had, what would you tell him about it?

Double-barreled questions are always to be avoided. The question, Do you like nurses or are doctors more helpful? is impossible to answer yes or no and does nothing but confuse the respondent. Questions should have a single focus. (The same principle is followed in nursing practice in avoiding the double-bind messages—Have you stopped beating your wife?) Ambiguous words should be vigorously edited out of both interviews and questionnaires. Responses to questions involving such words are impossible to analyze, since one doesn't know what particular meaning the patient has attached to the word. Stanley Payne lists forty-seven meanings for the word "fair" which suggests doing away with the word altogether (13). We once used the question, "Before you came to the hospital, did you expect nurses to be concerned about you personally?" The phrase "concerned about you personally" turned out to have four meanings: worried about you, concern only about *you*, concerned about your personal history, or concerned about you as a person instead of a thing. The last interpretation was the desired one, but analyzing responses to the question had to be done separately for each interpretation.

Another way to maximize the usefulness of the data is through the use of nondirective probes. This is specific to interviews and cannot be used in questionnaires. Obtaining the best information possible means not putting answers in the respondent's mouth. Therefore, certain phrases such as, Can you tell me more? or How come? or Why is that? or Oh? are often used to encourage the respondent to elaborate further on a response. Again, this same principle holds true in nursing practice.

Methods that help increase rapport between an interviewer and respondent include providing for privacy during the interview. This increases the respondent's perception of his importance and anonymity. Keeping the interview or questionnaire to a reasonable length shows respect for the respondent's contributions.

Allowing for free expression and a conversational atmosphere creates a sense of spontaneity and also helps build rapport. This is done in interviews by building in open-ended (free response) questions and then following them by closed-ended (fixed alternative) questions. For example, "How did you feel before you came to the hospital today?" allows the respondent to say anything he wants to say. Then following that up with, "Would you say you felt very nervous, moderately nervous, a little nervous or not at all nervous?" focuses the answer more. Such sequences of open-ended questions followed by closed-ended questions are called "funnels." (The same process occurs in nursing practice. The nurse may begin by asking general questions—"How do you feel?" "What made you think that?" and eventually sum up what she's heard by saying, "You sound as if you felt thus and so. Am I wrong?")

Still another way to increase the usefulness of the data is to make clear the sequence and relationship of one question to another. In interviews and questionnaires, this can be done by focusing sentences like, "Now I would like to have you think about something else." (14)

Even when devising an interview or questionnaire, steps have to be taken to prepare for analysis of data. Precoding answers to questions so that all the respondent or interviewer has to do is check a box make data analysis easier. Questionnaires may consist mostly of precoded categories, with a few write-in spaces left for comments.

Because interviews and questionnaires are usually used in studies at fairly high levels of inquiry, the data will be comparable from case to case. Deviations from the protocol or probes used should be written in, as well as respondent's answers. If the interviewer changes the wording of a question so that it asks for something different, the respondent's answer has to take into account the way the question was worded. After the data are all collected, one may be able to tell just how much difference question wording makes and decide how comparable answers were.

There are several ways to tell good questions from bad ones. One way is to count the number of don't know answers to a specific question. If there is a very large number of such answers, the question may have something wrong with it. In questions which have precoded categories, the number of other responses—answers that do not fit into the precoded categories—is often an indication that something is wrong with the categorization system or with the question. The amount of variation in the response to a particular question will help tell how good the question is. If the same answer is coming from all the patients even though there should be variation in response, there must be something in question that is putting words in the respondent's mouths.

Scales are a special case of questioning. Scaling means that for each question or item, the answers can be ranked in some way, and then for the whole instrument, the numbers of variously ranked items can be added up to form a "score" for each patient. Respondents are given a number of items and asked to indicate their feelings about the item through agreeing or disagreeing, or saying whether the item applies to them always, sometimes or never, or some variation of the two. Following is a small piece of a completed attitude scale administered to nurses:

	Agree Strongly	Agree Somewhat	Indifferent	Disagree Somewhat	Disagree Strongly
Patients don't often know what they need.					
One should care for a crying patient before taking care of a patient with a routine order.					
The most important thing is how patients feel about themselves and their treatment.					

The instrument contains a large number of such items, worded so that about half of them are positive and half negative. For example, there is a companion item to the first one but it reads: "Patients are quite able to say what they need." Each of the possible answers—agree, disagree, indifferent and so on—has a point score, in this case, ranging from -2 to $+2$. The total score for each respondent is then calculated. The distribution of the dimension being used is set in advance so that it is possible to tell what positive and negative scores mean. People can be rank-ordered in terms of their scores and the data analyzed as ordered-metric or interval data. In the above example, people with high scores would have positive attitudes toward patients, people with low scores, less positive attitudes.

Many attitude scales resemble this one, but may have different possible response categories—for example, "item definitely applies to me," "item definitely does not apply" or "item sometimes applies." There are usually an uneven number of possible responses, and each item must get a response.

This is called the "forced choice" approach and there is no possibility for the respondent to answer in anything but the categories provided.

Some attitude scales use a slightly different approach. Instead of providing boxes to be checked, a linear graphic scale is provided, as below:

Luck is the most important thing for getting up in the world.

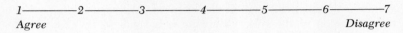

1————2————3————4————5————6————7
Agree   Disagree

The respondent is asked to circle the number that most closely approximates his opinion about the item. The answers are handled in the same way as in the earlier example, but the intervening step of using an answer sheet with the scores on it is eliminated. Scales such as the one above are also called "equal-appearing interval scales," and data are treated as if they were interval measurement, reasoning that the intervals between scale points are indeed "known" and "equal" because they are typed that way on the page. Sometimes one sees a variation in this kind of scale in which the numbers are removed and only dots used on the continuum, with an answer sheet giving the assignment of points to the anchor points of the scale.

An interesting variation on attitude scales is the "semantic differential" of Osgood (15). In this scale a particular stimulus is identified, and all the items consist of paired adjectives describing how the respondent views the stimulus. For example:

Patients with cancer are:

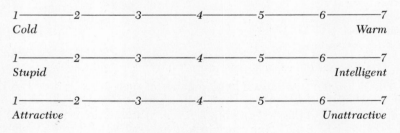

1————2————3————4————5————6————7
Cold   Warm

1————2————3————4————5————6————7
Stupid   Intelligent

1————2————3————4————5————6————7
Attractive   Unattractive

Etc.

Semantic differential-type scales have most recently been used in studies of sex-role stereotyping among health care practitioners (16). In these scales, there may be several dimensions. For example, one dimension might be "potency," and consist of adjective pairs connoting power—strong-weak and so on. Or, the two poles of the scale may be weighted in some way, when they reflect different ends of a continuum, such as in a scale of adjectives to describe men and women.

Making up items for attitude instruments and testing the instruments for reliability and validity does not differ much from constructing any other measure. In early stages of developing the instrument, logical validation and/or jury opinion are used to determine face validity. Logical validation simply means looking at each item from a common sense viewpoint to see if it looks useful. Jury opinion is the same thing but with more people, and usually people who have special qualifications for judging items. "Item analysis" is used as a specific validity test in attitude instruments. Each item is correlated with the total scores obtained from a number of people, and only those items with high correlations are retained in the scale.

Attitude scales are usually administered in questionnaire form—that is, self-administered. Occasionally they are included as part of an interview and read off to the respondent. The theory and practice of attitude scaling is treated in considerable depth in other books.

Self-reports are a special case of questionnaires. Most often, questionnaires are used to obtain opinions or attitudes, or sometimes other psychological phenomena, such as biases, preferences and so on. Self-reports are questionnaires used to obtain data on patient-perceived behavior, including sign and symptoms, comforts, discomforts and the like (17). Wolfer reviewed the literature on patient recovery and welfare and concludes that not enough use has been made of the promise of patient self-report, in contrast to other measures such as staff report, physiological behavior or chart data. He advocates devising measures that will reliably and validly get at how the patient perceives his own situation and argues that such data may be more valid than data obtained in other ways. Early studies of such patient reports in which patients were asked to rate their sleeping, eating, walking and other behavior, as well as their emotional states, are promising indeed.

PHYSIOLOGICAL BEHAVIOR

Collecting data on physiological phenomena is a special case of observation. Here, reliability is a matter of attention to the equipment to be used, or the procedure used to read laboratory tests or blood samples or whatever. Special precautions may be needed to be sure that the measurements are taken in the same way on every sample unit. If blood pressure is a measure, for example, it will be important to be sure that the same arm is used for every patient, the same cuff and stethoscope and the patient in the same position.

Initial calibration of equipment and repeated checks on accuracy of equipment or lab values is usually built into study designs. Since measurements of physiological phenomena are often interval or ratio levels of measurement, it may also be important to think through in advance the degree of precision appropriate to the topic and the measurement. In general, the highest degree of precision is aimed for in taking the initial measurements, knowing that later data analysis may group readings into larger intervals or round numbers up or down.

Problems of validity in measuring physiological phenomena come when the theoretical connections between the measure and the physiology aren't completely clear. For example, it is not at all determined how the peripheral nervous system might react to emotional stimuli, and, therefore, what a measure taken of peripheral nerve activity, such as palmar sweating, has to do with particular emotional states. The palmar sweat index is apparently an index of arousal, but whether that arousal is anxiety or anger or fear is not all that clear. There is yet a great deal to be known particularly about how psychosocial phenomena are displayed in physiology, and the researcher is wise to approach the use of physiological measures with caution and with full appreciation of the physiological research that may be necessary to understand fully what the body is doing.

RELIABILITY AND VALIDITY

Data are only as reliable and valid as the instruments used to collect it and the sources of data themselves. While most of the attention here has been on reliability and validity of measurements or instruments, a few words about reliability of data sources are in order.

Problems of reliability of data source are particularly apparent when data accumulated for another purpose (from the one in the present study) are used. A prime example is the use of the medical record or patient chart (18). Medical records are notoriously incomplete, and according to some, inaccurate, for research purposes. They are particularly unreliable sources of information about things other than medical diagnosis or treatment, such as nursing care, referrals, counseling and patient teaching. The medical record is highly dependent on the ability of the clinician and her/his time to accurately record information, as well as the pressures on the clinician that militate against being complete about information.

This kind of unreliability will be a consistent problem in studies which use the medical record as the primary source of data, and will be a systematic problem if there are systematic differences in charting practice or completeness of recording that might vary with independent variables in the study at hand. For example, if nurse practitioners routinely chart more completely or differently than a comparison group of physicians, the results of the study may show differences between the two groups of charts which are not measures of differences in patient care practice, but are measures of charting practice.

Other sources of data which may have built-in problems of reliability are various kinds of paper reports, such as annual reports of agencies, progress reports of various kinds, proposals for funds and the like. Since these reports are written to convince someone or some agency to refund a program or prove its continued usefulness, they may be overly positive about the services offered, and not so complete on the problems encountered. Archival materials of many kinds must be treated with a grain of salt, and, when possible, validated against other sources of information.

DATA REDUCTION/PRESENTATION

Once the data are collected, one has to make sense out of it all. The first step in data analysis is to reduce it to a manageable handful. Any basic statistics book will give the general principles of data reduction and they will not be elaborated upon here.

For studies at higher levels of inquiry, one usually describes the sample first, using the demographic variables that characterize it. Comparisons between or among sample groups (experimental, control) may also be made as an initial run. The next step is usually to analyze the data specific to the hypotheses or research questions. It is probably wise to use this particular order because it is all too easy to get caught up in the mountains of material any research project produces and forget what the data were collected for. When the hypotheses are tested, secondary analysis may be done to ferret out particular relationships, or to help explain anomolous findings.

The summary tables the researcher has invented as part of the study design will be an aide to conceptualizing the data analysis and findings. And the tables, if done well to begin with, may be easily translated into the report itself.

In general, tables should be used to simplify or amplify the text, but not to substitute for it. Similarly, the text shouldn't just repeat what is already obvious in the tables. And in general, tables of raw data are not as instructive as tables showing particular differences or patterns of relationship. Clearly labeled tables are a distinct boon to the reader, and, where appropriate, graphic figures that explain data analysis or particular patterns of responses are a great help, especially in correlational studies with large numbers of variables treated in relationship to each other.

Preparing data for presentation has two purposes: first, helping the researcher figure out what was really found, but second getting the data in shape to present to other audiences. Therefore, some more than cursory thought is in order, since the most common criticism of research reports by practicing nurses is that they are impenetrable, and, therefore, not useful where they could be most used.

CONFIDENTIALITY

Although the more general issue of ethics in research is covered in a later chapter, a few words about confidentiality are appropriate here. That the respondent's or patient's identity is carefully guarded is a basic principle of research. Only the investigator her/himself should know the patient's identity and such information is not for public consumption. Even in reporting case studies, initials of patients or pseudonyms are used instead of real names, for any other treatment of the data is an invasion of privacy.

Patients should be assured of the confidentiality of the data when it is collected from them if at all possible. Such assurance may involve showing the patient that her/his name does not appear on any of the data collection sheets (although a code number may appear), but it is probably conveyed more in the manner in which the investigator approaches the patient. If she genuinely respects the patient and feels her research is important, this will be conveyed as a professional commitment to guard the patient's welfare.

Patients' and respondents' names should never be written on the data collection sheets. Instead, the patient's code number can be written on the sheet, and the investigator may keep a master list of names and code numbers in a separate file. The Kinsey studies even had locked files of code numbers and names to which only the two senior investigators had keys and great precautions were taken so that no one respondent could be identified from her/his data.

Part of the introduction to an interview or an observation session includes telling the respondent or patient that the information is confidential and will be used only for research purposes. Some institutions have policies that require signed consent from patients, especially if the data involve audio or video tape recording. In addition, it is often wise to assure patients that the data will have no bearing on their subsequent stay in the hospital, for patients are often aware that their charts are available for personnel to read.

Research data should be destroyed as soon as it is possible to do so. Very often data are transferred to punched cards, and after being checked for accuracy, the original data sheets are burned. Summary tables of raw data should be preserved in case secondary analysis might be done, but raw data should be destroyed. Research data may be considered privileged information in some cases (depending on state laws) and covered by whatever legal statutes apply.

NOTES

1. Webb, E.J., et al.: *Unobtrusive Measures: Nonreactive Research in the Social Sciences.* Chicago: Rand McNally, 1966.

2. Pearsall, Marion: Participant observation as role and method in behavioral research. *Nursing Research,* 14:37–39, Winter 1965. Pearsall lists two other roles as well—participant-as-observer, and observer-as-participant.

3. Paulos, Evangeline S. and Gracia McCabe: The nurse in the role of research observer. *Nursing Research,* 9:137–140, Summer 1960; Malone, Mary: The research nurse and social science research. In Beenis, W.C., et al.: *The Role of the Nurse in the Outpatient Department.* New York: American Nurses Foundation, 1961, pp. 86–88; Benoliel, Jeanne: Research related to death and the dying patient, in Verhonick, Phyllis J. (ed.): *Nursing Research* (Vol. I). Boston: Little, Brown, 1975, pp. 189–228.

4. Hegyvary, Sue and R.K. Dieter Haussman: Monitoring nursing care quality. *Journal of Nursing Administration,* 5:17–26, June 1975.

5. Voda, Ann, Stanley Butts and Lucille Gress: On the process of involving nurses in research. *Nursing Research,* 20:302–308, July–August 1971.

6. Diers, Donna and Ruth L. Schmidt: Interaction analysis in nursing research. In Verhonick, Phyllis J. (ed.): *Nursing Research* (Vol. II). Boston: Little, Brown, 1977, pp. 77–132.

7. Downs, Florence S. and Joyce J. Fitzpatrick: Preliminary investigation of the reliability and

validity of a tool for the assessment of body position and motor activity. *Nursing Research,* 25:404–408, November–December 1976.

8. Griffin, Gerald, et al.: Clinical nursing instruction and closed circuit TV. *Nursing Research,* 13:196–204, Summer 1964. Wilcox, Jane: Closed circuit television: a tool for nursing research. *Nursing Research,* 13:211–216, Summer 1965. Two recent research projects have accumulated continuous video tape recordings of patients in intensive care: see Rita Chow: Postoperative cardiac nursing research. *Nursing Research* 18:4–13, January–February 1969; also Chow, Rita: Identifying professional nursing practice through research. *International Journal of Nursing Studies,* 9:125–136, August 1972; Daubenmire, Jean et al.: Methodologic framework to study nurse-patient communication. *Nursing Research.* 27:303–307, September–October, 1978.

9. See Note 5.

10. Wallston, Kenneth, et al.: Increasing nurses person-centeredness. *Nursing Research,* 27:156–159, May–June 1978.

11. See Note 1, p. 13.

12. Webb, et al., see Note 1. Webb includes sampling error which is here discussed in Chapter 3.

13. Payne, Stanley: *The Art of Asking Questions.* Princeton: University Press, 1964.

14. General references on interviewing include Barton, Allen H.: Asking the embarrassing question. *Public Opinion Quarterly,* 22:67–68, Spring 1958; Berengarten, Sidney: When nurses interview patients. *American Journal of Nursing,* 50:13–15, January 1950; Hyman, Herbert H.: *Interviewing in Social Research.* Chicago: University of Chicago Press, 1954; Kahn, Robert L. and Charles Connell: *Dynamics of Interviewing.* New York: John Wiley & Sons, 1957; Meadow, Lloyd and Gertrude Goss: Problems of the novice interviewer. *American Journal of Nursing,* 6:97–99, February 1963; Owens, Charlotte: Concepts of interviewing. *Nursing Outlook,* 1:10–12, October 1953; Selltiz, Claire, et al.: *Research Methods in Social Relations.* New York: Holt, Rinehart & Winston (1st edition), 1960, especially Appendix C.

15. Osgood, C.E., G. Suci and P. Tannenbaum: *The Measurement of Meaning.* Urbana, Ill: University of Illinois Press, 1957.

16. Kjervik, Diane K. and Mari Palta: Sex-role sterotyping in assessments of mental health made by psychiatric-mental health nurses. *Nursing Research,* 27:166–171, May–June 1978.

17. Wolfer, John A.: Definition and assessment of surgical patients' welfare and recovery. *Nursing Research,* 22:394–401, September–October 1973.

18. Jones, Louis and Nancy V. Rude: Research Q and A. *Nursing Research,* 27:195–196, May–June 1978; Lyons T. and B. Payne: The relationship of physicians' medical recording performance to their medical care performance. *Medical Care,* 12:463–469, May 1974.

11

Rights of Human Subjects

INTRODUCTION

The protection of the rights of human subjects in research has received considerable attention recently in the professional and the lay press. The dramatic excesses of the Tuskegee case, the Jewish Chronic Disease Hospital and the University of Chicago case involving experimentation with diethylstilbesterol (DES) are all examples of untoward risks to which human beings were put, without their informed consent. The discovery of such cases has produced a climate of concern in research communities—concern not only that such events not occur again, but a similar concern that the protection of human subjects not be placed in opposition to society's need for scientific knowledge.

At the same time, it has been pointed out that in clinical research in nursing and medicine, we have a double standard: we enforce rigorously procedures for informed consent in research activities, but when those same activities are done as part of clinical practice, no such rigor applies (1). Even the right to privacy is defined differently in everyday practice than in research. Investigators will go to considerable lengths to assure the confidentiality of research data, while discussing cases by name over coffee in public hospital cafeterias.

Federal funding agencies, institutions and universities now have in place systematic procedures for assuring that the rights of human subjects are protected. Applications for federal funds will not even be reviewed until and unless there has been clearance of the project at the local level by an institutional review committee which must include representation of consumers.

Some have criticized the bureaucracy of institutional mechanisms for protection of human subjects as "system over-correction," (2) and, indeed, sometimes the procedures seem overly tedious. More troublesome to nurse researchers, however, has been the lack of distinction between protection of the rights of human subjects and methodological or administrative clearance of a project.

264

INFORMED CONSENT

Decisions on the protection of individual rights in research are based on the Articles of the Nuremberg Tribunal. These Articles were drawn up after it became known that the major defense to be offered in the "doctor trials" would be that the Nazi doctors were engaged in important research. Some standards against which their conduct could be judged were necessary, so the Secretary of State and the Secretary of War requested the American Medical Association to appoint a group to formulate standards for this kind of experimentation and clinical research. Dr. Andrew Ivy was appointed Chief Consultant to the attorneys prosecuting the trial. He prepared a code of ethics which was accepted by the Court and has now become the "Nuremberg Laws."

Articles of the Nuremberg Tribunal (3)

1. The voluntary consent of human subject is absolutely essential. This means that the person involved should have legal capacity to give consent; should be so situated as to be able to exercise free power of choice, without the itervention of any element of force, fraud, deceit, duress, overreaching, or other ulterior form of constraint or coercion; and should have sufficient knowledge and comprehension of the elements of the subject matter involved as to enable him to make an understanding and enlightened decision. This latter element requires that before the acceptance of an affirmative decision by the experimental subject, there should be made known to him the nature, duration, and purpose of the experiment; the methods and means by which it is to be conducted; all inconveniences and hazards reasonably to be expected; and the effects upon his health or person which may possibly come from his participation in the experiment.

The duty and responsibility for ascertaining the quality of the consent rests upon each individual who initiates, directs, or engages in the experiment. It is a personal duty and responsibility which may not be delegated to another with impunity.

2. The experiment should be such as to yield fruitful results for the good of society, unprocurable by other methods or means of study, and not random and unnecessary in nature.
3. The experiment should be so designed and based on the results of animal experimentation and a knowledge of the natural history of the disease or other problem under study that the anticipated results will justify the performance of the experiment.
4. The experiment should be so conducted as to avoid all unnecessary physical and mental suffering and injury.
5. No experiment should be conducted where there is an *a priori* reason to believe that death or disabling injury will occur; except, perhaps in those experiments where the experimental physicians also serve as subjects.

6. The degree of risk to be taken should never exceed that determined by the humanitarian importance of the problem to be solved by the experiment.
7. Proper preparation should be made and adequate facilities provided to protect the experimental subject against even remote possibilities of injury, disability, or death.
8. The experiment should be conducted only by scientifically qualified persons. The highest degree of skill and care should be required through all stages of the experiment of those who conduct or engage in the experiment.
9. During the course of the experiment the human subject should be at liberty to bring the experiment to an end if he has reached the physical or mental state where continuation of the experiment seems to him to be impossible.
10. During the course of the experiment the scientist in charge must be prepared to terminate the experiment at any stage, if he has probable cause to believe, in the exercise of good faith, superior skill, and careful judgment required of him, that a continuation of the experiment is likely to result in injury, disability or death to the experimental subject.

The terms used in the Nuremberg Articles are not defined: "voluntary," "legal capacity," "sufficient understanding," "enlightened decision." Thus, there have been numerous thoughtful pieces by lawyers, ethicists and others arguing various interpretations of the intent of the Articles (4). The legal grounding for informed consent is based almost exclusively on litigation in the context of the practice of medicine. There is very nearly no case law in any other field (5).

Abdellah points out that "clinical nursing research may differ from medical research in the degree and kind of risk to patients." (6) In recent years, "risk" has become the central concept around which informed consent procedures have evolved. The Department of Health, Education and Welfare (DHEW) regulations define "subject at risk" as "any individual who may be exposed to the possibility of injury, including physical, psychological, or social injury, as a consequence of participation as a subject in any research, development, or related activity which departs from the application of those established and accepted methods necessary to meet his needs, or which increases the ordinary risks of daily life, including the recognized risks inherent in a chosen occupation or field of service." (7)

Federal regulations require a fair explanation of procedures; disclosure of risks; explanation of benefits; description of alternatives; an offer to answer questions; and a statement that the subject may withdraw at any time. It is the job of the institutional review committee to make an independent assessment of the degree to which these assignments have been considered and the procedures designed to implement them. Lebacqz and Levine suggest that some additional standards of disclosure also be added: a statement of the overall purpose of the research; a clear invitation to participate, distinguishing maneuvers required for research purposes from those necessary for therapy; an explanation of why the particular person is invited (selected); a suggestion that the prospective subject might wish to discuss the research with another person; and an explanation (when appropriate) of the fact that the risks are unknown (8).

Institutional review committees may adopt their own outline of material to be submitted on any proposed project, and such guidelines may or may not include all of the conditions above. In general, a proposal to be submitted to an institutional review committee specifies in detail the procedures that will be used to obtain informed consent, including often, the actual "script" the investigator will follow for each person. Whether the consent to participate may be verbal or must be written is usually determined by institutional practice or administrative desire.

When obtaining fully informed consent prior to participation in a study would invalidate the study, institutional review committees may approve a method which would allow for full "debriefing" of participants later. In experimental studies, it is generally understood that potential subjects must be informed before they are entered into the sample and before they are assigned to groups. They may simply be told that if they agree to participate, they may be selected for a group in which particular procedures will be used (experimental group) or another group, but permission to participate should be gotten in advance. The reasoning is that the patient has the right to be informed not only of what will happen to her/him, but of what participating in the study altogether will mean, regardless of which treatment group the patient ends up in.

Where there is no risk to the subject, in general, no consent procedures are followed. Retrospective chart reviews are thought to carry no risk (except, perhaps, violation of confidentiality) so studies may be done without the permission of the patients whose charts are used. On the other hand, access to chart data of patients who are currently hospitalized is thought to be a different matter, governed by state statute which may define, as it does in Connecticut and Massachusetts, that the patient "owns" her/his chart and, therefore, must give permission for its use.

Institutional review procedures vary from committee to committee, and place to place, so the investigator is wise to consult with the committee in advance, to avoid hassle and potential lack of permission to conduct the study.

RIGHT TO PRIVACY

Another aspect of the rights of human subjects is the right to privacy.

The claim to privacy—in this case one's personality and private thoughts—has not yet been recognized or protected by law in a technical legal sense other than indirectly through the First, Fourth, and Fifth

Amendments to the Constitution. The process has been slow because privacy is in conflict with other valued social interests, such as informed and effective government, law enforcement and free dissemination of information. (9)

Recent revelations that big companies, school systems, and certain governmental agencies use psychological tests in hiring employees or diagnosing student problems have dramatized the right-to-privacy issue. Invasion of privacy has been defined: "[the human subject] is not aware of the nature of the information being elicited and the use to which it will be placed." (10)

Part of the procedure of institutional review of proposals for research includes the requirement that the investigator state the precautions that will be used to protect the confidentiality of the data and the anonymity of the subjects. At a minimum, it should be stated that the patient's name will not be recorded on data collection forms, and that to the extent possible, no personally identifying information will appear on the data sheets. A master list of names may be kept securely in another place, but this is rarely necessary unless for some reason names are the only way to retrieve information later. Instead, code numbers or unit numbers may be used without the necessity even to record patient names. The extent to which persons other than the investigator her/himself will have access to the data is also part of the procedure for informed consent. In general, there should be no need for anyone other than the investigator to have access to the raw data, though research advisors may have access to coded or otherwise disguised printouts.

Again, particular procedures for protection of privacy may vary from institution to institution. And it is standard operating procedure that reports of research never contain personally identifiable information.

RESEARCH CLEARANCE PROCEDURES

Investigators submit their proposals for how the rights of human subjects will be protected to an institutional review committee. In some universities, this is a large committee which acts on all research. In other places, there may be separate committees for behavioral research, for medical research and for nursing research. If the committee is one approved by DHEW, it must have on it qualified researchers, consumers, a lawyer and various others depending on the field of study. The members of the committee must not be involved in the particular study under review, or at least must not participate in the decision on that study, since they are to reach an independent determination of the extent to which the rights of human subjects are protected. Usually such committees have sets of instructions for potential investigators, giving an outline of the steps to be taken, number of copies, timing of the review and so on, obtainable from the chairperson of the committee. When the committee signs off on a proposal, it is accepting responsibility for protection of human subjects, so it is likely to be rather cautious in interpreting guidelines and procedures.

Usually, the proposal for protection of the rights of human subjects is not the same as the research proposal itself. The committee does not need all the theoretical material and research design information, but it does need exact details of what it is that is being asked of human subjects. Copies of interviews, questionnaires and test forms must be included, along with data collection sheets and procedures for obtaining consent.

Nurse-researchers have sometimes felt, with some reason, that their research is reviewed with different standards than the research of physicians who may use the same clearance committee. There has been a tendency in some places in which nurse-researchers go through a medical school committee, for there to be considerable unwarranted attention paid to the social science methodology of the nursing studies, with the result that nursing studies which do not put the patient at risk are disapproved, while other studies which put the patient at considerable risk are passed through.

This kind of problem results when there is not a clear distinction among the kinds of research clearance that might be needed.

The first kind of "clearance" is methodological. The rigor of the design and the methodological issues of the study are the responsibility of the investigator, sometimes shared, in the case of student studies, with a committee of advisors.

Then there are administrative clearances, the grant of access to patients or subjects by an institution such as a hospital, nursing home, health agency or whatever. Here, the clearance is given based on the extent to which the agency feels the study can be accommodated in its environs, the burdens it will put on agency staff, as well as patients, and the priority the agency gives to research.

Finally, there is the protection of human subjects clearance, as discussed before. These three kinds of clearance tend to become mixed together, since there are some inevitable overlaps. For example, in determining a risk/benefit ratio for human subjects protection, one criterion may well be how good (methodologically sound) the study is. But there can be vast disagreements among disciplines about what constitutes a "good" study, and it is in this arena that interprofessional relationships touch on protection of human subjects. Similarly, a study may be "good," it may have well-thought-through procedures for protection of human subjects, but still not be approved by a clinical agency if the agency has other priorities.

When and where possible, it is useful to keep these three aspects of research clearance separate conceptually, as well as operationally. For example, a human investigations committee should be responsible only for the protection of human subjects, not for administrative clearance for research, but very often, especially in university medical centers, the clearance of human subjects means automatic access to clinical facilities. Nurses have encountered this problem when they may suddenly be told that they must participate in some research project by collecting specimens or something, without having had the chance to participate in the decision that the project should go on in the setting, given the staffing constraints or other responsibilities.

It should be the case that institutional review committees have representation, with real authority, of nurses when either the research reviewed is nursing research, or when access to subjects will hit nursing practice. Such is too rarely the case now, but something to be worked toward.

The American Nurses Association guidelines on the nurse in research, is a useful outline of some of the points made here (11). But even in the ten years since the guidelines were published, there have been enough advances in the profession and its interprofessional stands to suggest that it may be time for an update. MacElveen has usefully summarized critical issues in access to data in a model of a dynamic interactional system which includes the issues regarding rights of human subjects as well as administrative access as discussed here (12).

Prescribing commitment to the rights of human subjects is a lot more complicated than prescribing good will or peace. Nurses have no special monopoly on respecting the rights of patients nor any special qualifications of service that guarantee their patients' rights. Research in nursing practice, as presented here, poses especially interesting questions that will be resolved as more clinical research to improve patient care is conducted, and as we get surer about the theoretical bases that lie under thoughtful practice (13).

NOTES

1. Feinstein, Alvan: Medical ethics and the architecture of clinical research. *Clinical Pharmacology and Therapeutics*, 15:316–334, 1974; Downs, Florence: Ethical inquiry in nursing research. *Nursing Forum*, 6 (1):12–20, 1967; Conant, Lucy: Reader response to "ethical inquiry in nursing research." *Nursing Forum*, 6 (2):164–170, 1967. Also, subsequent articles by Mary Neal and Luther Christman, same journal, same citation.

2. Stevenson, Joanne: Protection of human subjects and the phenomena of overcorrection. *CNR Voice*, Ohio State University School of Nursing Newsletter, (3):1–3, 1974.

3. Cited in panel discussion: moral issues and clinical research. Paul Beeson, Philip Bondy, Richard Donnelly, and John Smith: *The Yale Journal of Biology and Medicine*, 36 (6):455–476, June 1964.

4. Lebacqz, Karen and Robert J. Levine: Respect for persons and informed consent to participate in research. *Clinical Research*, 25:101–107, 1977; Katz, Jay: *Experimentation with Human Beings: The Authority of the Investigator, Subject Professions and State in the Human Experimentation Process.* New York: Russell Sage, 1972. Mechanic, David: Social psychology of informed consent in experimentation and therapy. In *The Growth of Bureaucratic Medicine.* New York: John Wiley & Sons, 1976, pp. 255–277. The *Hastings Center Report* (publication of the Institute of Society, Ethics and the Life Sciences, 360 Broadway, Hastings-on-Hudson, New York, 10706) regularly publishes papers on aspects of informed consent in biomedical research, and collected bibliographical citations of articles published elsewhere as well.

5. Lebacqz and Levine, *Ibid.*, especially footnote a, p. 101.

6. Abdellah, Faye G.: Approaches to protecting the rights of human subjects. *Nursing Research*, 16:316–320, Fall 1967.

7. DHEW. Protection of human subjects: technical amendments. *Federal Register*, 40 (50):11854–11858, March 13, 1975.

8. Lebacqz and Levine, see Note 4, footnote g, p. 105.
9. Abdellah, see Note 6.
10. *Ibid.*, p. 317.

11. American Nurses Association: The nurse in research: ANA guidelines on ethical values. *American Journal of Nursing*, 68:1504–1507, July 1968.

12. MacElveen, Patricia: Critical issues in access to data. In Batey, Marjorie V. (ed.): *Communicating Nursing Research*. Boulder: WICHEN, January 1975, pp. 1–16.

13. Two useful summaries of ethical and legal issues in nursing research are Armiger, Sr. Bernadette: Ethics of nursing research: profile, principles, perspective. *Nursing Research*, 26:330–336, September–October 1977; Creighton, Helen: Legal concerns of nursing research. *Nursing Research*, 26:337–341. September–October 1977. Sr. Bernadette's article contains useful citation to the Helsinki declaration, which updated the Nuremberg Laws, as well as a comprehensive analysis of the sparse nursing literature on the topic of rights of human subjects.

Various legal and ethical concerns in clinical practice and research are dealt with in Holder, Angela R.: *Medical Malpractice Law*. New York: John Wiley & Sons, 1975 and Holder, Angela R.: *Legal Issues in Pediatrics and Adolescent Medicine*. New York: John Wiley & Sons, 1977. Despite their titles, these books contain highly relevant material on ethics and legal issues in informed consent as they apply to nursing as well as medicine.

12

Evaluating and Writing Research

INTRODUCTION

A research project isn't done when the data are all in, and analyzed and some sense has been made of it all. Nursing will not progress as an intellectual discipline, much less a practice profession, until research is reported, used, tested in practice, reformed, redone and tested again and again. In a study of why research is not implemented in practice, Miller and Messenger report that the greatest obstacles to applying research findings are the need for wider distribution of reports and "more and clearer articles." (1) So evaluating research reports and writing them require a little attention here.

EVALUATING NURSING RESEARCH

Evaluating research is a whole lot easier than conducting it. There are always things in the reports of studies that an astute reader can quarrel with. From the identification and analysis of the problem and through its implications for future research and practice, every study is a personal endeavor and the ideas that go into the study may or may not be shared by other readers. The purpose of evaluating research is not so much to show off one's critical ability and prove what a dunce the investigator was as to evaluate the report for how well it fulfills its purposes in terms of its function for further nursing studies or for the profession in general (2). In one sense, research is never finished. Each study builds on previous work, sometimes taking off on new areas of investigation. Therefore, evelution of research means asking not only how good the evidence is for the author's conclusions, but also what can be learned from the report that might help another study come closer to the solution or resolution of a problem.

There are three aspects of a research report that are evaluated: nursing significance, methodology and exposition. The evaluation of each becomes a matter of emphasis, since the three are all closely related and overlapping.

272

Nursing significance means the relevance of the study for nursing as it is now, or as it could or should be. Methodology is the way in which the study was carried out, including the gathering and analyzing of information. Exposition is the way in which the study is reported.

Both nursing significance and methodology can be examined in each of three areas: the problem, the study design and the results. That is, we can look at the nursing significance of the problem, the study design and the results, and the methodology of the presentation of the problem, the study design and the analysis of data. Exposition applies to the whole study.

Nursing Significance

The first question to be asked of any reported study is, What evidence is there that the problem is conceived as a *nursing* problem? This information should be supplied to the reader formally in an early part of the report; if the problem is indeed a nursing problem, the evidence will pervade the whole report. Is the problem being studied explicitly related to nursing practice? To nursing theory? To a more general problem in nursing? For example, a study on the effect of nursing on patients' abilities to follow medically prescribed diets can be an instance of the more general problem of following any medical prescription. Is the investigator aware of where the problem fits into the whole of nursing practice? Does the investigator present evidence of the importance of the problem and therefore the purpose of doing the study? Is the problem a discrepancy *that matters*? What does it matter to nursing if the problem is ignored? Where did the problem originate and does the investigator trace the development of her interest and her thinking about the problem?

The nursing significance of the study design is evaluated by asking such questions as: does the design relate to the problem? Is it appropriate to the nursing situation from which the problem arose? Is there evidence of an awareness that the problem is a nursing problem and the design tailored to nursing practice? Does the investigator seem to consider the implications of the design for possible implementation of the findings? Does the study approximate practice in its conduct? If so, how? If not, why not, and does the investigator recognize the importance of approximating practice?

Other questions that are asked about the study focus on the other parts of the study design: is the sample appropriate? Is it representative of patients in general? What is the setting and how representative is it? Are the sources of information realistic in terms of practice? Are the variables studied accessible or controllable in nursing? Are the measurements meaningful, reliable and so on? Is use of the measurements possible or relevant in practice? Are the data collection instruments related to the practice phenomena? Is there any evidence of a lack of concern for nursing in the study? That is, would the study be detrimental either to the patients sampled or to the nurse (in terms of nursing costs, time, energy and so on) or to relationships between the research and the practice setting? Does the study interfere with ongoing patient care? Could the study give patients a negative impression of nursing even though patients might not be actually harmed by participation in the study?

Are any or all of the sources of information, data collection, measurements, analysis procedures and so on, seen by the researcher as having significance for nursing? Is the researcher even aware that they might be seen as significant?

The findings of the study and the suggested implications come in for particular scrutiny. The major question is how are the findings related (explicitly) to the original problem? Is the researcher aware of how far she has come toward the solution or resolution of the problem, or even toward a redefinition of the problem? What evidence is there that the researcher is concerned about the resolution of the problem, not just about collecting data? Has the researcher considered the implications of the results for the original problem? For nursing practice? For nursing theory? For the more general problem? For her own learning experience or her own clinical practice?

Studies should report how the results contribute to the solution of resolution of the problem and what remaining steps need to be taken for such solution or resolution. Included in such a report would be a discussion of whether the problem is still a discrepancy that matters and, therefore, warrants further study. Does the researcher go beyond mere reporting of the facts to draw out any interesting creative, new or novel implications? Does the research indicate a *nursing sense* about the data and the study?

Just as the researcher has to present the evidence on which conclusions are based, the reader or evaluator of a research report should present the evidence on which the evaluations are made. It is not enough merely to say that the nursing significance of a report is outstanding. One should also be able to say why that judgment was made; for example, the investigator clearly outlines the development of the problem, is sensitive to practice considerations throughout the report and draws out interesting implications for future research and for present nursing practice. The specific items in the report that lead to such statements should be a part of any evaluation whether the evaluation is written or not.

Methodology

Methodology is evaluated from two points of view: the nursing problem under study and the standards of the scientific community. The reported research methodology is examined both as it relates to nursing practice and the particular nursing problem, and as it meets or does not meet the standards usually considered acceptable for designs, data collection, measurements, analysis and so on. The two evaluations are separate only analytically.

The evaluation of methodology of a study begins with the following question: what evidence is there that the investigator made appropriate use of available resources in planning and executing the study? Has she considered her own experience and the (unreported) experience of others? Has she made appropriate use of pertinent literature in nursing or elsewhere? Has she made imaginative use of theory or research done previously? Does she merely cite reams of material or has she been selective and critical in her choice of supporting data? Considering all the prestudy resources, is it clear why the investigator still considers the problem a problem? In some areas there has been a great deal of work. For example, the effects of nursing on pain has been studied by many people recently. Yet this area is still considered important because people have used so many different approaches from so many different theoretical frameworks with conflicting results that it is still not possible to draw general implications for nursing practice. The investigator should present the thinking behind why the area is still considered important.

The study design, sample, measurements, data collection procedures are all reviewed from the same two points of view—the problem and the scientific standards. Is the design adequate for the problem? Is the design appropriate to the level of inquiry of the problem? Is the design economical of research time, patient time, energy, expense and so on? Is the setting appropriate to the design; that is, does it contain the phenomenon being observed in sufficient quantity? Is the sampling and/or assignment procedure appropriate to the design? For example, if the study is a causal hypothesis-testing study, random assignment to treatment groups is essential to meet the conditions for inferring a causal relationship.

Does the researcher include evidence to support the selection of measures or indicators used? Is evidence of validity (conceptual and empirical) presented? Is there an attempt to assess the reliability of measures? Are measures meaningful, accessible, controllable, appropriate to practice? Is the rationale behind the selection of measurements clear? Does the investigator recognize the possibility of bias in the measurement? Does the investigator recognize the possibility of the measurement procedure itself affecting the phenomenon involved? If evidence of the reliability or assessment of bias is not presented, is there at least an indication that the investigator considered these questions even if they weren't empirically examined?

Evaluation of analysis procedures does require some knowledge of statistics, but even the most nonstatistically inclined reader can often make important evaluations of analysis techniques. For example, are the tables, graphs or other presentation devices understandable and clear? Do they seem rational? For example, one study indicated that a series of observations of nurses was made, yet the summary tables presented only one "score" per nurse without telling how such a score was arrived at. Is it clear what the units are that were analyzed, and are the analysis procedures appropriate for the units involved? Are the assumptions underlying the statistical tests met?

Were the data for the study exploited? That is, were the data analyzed fully, or if not, is it clear why not? Were possibilities overlooked or omitted?

Do the analysis procedures help answer the original questions; that is, are they designed so that the questions could be answered? Were the data used creatively to derive insights? Did the investigator capitalize on information available? For example, if data that did not fit the categories of a measurement were collected, were they analyzed to redefine the categories or reconceptualize the measure? Did the researcher carry out the analysis beyond the point of merely answering the study questions? Often, the most fruitful analysis comes out of questions that come up during data collection and couldn't have been anticipated.

Did the researcher draw appropriate conclusions? Is it clear from the report what conclusions are drawn from the data, which ones are supported by the data, which ones are merely suggestions? Is the evidence for each conclusion clearly presented? Does the investigator go on to speculate about hunches which may not be supported by the data but are interesting anyhow? And finally, is the investigator appropriately aware of the limitations of the study with neither excessive humility or braggadocio?

Exposition

Evaluation of exposition begins with consideration of the appropriate audience to which the report is aimed. The journal in which a report appears will, of course, determine the audience to some extent, but the reader will also evaluate how well the report is likely to be received by the specified audience. Is it overly technical so that a nonresearch audience would be baffled? Is it overly simplified so that the tone is condescending? Is it overly rabble-rousing so that the content gets lost in emotion? Is it overly precise so that it is dull to read?

The same standards that apply to research to be evaluated also apply to evaluations themselves. Evaluations should contain the evidence used in reaching conclusions and should be acceptably written for the appropriate audience. The purpose of evaluation is to further the cause of research; therefore, evaluations that are thoughtful, not overly negative, but make appropriate use of the reader's subjective impressions are most valuable.

Figure 12-1 is a suggested outline for evaluation research.

The written evaluation of a study emerges as a "research critique." Its purpose is to illuminate aspects of the study that might be suggestive of future research, deserving of replication or those which might suggest alternative design or interpretation. A well-conceived research critique is a valuable step forward in a line of inquiry (4).

WRITING RESEARCH

Whether research is presented orally or in writing, there are certain common considerations. Research reports have to provide enough informa-

Figure 12-1: *Guide for Evaluation of a Nursing Study (3)*

I. Nursing significance
   A. Of the problem
      1. Is the problem seen as a *nursing* problem?
      2. Is the problem explicitly related to nursing practice?
         To nursing theory?
         To more general problem(s)?
   B. Of the study design
      1. Is the problem conceived as a *nursing* problem?
      2. Is the study design appropriate to nursing?
         Is the sample?
         The measurements?
         Data collection procedures?
         Data analysis?
      3. Is there concern for nursing shown?
   C. Of the results
      1. Is the analysis and interpretation of the results seen in light of the orginal problem?
         Nursing practice?
         Nursing theory?
         More general problem(s)?
      2. Is it clear how the results contribute to the solution or resolution of the problem?
II. Methodology
   A. Of the problem
      1. Are the prestudy resources appropriately used? (Experience, literature, research and soon)
      2. Is the analysis of the problem adequate?
   B. Of the study design
      1. Is the design appropriate to the level of inquiry of the problem?
      2. Is the design carried out appropriately?
      3. Are the setting, sample, measurements, data collection procedures adequate, appropriate to the problem and the scientific standards?
      4. Are the data analysis procedures appropriate to the data?
   C. Of the results
      1. Are analysis and interpretation adequate to the problem?
         To scientific standards?
      2. Were the data fully exploited?
III. Exposition
   Consider the adequacy of the exposition with respect to the intended audience and the standards of good writing.

tion to the audience for them to decide whether the evidence is good enough for them to make the indicated changes in practice. The kind of information needed to evaluate the quality of the evidence includes the description of the problem and how the researcher arrived at the specification of the problem. The reader needs to know the theory behind the problem and how the researcher sees the problem fitting in with other important problems in practice. (The analysis of the problem covers this point.) The reader needs to know how the researcher is using the concepts and terms in the study and the assumptions behind their use. The researcher should also indicate his intellectual debts to earlier investigators and other writings.

Other aspects of the research that are included so that the reader can judge the validity of the evidence are the research design, sample, setting, operational definitions, data collection, processing and analysis procedures, including evaluation of bias, reliability, validity and so on, of any measurements used. The report should also include the inferences the investigator has drawn from the data and the basis on which the inferences were drawn. Implications for nursing practice, implications for further research into the problem and for the development of nursing theory are important too. Of course, any one study and any one researcher cannot possibly draw out all of the possible implications of a project and some drawing out of inferences must be left for the reader. Nevertheless, the reader must be provided with enough information on which to evaluate what contributions any particular study makes to her own nursing practice and research.

The form the research report takes may be any one congenial to the writer. Some logical order should guide the content. The report might be organized in various ways:

1. What I intended to do
2. What I did
3. What I learned

or

1. What I wanted to find out
2. What I did find out
3. How much confidence I place in the results

or

1. What I found out
2. What I did to find it out
3. What needs to be done next

The reporting order should be the order of understanding for the reader and may or may not reflect the temporal sequence of the study's production. A report should be as short as possible as long as all the important aspects have been covered. Redundancy and needless repetition should be decisively edited out.

There is no rule that says research reporting has to be dull. The reader should be stimulated to continue reading the report (or listening to the presentation). Overly dramatic phrases probably are a bit much, but examples, illustrations, thought-provoking statements all increase the readability of a written presentation. Tables and graphs, which in themselves aid understanding, should be discussed, not just summarized in the text. Tell us what the table *means*, not just what's in it.

Although it is important to review pertinent literature, a section called "Literature Review" is very boring to read. If the literature citations can be integrated throughout the text whenever pertinent, the report is both more interesting and shows the researcher's grasp of the study better.

Any good creative writing book will give a potential author clues about how to write interesting research reports. I do not believe it is imperative to use the objective editorial third person (the researcher) when it is more interesting to say I or we. Active voice verbs and general adherence to standards of good writing are indicated.

There are any number of books on good writing, as well as amusing critiques of poor writing (5). I have a particular fondness for Edwin Newman's way of approaching the language, and especially his distaste for -ize words, of which research reports are full (6).

A few words about titles for studies are in order. In general, the briefer the title, the better, as long as it conveys some sense of what the study is about. The title, "A Study of the Process of the Nurse's Activity as it Affects the Blood Pressure Readings and Pulse Rates of Patients Admitted to the Emergency Room" certainly contains all the information, but it is far too elaborate and lengthy. Perhaps, "The Effect of Nursing During Emergency Admission" would be an appropriate short title. The kind of study that is conducted can be determined from a cleverly written title. "The Effect of . . ." usually indicates a causal hypothesis-testing study. "Relationship Between . . ." usually indicates either an association-testing study or a relation-searching study, etc. "An Exploratory Study of . . ." or "A Descriptive Study of . . ." suggests factor- or relation-searching. It is important to convey the sense of the study in the title because others who may want to look at studies will select the ones to review by looking through the titles printed in a series of abstracts, a bibliography, a list of theses, a nursing studies index and the like.

PUBLICATION

There is a great need for quality writing in nursing (as any quick scanning of the journals will indicate). This need is almost as great as the need for nursing practice research. Practitioners as well as researchers should feel the obligation to spread the knowledge gained and not be intimidated about submitting material to journals. Editors are always looking for good writing and interesting content.

Each journal has its own particular focus, usually stated somewhere in the magazine. For nontechnical journals, a review of a recent year of a journal will indicate whether the magazine has already published a number of articles on the same subject and, therefore might not want any more. Every journal has its own requirements for submitting of manuscripts (number of lines per page, footnoting, content, number of copies) and their regulations are usually printed on the inside front cover or somewhere in the magazine. If a nurse has an interesting idea for an article, but doesn't yet have it written or doesn't know whether a journal might be interested, she can always write a query to the editor to find out.

All journals require that any manuscript submitted to them not be submitted simultaneously to any other journal. Some journals even require a signed statement to this effect. Not only is the practice of submitting a manuscript to a number of places at the same time discourteous to all those editors who have to read it, but if the article is accepted for publication, journals can get into huge copyright difficulties by simultaneous publication. Journal editors move in the same circles, so it is not difficult at all for them to discover that the same article has been submitted several places. If an author is revealed to have done this, chances are an editor will think three or four times before ever accepting another manuscript from him; and if an author really has so little faith in a manuscript's worth that he submits it indiscriminately in the faint hope of its being published somewhere, chances are it's not worth publishing anywhere.

Nurse Educator has published a very useful list of the nursing journals, complete with editor's name, deadlines, information on payment and reprints, publication criteria and the like (7). There are now a fairly large number of sources of presentation and publication of research reports. Carnegie summarized the major avenues for research reporting in an editorial in *Nursing Research* (8).

There is a distinction in scientific journals between "refereed" or "juried" and "nonjuried" journals. A juried journal is one in which manuscripts are circulated to members of a review panel, usually two or three people, for their opinions on the worth of the study. A nonjuried journal is one in which editorial decisions are made by the editors themselves, without referring the manuscript to a peer review panel. In general, juried journals may take longer to review a manuscript. An author may expect to hear immediately that a manuscript has been received, and should follow-up if no acknowledgment arrives. Manuscripts have been known to disappear in the postal system.

Different journals have different audiences, and a researcher may decide that for a particular piece of work, an interdisciplinary audience is indicated rather than an audience composed primarily of nurses. While it is not at all ethical to submit exactly the same manuscript to more than one journal, it is wise to think about writing several articles from a study, highlighting different data, or writing for different audiences. A nontechnical article for a general nursing audience can often be done, along with a more technical article for a research audience.

Along with the more public obligation to disseminate research information, the researcher has a responsibility to fill in the data collectors, staff nurses or others who have either been directly involved in the project or whose facilities have been used. Efforts made to let interested people know how the research was conducted and what was learned helps interest other people in conducting research or using the results of research to improve their practice.

Generally, the most appropriate audience for communication of research is the personnel in the setting in which data were collected. They should already have a vested interest in the study and the results would be most meaningful to them. But any scholar or researcher has the obligation of communicating whatever information she/he believes important in a way that will reach whatever audience is appropriate. In part, the decision on how best to communicate research depends on the problems selected for the study, the methods, and the results of the investigation. For example, a very technical measurement study might be most important for a group of researchers; a content study could be useful to almost anyone.

Publication is only one way of communicating research, albeit a very important way.

As nursing continuing education becomes established, more and more avenues for reporting research are available. The "research days" sponsored by nearly all Sigma Theta Tau chapters are an excellent vehicle, as are the ANA clinical sessions and research sessions sponsored by various university schools of nursing. There are frequent calls for abstracts appearing now in the nursing literature, so researchers should rarely feel blocked from presenting their ideas.

AUTHORSHIP

Writing a paper with others can be a good way to get started in publishing. But there are some conventions about authorship it may be well to state.

In general, the senior (first) author is the one who writes the first and last draft. The collaboration with other authors should be negotiated in advance, to prevent fallout of friendships at some later point. It was once the case that when a graduate student published with a faculty member, the faculty member's name always went first. It appears that this custom is dying out, especially when the research is really the student's, and the faculty member is facilitating its conduct and publication.

It was once also conventional that when authors of different disciplines published together (a nurse and a psychologist, say), the one in whose discipline the article would be published was listed first. If the article went to a nursing journal, the nurse went first, if to a psychology journal, the psychologist went first. This convention too seems to be disappearing, and probably wasn't necessary in the first place.

Usually it is also the senior author who takes responsibility for correcting and signing off on page proofs and galley proofs and for answering requests for reprints, though this may vary as well.

Since academic reputations often rest on authorship matters, and author order, these points are not as trivial as they may seem.

Finally, it is simply a matter of courtesy to acknowledge in a footnote, the help of other colleagues on a project, when they are not themselves authors. Graduate students might acknowledge their advisors, or authors may wish to name persons who have read and reviewed and commented upon earlier drafts of the manuscript. Sources of financial support for the study should always be acknowledged.

NOTES

1. Miller, Jean R. and Susan R. Messenger: Obstacles to applying nursing research findings. *American Journal of Nursing*, 78:632–634, April 1978.

2. Stetler, Cheryl B. and Gwen Marram: Evaluating research findings for applicability in practice. *Nursing Outlook*, 24:559–563, September 1976.

3. This guide was originally the work of Joyce Semradek, then revised by members of the Nursing Theory Seminar, Yale School of Nursing, 1966, especially Patricia James and James Dickoff.

4. Downs, Florence: Elements of a research critique. In Downs, F. and M. Newman (eds.): *A Source Book of Nursing Research*. Philadelphia: F.A. Davis, 1973, pp. xi–xvi; Leininger, Madeleine: The research critique: nature, function and art. In Batey, Marjorie V. (ed.): *Communicating Nursing Research: The Research Critique* (Vol. I). Boulder, Colorado: WICHEN, 1968, pp. 20–32; Fleming, Juanita and Jean Hayter: Reading research reports critically. *Nursing Outlook*, 22:172–175, March 1974.

   Excellent examples of research critiques may be found in the series *Communicating Nursing Research*, edited by Marjorie Batey, Boulder, WICHEN, Vol. I–IX.

   Gortner has written a fine review of research proposals, as opposed to completed studies. Gortner, Susan: Research grant applications: what they are not and should be. *Nursing Research*, 20:292–295.

5. Merrill, Paul: The principles of poor writing. *Scientific Monthly*, 64(1):72, January 1947; Marriott, Henry J.L.: Balm for writer's itch. *American Journal of Cardiology*, February 1961 (reprinted by F.A. Davis, Philadelphia as a pamphlet); Flesch, Rudolf: *How to Write, Speak and Think More Effectively*, and *The Art of Plain Talk* (paperback); Quiller-Couch, Arthur: *On the Art of Writing*. New York: Putnam, 1928; Strunk, William and E.B. White: *Elements of Style*. New York: Macmillan, 1959; Zinsser, William: *Writing Well*. New Haven: Yale Press, 1975.

6. Newman, Edwin: *Strictly Speaking*. New York: Random House, 1976, and *A Civil Tongue*, 1977.

7. McClosky, Joanne Comi: Publishing opportunities for nurses: a comparison of 65 journals. *Nurse Educator* 2(4):4–12, July–August, 1977.

8. Carnegie, M. Elizabeth: Editorial: avenues for reporting research. *Nursing Research*, 26:83, March–April 1977.

Index